Medicine, Health and the Public Sphere in Britain, 1600–2000

Medicine is concerned with the most intimate aspects of private life. Yet it is also a focus for diverse forms of public organization and action. In this volume, an international team of scholars use the techniques of medical history to analyse the changing boundaries and constitution of the public sphere from early modernity to the present day.

Following the pathbreaking work of Jürgen Habermas, historians and sociologists have tended to think of the public sphere primarily as a site of discourse and opinion formation. The medical historians collected here expand this perspective to include other kinds of social action, ranging from the redefinition of doctor–patient relations in the seventeenth century to the regulation of *in vitro* fertilization in the 1990s.

In a series of detailed historical case studies, contributors examine the role of various public institutions – both formal and informal, voluntary and statutory – in organizing and co-ordinating collective action on medical matters. In so doing, they challenge the determinism and fatalism of Habermas's overarching and functionalist account of the rise and fall of the public sphere.

Of essential interest to historians and sociologists of medicine, this book will also be of value to historians of modern Britain, historical sociologists, and those engaged in studying the work of Jürgen Habermas.

Steve Sturdy is lecturer in the History of Medicine at the Science Studies Unit, University of Edinburgh. With Michael Barfoot and Christopher Lawrence he is currently writing up a project on clinical science in inter-war Edinburgh. His publications include *War, Medicine and Modernity* (Sutton, 1998) and *Medicine and the Management of Modern Warfare* (Rodopi, 1999), both jointly edited with Roger Cooter and Mark Harrison.

Routledge Studies in the Social History of Medicine

Edited by Bernard Harris, Department of Sociology and Social Policy, University of Southampton, Joseph Melling, University of Exeter and Anne Borsay, University of Wales at Lampeter.

The Society for the Social History of Medicine (SSHM) was founded in 1969, and exists to promote research into all aspects of the field, without regard to limitations of either time or place. In addition to this book series, the Society also organizes a regular programme of conferences, and publishes an internationally recognized journal, *Social History of Medicine*. The Society offers a range of benefits, including reduced-price admission to conferences and discounts on SSHM books, to its members. Individuals wishing to learn more about the Society are invited to contact the series editors through the publisher.

The Society took the decision to launch 'Studies in the Social History of Medicine', in association with Routledge, in 1989, in order to provide an outlet for some of the latest research in the field. Since that time, the series has expanded significantly under a number of series of editors, and now includes both edited collections and monographs. Individuals wishing to submit proposals are invited to contact the series editors in the first instance.

1. Nutrition in Britain
Science, scientists and politics in the twentieth century
Edited by David F. Smith

2. Migrants, Minorities and Health
Historical and contemporary studies
Edited by Lara Marks and Michael Worboys

3. From Idiocy to Mental Deficiency
Historical perspectives on people with learning disabilities
Edited by David Wright and Anne Digby

4. Midwives, Society and Childbirth
Debates and controversies in the modern period
Edited by Hilary Marland and Anne Marie Rafferty

5. Illness and Healing Alternatives in Western Europe
Edited by Marijke Gijswit-Hofstra, Hilary Marland and Hans de Waardt

Medicine, Health and the Public Sphere in Britain, 1600–2000

Edited by Steve Sturdy

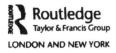

Routledge
Taylor & Francis Group

LONDON AND NEW YORK

First published 2002
by Routledge
2 Park Square, Milton Park, Abingdon, Oxon OX14 4RN

Simultaneously published in the USA and Canada
by Routledge
711 Third Avenue, New York, NY 10017

Routledge is an imprint of the Taylor & Francis Group

Typeset in Baskerville by Taylor & Francis Books Ltd

First issued in paperback 2013

British Library Cataloguing in Publication Data
A catalogue record for this book is available from the British Library

Library of Congress Cataloging in Publication Data
A catalog record for this book has been applied for

ISBN13: 978-0-415-86304-9 (pbk)
ISBN13: 978-0-415-27906-2 (hbk)

Contents

Contributors

Logie Barrow has taught the social history of the 'British' archipelago, of Anglo-British slavery and of South Africa at the University of Bremen since 1980. Since 1966, his research areas have been labour history and intellectual dis/empowerment. His publications include *Independent Spirits: Spiritualism and English Plebeians 1850–1910* (Routledge & Kegan Paul, 1986).

Deborah Brunton is lecturer in the History of Medicine at the Open University. She has published on smallpox inoculation and vaccination, and is completing a book on vaccination policy in nineteenth-century Britain. She is currently researching into sanitary reform in Victorian Scotland.

David Cantor works at the National Cancer Institute, Bethesda, Maryland, where he is researching a history of diet, nutrition and cancer. He has previously published on the histories of cancer, the rheumatic diseases and neo-hippocratism. He is the editor of *Reinventing Hippocrates* (Ashgate, 2001).

Pamela K. Gilbert is Associate Professor of English at the University of Florida. Her books include *Disease, Desire and the Body in Victorian Women's Popular Novels* (Cambridge, 1997); *Imagined Londons*, an edited collection (SUNY, 2002); and *Beyond Sensation, Mary Elizabeth Braddon in Context*, a collection co-edited with Marlene Tromp and Aeron Haynie (SUNY, 2000). She is finishing a book on the social body and public health in England, 1832–67.

Martin Gorsky is Senior Lecturer in British History at the University of Wolverhampton. His research interests lie in the history of philanthropy and mutual aid, and recent publications include studies of the geography and finance of British voluntary hospitals. He is currently working, along with John Mohan, on a study of hospital contributory schemes in the twentieth century.

Christopher Hamlin is Professor of History at the University of Notre Dame. His publications include *A Science of Impurity: Water Analysis in Nineteenth-Century Britain* (University of California Press, 1990) and *Public Health and Social Justice in the Age of Chadwick: Britain 1800–1854* (Cambridge University Press, 1998).

Bill Luckin is Professor in Urban History at Bolton Institute. The author of *Pollution and Control: A Social History of the Thames in the Nineteenth Century* (Hilger, 1986) and *Questions of Power: Electricity and Environment in Inter-War Britain* (Manchester University Press, 1990), he is also co-author with Graham Mooney and Andrea Tanner of *Death in the Metropolis: Patterns of Mortality in London 1860–1920* (forthcoming). His main interests lie in the fields of environmental and epidemiological history.

John Mohan is Professor of Geography, University of Portsmouth. His research interests are in historical and contemporary geographies of health and health care. He is author of *A National Health Service?* (Macmillan, 1995), *Planning, Markets and Hospitals* (Routledge, 2002) and co-author (with Martin Gorsky) of *Don't Look Back? Voluntary and Charitable Finance of Hospitals in Britain, Past and Present* (Office of Health Economics, 2001).

Andrew A.G. Morrice currently works as a General Practitioner in Midsomer Norton near Bath. He is a graduate of the Wellcome Institute for the History of Medicine's intercalated BSc course, and after medical qualification spent a further two years as a Research Fellow at the Institute. His MD thesis (1999) concerned the medical ethics work of the BMA in the early twentieth century.

Margaret Pelling is Reader in the Social History of Medicine at the University of Oxford. Recent publications include *The Common Lot: Sickness, Medical Occupations and the Urban Poor in Early Modern England* (Longman, 1998). A monograph, *The College of Physicians and Irregular Medical Practitioners in Early Modern London* is in press with Oxford University Press.

Naomi Pfeffer has published widely on reproductive medicine, including *The Stork and the Syringe: A Political History of Reproductive Medicine* (Polity, 1993). She teaches health policy at the University of North London.

Martin Powell is Senior Lecturer in Social Policy in the Department of Social and Policy Sciences, University of Bath. His research interests include historical and contemporary perspectives on health policy. He has published a number of articles on British hospitals in the 1930s, and is the author of *Evaluating the National Health Service* (Open University Press, 1997).

Steve Sturdy is lecturer in the History of Medicine at the Science Studies Unit, University of Edinburgh. With Michael Barfoot and Christopher Lawrence he is currently writing up a project on clinical science in inter-war Edinburgh. His publications include *War, Medicine and Modernity* (Sutton, 1998) and *Medicine and the Management of Modern Warfare* (Rodopi, 1999), both jointly edited with Roger Cooter and Mark Harrison.

Elaine Thomson received her PhD in the Social History of Medicine from Edinburgh University in 1998. She has published a number of articles on women doctors in late nineteenth- and early twentieth-century Edinburgh. She is currently a lecturer at Napier University, Edinburgh.

Adrian Wilson is lecturer in the History of Medicine in the School of Philosophy, Division of History and Philosophy of Science, at the University of Leeds. He is the author of *The Making of Man-midwifery: Childbirth in England, 1660–1770* (UCL Press and Harvard University Press, 1995) and editor of *Rethinking Social History: English Society 1570–1920 and its Interpretation* (Manchester University Press, 1993).

Acknowledgements

Most of the chapters in this volume are based on papers given at the annual conference of the Society for the Social History of Medicine (SSHM) held at the University of Edinburgh, 17–19 July 1998. Our thanks are due to all the contributors and participants who made that conference so stimulating and enjoyable. The conference benefited from the generous financial support of the Wellcome Trust and of the Humanities Research Board of the British Academy, from the assistance of the staff and postgraduate students of the Science Studies Unit, University of Edinburgh, and from the administrative support of the SSHM, particularly the Society Treasurer David Wright. We are greatly indebted to the SSHM series editor Bernard Harris for his invaluable advice and encouragement throughout the preparation of this volume, and to Joe Whiting, Yeliz Ali, Annabel Watson and Simon Bailey at Routledge for seeing the project through to publication.

Introduction

Medicine, health and the public sphere

Steve Sturdy

Questions about the structure and function of the public sphere have never been more pressing than at present. At a time when many public services are being transferred into private hands, when states have unprecedented powers of surveillance over their citizens' private affairs, when the media thrive by publishing exposés of the private lives of celebrities and non-entities alike, and when private corporations increasingly operate beyond the control of elected governments, we face urgent issues of how to reconcile the legitimate pursuit of private interest with the negotiation, formulation and assertion of a common public good. A good deal of academic ink has been expended on such issues, particularly over the past twenty years or so – much of it flowing from the pens of historians, who have done a great deal to clarify our understanding of the constitution of the public sphere from past to present. Remarkably little has been contributed to this endeavour by historians of medicine, however. This is surprising in view of the fact that medicine, and health care more generally, has long been a key site for the provision of public services and the pursuit of the public good. The present volume is intended to explore some of the ways that the history of medicine might add to our understanding of the changing nature of the public sphere.

Recent academic writing about the public sphere tends to characterize it as a sphere of discourse, aimed primarily at influencing and legitimizing the actions of government and the state. The *locus classicus* of this characterization, and the starting point for much subsequent theorizing, is Jürgen Habermas's *The Structural Transformation of the Public Sphere*, first published in German in 1962 but only translated into English in 1989.[1] Habermas locates the emergence of the democratic public sphere within the broader social and economic context of the rise and decline of bourgeois capitalism. He argues that the growth of capitalism during the late seventeenth and eighteenth centuries led in the first instance to the development and valorization of new forms of privacy, based in the household as the primary site for the ownership of private property, and in private business between heads of households as the favoured means of conducting economic transactions. According to Habermas, the circumstances of private life both in the home and the marketplace fostered a subjective sense of individual self-determination and autonomy that made possible new and essentially private forms of sociability that he identifies, following Hannah Arendt, with the distinctively modern sphere of civil society. Within this essentially private sphere, however, there emerged new sites and media of public communication – notably the salon, the coffee house and the popular press – that constituted a novel bourgeois public sphere distinct from the pre-existing public sphere of the state.

Crucially, Habermas argues, the conduct of discourse within the bourgeois public sphere was no longer informed by appeals to older forms of public status and authority, but rather presupposed parity of citizenship among the participants. As a result, the outcome of debate in that sphere could now be determined according to purely rational criteria, such that 'the authority of the better argument' would prevail.[2] Bourgeois public discourse thus provided a uniquely effective means for the community of private individuals to reflect upon, debate and agree the forms of public and private life that best suited their common interest. Only belatedly did such public opinion come to exert any significance on affairs of state, however – most notably in what Habermas takes to be the model case of Britain. With the emergence and institutionalization of faction and party in Parliament during the eighteenth century, politicians looked increasingly to public opinion to legitimize their actions and policy decisions. This relationship between public and state was formalized with the extension of the franchise and the establishment of more representative forms of parliamentary democracy, until by the 1840s the bourgeois public had effectively become an organ of government in its own right.

Subsequently, however, with the growth of an increasingly organized and assertive working class on the one hand, and with accelerating concentration of capital and economic power in the hands of wealthy individuals and corporations on the other, civil society itself began to polarize around conflicting sectional interests. According to Habermas, such polarization militated against the rational negotiation of a common political purpose in the public sphere. In response, the state intervened to mediate and reconcile these conflicts, on the one hand by assuming new powers to restrict the pursuit of various forms of private action, and on the other by providing services such as social insurance and medical care, responsibility for which had hitherto been assumed to rest primarily with private citizens. By the mid-twentieth century, the private sphere was thoroughly permeated by the agencies of the state. One effect of this, on Habermas's view, was to undermine the conditions of economic and social autonomy that had made possible the social and discursive relations of the bourgeois public sphere. Instead of actively engaging in rational-critical political debate and opinion formation, the public now increasingly became passive consumers of commodified forms of culture and opinion produced by public and private agencies of mass communication. The bourgeois public had become a mass public, in other words, whose power to direct and legitimize state action had been reduced to little more than plebiscitary approval of policies initiated by government and publicized through the mass media.[3]

Habermas's *Structural Transformation* appeared in English at a time when neo-conservative governments in Britain and the United States were privatizing state welfare services, challenging the power of organized labour, and conniving at the evasion of the regulatory powers of nation states by trans-national corporations. At the same time, the growth of democratic movements in communist countries brought hopes that a revitalized public sphere might provide a site for the negotiation and advancement of political reform. To sociologists anxious to understand such processes, and in particular to examine how democratic public opinion might still be brought to bear on the actions of governments, Habermas appeared to provide an appropriately global framework within which to rethink the nature of public politics. Consequently, his theorization of the public sphere was quickly adopted and put to use, for instance in studies of the role of the media in modern democracy,[4] and of the emergence and significance of new social movements.[5]

Meanwhile, social and sociologically inclined historians picked up Habermas's project of elucidating the circumstances under which democratic forms of public discourse first emerged and flourished. Such work soon began to suggest the need for significant revisions to Habermas's account of the history of the public sphere. Habermas himself recognizes that, while members of the bourgeois public argued that in principle the public sphere should include all members of society, in practice only those who conformed to bourgeois expectations of property and education were allowed to participate.[6] But more detailed historical investigations have made clear the sheer extent of the exclusionary practices and dominance relations which ensured that women and the poor, to name two of the most obvious groups, were denied a place in bourgeois public discourse, or at best consigned to a position of subordination.[7] Moreover, historians have shown that such groups were not simply silenced, but often constituted their own counter-publics as sites for debating and asserting their own sectional identities and interests within the wider sphere of civil society and politics.[8] Finally, historical analysis of such counter-publics has indicated that the formation and assertion of public opinion was not necessarily pursued solely through bourgeois forms of rational discourse, but might also involve a variety of alternative discursive, dramaturgical and performative practices.[9]

Such arguments have had a considerable impact on how the public sphere is theorized. Historians and sociologists now tend not to think of some unified public or some singular form of public discourse, but rather of a multiplicity of more-or-less localized, partial and often transient publics and discourses. Indeed, Nancy Fraser has argued that such multiplicity should be welcomed. Since exclusionary practices and dominance relations are likely to be a feature not just of the bourgeois public sphere but of any public that incorporates an element of identity politics, a diversity of publics should be welcomed by all who aspire in principle to the establishment of a universally inclusive public sphere.[10] This is distinctly at odds with Habermas's own account of the public sphere. For Habermas, it is precisely the critical-rational nature of bourgeois public discourse, and its claim to represent the public as a whole, that makes possible the articulation of an authoritative body of public opinion that can effectively legitimize the actions of government. Consequently, he tends systematically to exclude from his purview the kinds of non-bourgeois counter-publics that have been the focus of more recent historical scholarship.[11] Nonetheless, historians of the public sphere have generally persisted in asserting the historical importance not just of the bourgeois public, but also of various counter-publics and non-bourgeois forms of political expression.[12]

Despite disagreeing with Habermas over the identity of the public and the ways in which it might legitimately express itself, however, most historians continue to follow him in regarding the public sphere primarily as a sphere of discourse and opinion formation, and in supposing that the most significant function of such discourse is to guide and legitimize the actions of government and the state. On this view, the public sphere is best understood as 'the structured setting where cultural and ideological contest or negotiation among a variety of publics takes place',[13] or as 'a theatre for debating and deliberating' about matters of political and social import.[14] Within this setting, diverse and more-or-less local publics endeavour to propagate their views and opinions among other participants in the public sphere; indeed, it is precisely this proselytizing orientation, rather than any principled claim to universality, that now tends to be regarded as distinguishing public discourse from more private forms of communication.[15] Despite this acknowledgement of the existence of multiple contending publics within the public sphere, however, there is nonetheless a tendency, particularly among sociologists, to regard the public sphere itself as constituting, at least potentially, a universal community of interest.[16] Others, meanwhile, have suggested that we should see the public sphere as not constituted in particular institutional settings, but rather in shifting networks of communication that span the institutional structures of society.[17]

But this is to neglect the extent to which institutions of various kinds were implicated in the structuration of the public sphere itself. Habermas himself acknowledges this when he points to the formative role of a number of key 'institutions of the public sphere' – the salon, the coffee house, the press and the concert hall – in the emergence of what he regards characteristically public modes of association and discourse.[18] To medical historians, conscious of the institutional structures of profession and practice that were crucial to the identification of medicine as a public activity, this neglect of institutions is all the more striking. We only have to glance at the eighteenth-century hospital movement to realize the extent to which institutions, in the most obvious sense of the word, were implicated in the formation of the bourgeois public sphere.[19] It is thus no surprise that the medical historians who contribute to the present volume choose to focus on particular public institutions, or on public debates or practices that can be located in particular institutional settings. This focus on institutions gives a rather different slant to our thinking about the structure and function of the public sphere, and about specific publics within it, from that taken by Habermas and others who concentrate primarily on public discourse. In the following pages I will discuss some of the ways in which the individual chapters help us to rethink the history of the public sphere, and will conclude with some general remarks about the light this throws on Habermas's account of the rise and decline of the bourgeois public sphere and its consequences for public politics more generally.[20]

Public–private interactions

Until recently, historians and sociologists have tended to adopt a rather simplistic view of the relationship between public and private spheres, privileging the former as the site of the important business of politics while regarding the latter as merely a secondary and relatively deprived site concerned with little more than the work of demographic reproduction.[21] It is one of the virtues of Habermas's *Structural Transformation* to have added an extra layer of functionality to this relationship. Habermas sees the consolidation of bourgeois privacy and especially domesticity during the eighteenth century as creating a vitally important site for the cultural formation of the autonomous and individuated citizens who populated the bourgeois public sphere. He also notes a reciprocal relationship, in that the new genres of popular literature – the novel, for instance – that circulated in the bourgeois public sphere were at least partly concerned with articulating idealized models of private and domestic life for others to emulate.[22] Habermas spends little time in developing this latter observation, however. Since, his chief interest is in the public sphere as a locus for conferring public legitimacy on government action, he pays little attention to the ways in which public discourse or activity might also have impacted directly on the organization and regulation of private life. But as the papers collected in the first part of the present volume make clear, concerns about configuring the private were central to many areas of public activity, and might even be regarded as one of the primary purposes of public association.

In this respect, it is notable that Habermas's recognition of the role of the private sphere in preparing individuals for public life leads him to assume that bourgeois privacy must have preceded the bourgeois public sphere both logically and chronologically – hence his invocation of the economic demands of early capitalism to explain the privatization of the bourgeois household. As Margaret Pelling's contribution to the present volume makes clear, however, the forms of sociability and discourse that characterize the Habermasian public sphere may also have had their own institutional history, independent of and perhaps even prior to the valorization of bourgeois privacy.[23] Pelling takes as her example the case of the early seventeenth-century College of Physicians of London. Early modern physicians occupied an ambiguous social position. Though they aspired to be regarded as learned gentlemen, their role as attendants of the sick located them in what was still a residual and deprived sphere of domestic privacy, remote from the structures of rank and status that centred on the public world of court and state, and uncomfortably close to women and servants. Likewise, the contractual nature of much of their practice associated them more closely with trade than with the gentlemanly relations of patronage. The College of Physicians provided them with a site in which to explore new forms of sociability that they associated with a more congenial public identity. The homosocial life of the College, made up of late-marrying men who collectively eschewed the public responsibilities that normally devolved onto heads of households, served to distance the physicians from the feminized realm of the domestic. But at the same time the forms of life adopted within the College distinguished it from public bodies such as the guilds and companies that oversaw matters of craft and trade. While these older institutions represented themselves with the pomp of public ceremony and the trappings of office, the College avoided appearing in public as a body, and instead stressed the sobriety and dignity of its individual members. Within the College, meanwhile, the physicians' desire to publicize the transparency of their proceedings and the rectitude of their membership led them to deplore impassioned utterances in favour of more measured and reasoned forms of exchange, and to abandon Latin for the vernacular.

In these respects, the College of Physicians anticipated – albeit within a relatively closed and circumscribed institutional setting – particular forms of interaction that Habermas sees as characteristic of the bourgeois public sphere, most notably the pursuit of rational and transparent debate within a community of equals. But the emergence of such novel social forms within the College was not dependent upon any prior valorization of the private sphere. Rather, it came about simply through the physicians' efforts to reconcile the ambiguities of their public identity. Indeed, if anything, these reconfigurations of public life conduced to the establishment of more modern forms of privacy relations, as where physicians sought to cultivate a role as privileged and confidential medical advisers to their elite patients. In this instance, then, the pursuit of proto-bourgeois forms of public life for the purpose of local institutional and occupational advancement not only preceded but also actually helped to achieve the privatization of social and economic intercourse.

If a concern to reconfigure private life can be discerned in the emergence of proto-public institutions like the College of Physicians, that concern would come to dominate certain bourgeois public institutions that emerged during the nineteenth century. It is important in this regard to recognize that the demarcation between public and private was not clear-cut and absolute. Rather, as a number of recent writers have shown, even the circumscribed realm of the bourgeois household was divided into areas of more or less public space. Control over the admission of outsiders to such spaces – a control exercised especially by the women of the household – provided a means of monitoring and regulating appropriate forms of behaviour.[24] 'Public' and 'private' thus did not simply denote discrete spheres of civil society; more than this, they identified hierarchies of accessibility that structured social interaction in ways that were vitally important for the organization and regulation of social life.[25] And as Pamela Gilbert shows in her contribution to the present volume, judicious navigation of these hierarchies of publicness and privacy could provide a means by which rules of domestic life articulated and negotiated in the public sphere might be carried into private life, particularly among the poor.

Gilbert looks at how the nineteenth-century philanthropist and housing reformer Octavia Hill was able to bring publicly approved knowledge of healthy forms of private existence to bear on day-to-day decisions about the conduct of domestic life among the poor. Deploring the absence of recognizably bourgeois standards of domestic privacy among her tenants, Hill sought to coax and coerce them into reproducing in their own homes some semblance of the middle-class domesticity that she thought necessary to their development as healthy individuals and responsible citizens. She addressed herself particularly to her women tenants, claiming equality with them in their feminine remoteness from the public world of politics and in their intuitive understanding of domestic life. But this claim to equality was disingenuous. In her capacity as landlady, Hill was in a position to exert very real coercive power over her tenants. As an educated member of the middle class, moreover, she had far greater access than her tenants to the public sphere of medical knowledge, while her efforts to impose middle-class standards of domesticity were reinforced, both morally and financially, by public support for her philanthropic activities. Much of that support in turn derived from the information and opinion she brought back to the bourgeois public from her excursions into the private lives of the poor. Hill was thus able to exploit the feminine networks of domestic social life to provide a channel through which public knowledge of working-class privacy could be garnered, and through which the social and economic power of the bourgeois public could in turn be applied directly to the work of reshaping working-class privacy.[26]

We should not suppose that the bourgeois public's concern with regulating private life was directed solely towards the poor, however. Their own private affairs were likewise matters of scrutiny and discipline. But charitable assistance did not provide the same coercive purchase on the behaviour of their own class as it did on those less well-off than themselves. Consequently, in so far as the bourgeoisie saw the need to exert direct forms of compulsion over their peers, they tended instead to act through the machinery of public authority, especially the courts. Habermas is well aware of the importance of the law in providing a framework within which private affairs, particularly commercial relations, could be ordered around publicly agreed norms.[27] But his understanding of the public sphere chiefly as a sphere of discourse and opinion formation inclines him to think of public influence over the law primarily in terms of legitimation of the legislative process. There is also a case to be made for thinking about the courts themselves as a site of public action, however – the public in this instance being constituted not primarily through discourse but through common patterns of practice based on legal precedent. Looked at in this way, the courts belonged not just to the sphere of public authority vested in the state, but also to a bourgeois public sphere of private individuals acting collectively in pursuit of a common public interest.

During the early years of the twentieth century, as Andrew Morrice shows in the third chapter of the present volume, a growing proportion of the courts' time began to be taken up with cases involving questions of sexual and marital propriety, particularly once public access to the divorce courts began to be made easier in the years after the First World War. In such cases, doctors increasingly found themselves called to give evidence concerning their patients' private affairs, for instance where venereal infection or the after-effects of an abortion could be taken as evidence of infidelity. In effect, doctors now found their intimacy with their patients exploited by those who wished to bring private matters of sexual conduct into the public arena of the courts. Doctors were understandably reticent about providing information that had such profound implications for their patients' public reputations. Elite private practitioners, in particular, feared that disclosure would undermine the trust and confidentiality that they regarded as central to their relations with their wealthy clients. Consequently, they responded by arguing that medical secrecy was itself a public good, since it encouraged patients to seek treatment for conditions such as venereal disease that might otherwise be passed on to others in the community. That being the case, doctors claimed that they should be given immunity from the duty incumbent on other citizens to disclose whatever evidence the courts deemed relevant to resolving the cases brought before them. Such arguments carried little weight with the judiciary, who regarded public health concerns as secondary to their own duty to see that justice was served. The judges' view was evidently shared by those members of the public who brought divorce suits and by their legal representatives. As a result, doctors' knowledge of some of the most intimate aspects of their patients' health and behaviour became a matter of legitimate and routine public interest in the divorce courts, and thus an important element in the enforcement of publicly accepted norms of private conduct.

As these chapters make clear, public institutions were concerned with far more than simply debating and legitimizing the work of government. However they were constituted – as professional bodies within pre-bourgeois structures of status and authority, as voluntary associations of bourgeois individuals, or simply through the informally co-ordinated activities of individual citizens exercising their legal rights in the courts – they also provided the means of imposing collectively agreed norms of conduct, including private conduct, on their members and on others. The public sphere should thus not be seen simply as a site for the discursive projection and negotiation of universal or local private interests. It is also – and perhaps above all – a site for the pursuit of various forms of collective action. If we neglect this, we neglect one of the most important reasons for individuals to come together as publics.

Voluntary institutions and the public sphere

Attention to institutional structures and practices can also help to sharpen our thinking about other aspects of the functioning of the public sphere, including issues of inclusion and representation that have arisen from historians' recognition of the often local and partial nature of specific publics. Who participated in public institutions and on what terms? How far did those institutions correspond to Habermas's ideals of equality, transparency and openness? Did the activities of those institutions really represent the common interest of all their members?

It is convenient to begin by considering voluntary institutions. Habermas is strongly of the view that, if public discourse is to express an autonomous popular will, unconstrained by structures of authority and compulsion, it must be constituted on a purely voluntary basis. This association between voluntarism and publicness has been reinforced by historical research into the enormous growth of voluntary philanthropic activity that occurred during the eighteenth and nineteenth centuries, which identifies such activity as a major contributory factor in the formation of the bourgeois public sphere.[28] The so-called voluntary hospitals, in particular, have been singled out for historical attention. On the whole, the results of such research have tended to vindicate Habermas's analysis of the bourgeois public sphere. Involvement in the organization and management of the new voluntary hospitals was based less on older forms of social identity or status than on the ability to contribute financially to the philanthropic enterprise. As a result, the hospitals provided a site where the aristocracy and gentry could combine with the emerging bourgeoisie in pursuit of a common social project, namely the relief and domestication of the poor.[29] Indeed, some authors have gone so far as to suggest that the hospitals actually served an eirenic as much as a philanthropic function, by reconciling hitherto divergent social, political and religious interests within a single institutional endeavour.[30]

Adrian Wilson's contribution to the present volume reveals that the reality may have been more complicated than this peculiarly pacific picture suggests. Wilson takes as his example the events leading to the establishment of the Birmingham General Hospital in 1779. The hospital campaign was first launched in 1765, at least partly with the aim of consolidating an exclusive but rather fragile alliance between Tory interests in the town of Birmingham and the county of Warwickshire, and of winning wider support for those interests from the town's electorate. However, the very publicness of this first hospital campaign would prove its undoing. The decision by a number of Whigs and Dissenters to involve themselves in the campaign was too much for the Church-and-King contingent of landed Tories, who abandoned the hospital. The town Tories now found themselves deprived of their main incentive to participate, and withdrew in their turn. The Dissenters' interest in this Tory-inspired campaign was not strong enough to carry the hospital to completion, and the project collapsed in 1769. Only when the campaign was relaunched in 1776, with overwhelming representation from among the town's Dissenters, was a sufficiently robust coalition of town interests formed to complete the project – this time without significant support from the county Tories. The hospital had come to represent a predominantly urban and Dissenting public – not because of any deliberate act of exclusion, but because the county Tories, finding the institution politically and religiously uncongenial, excluded themselves. Whatever commonality of public interest the hospital might have represented, it was insufficiently attractive to overcome deep-seated divergences of political and religious inclination.

If some chose to exclude themselves from the bourgeois public sphere of the hospitals, others found themselves actively excluded. These included the poor, who were cast as passive recipients of charity rather than active participants in the hospitals' philanthropic project. They also included women, who were generally accepted as contributors but were often excluded from positions of particular responsibility. Thus, from their beginnings in the eighteenth century, the voluntary hospitals provided a site where male medical practitioners could offer their services, and thereby advance their professional interests and enhance their public standing. When middle-class women began to seek access to the profession from the mid-nineteenth century, however, they were denied similar privileges in the hospitals.

Nonetheless, as Elaine Thomson shows in the present volume, women doctors were in some instances able to establish their own hospitals for that purpose. Thomson looks at the case of the Edinburgh Hospital for Women and Children, founded in 1878 as a site where a small group of women doctors could begin to define a public medical role for themselves. They justified this initiative by laying claim to a similarly hybrid gender role to that which Octavia Hill defined for herself in her housing work. As doctors, they argued, they possessed the same knowledge of health and illness as their male counterparts. But as women, they were peculiarly well suited to convey such knowledge to their women patients, and to impart a measure of hygienic self-knowledge that would carry over into their patients' management of their domestic affairs. Such claims were sufficient to win the medical women the measure of public support – chiefly from other women, though a minority of male doctors and laymen also lent their backing – that they needed to set up the Edinburgh Hospital and thereby secure for themselves an institutional base in the public sphere.

It is notable, however, that the Edinburgh medical women departed in important ways from the philanthropic paternalism that characterized more male-dominated institutions. The Edinburgh Hospital did not operate solely as a charity. Those patients who could afford to do so were asked either to pay for their treatment outright, or to pay a monthly contribution into what was effectively a provident insurance scheme. The hospital's patients were thus encouraged to demonstrate the kinds of moral qualities – of thrift, forethought and self-sufficiency – that would help to identify them as active and independent providers of their own health care. Thus, unlike the voluntary general hospitals, which served to reinforce the economic and social distinctions between the donors and recipients of charity – and hence between those who qualified for membership of the public and those who did not – the Edinburgh Hospital tended to enhance working-class women's claim to membership of the public by linking them into an alternative network of feminine solidarity that included the middle-class women who staffed, managed and donated money to the hospital. This distinctiveness would eventually be eroded. As financial difficulties compelled the medical women to link the Hospital with more male-dominated medical campaigns – for instance that against venereal disease – so the tenor of their medical rhetoric, and ultimately of their institutional practice, began to shift towards the kind of paternalistic moralizing that prevailed elsewhere in the profession. But for a while, at least, the Edinburgh medical women and their supporters were able to maintain a public institution that departed significantly from the forms of exclusion by class and gender that prevailed elsewhere in the bourgeois public sphere.

Meanwhile, as the chapter by Martin Gorsky, John Mohan and Martin Powell makes clear, the exclusionary practices that typified the majority of voluntary hospitals not only persisted, but if anything were reinforced. Gorsky and his colleagues look at the changes that occurred in the funding and management of the voluntary hospitals from the mid-Victorian period to the Second World War. During that time, the hospitals experienced a marked decline in the relative importance of individual donations to their funds. Instead, they came increasingly to rely on the collective wealth of the working class, which they tapped through contributory schemes organized in local workplaces. Ostensibly, this led to a widening of democratic accountability, as representatives of the contributory schemes were granted seats on the boards of management. The numbers of such seats did not match the scale of the financial input from the contributory schemes, however. Consequently, when conflicts of interest occurred, the middle-class members of the boards were able to close ranks and vote down working-class representatives. Actual decision-making came increasingly to be dominated by small cliques of elite subscribers, managers and doctors, while decisions about the day-to-day running of the hospitals were reallocated to other sections of the institutions' burgeoning administrative and medical hierarchies. In effect, during the inter-war years the voluntary hospitals ceased to be managed and directed by their contributing publics, and came more closely to resemble private corporations providing medical services for a public of paying consumers.

The lesson is even starker if we look at the medical research charities, which displaced the hospitals as the major medical beneficiaries of public giving from the 1890s onwards. David Cantor's contribution to the present volume examines the case of the Empire Rheumatism Council – later the Arthritis and Rheumatism Council for Research (ARC) – established in 1936 to promote research into the rheumatic diseases. From the beginning the Council was an exclusive and elite body, dominated by a handful of leading doctors and businessmen who made up its governing council. These men regarded themselves as public figures and the Council as a public body, serving the public good. But like so many of the intellectual elite at that time, they also distinguished themselves sharply from 'the public', whom they portrayed as an ignorant, irrational and undisciplined mass in need of intelligent leadership in the fight against disease. Nevertheless, the ARC depended on that public not just to make donations but also to organize countless local fund-raising events, particularly after the establishment of the National Health Service (NHS) led to a rapid decline in large financial contributions from wealthy businessmen. Consequently, by the 1960s the Council had begun to adopt a more differentiated view of the public, primarily in order to identify specific target groups at which to aim its publicity material. It also began to credit the public with a degree of foresight and rational self-interest that the Council sought to mobilize in support of its medical research. None of this meant that members of the public were given any say in planning or organizing publicity campaigns, however, let alone in the direction or interpretation of research into rheumatic disease and its treatment. On the contrary, the many unsolicited proposals and suggestions received by the Council were routinely dismissed as ill informed, unhelpful and a hindrance to the work of the Council itself. In so far as the ARC sought to understand the public, then, it was solely in order to facilitate the manipulation of public sentiment in support of the Council's own initiatives. For all that the ARC regarded itself as a public voluntary body, active among and reliant upon the goodwill of a wide public of supporters, its institutional structures and managerial activities were essentially private.

As these chapters together make clear, the voluntary institutions that made up the bourgeois public sphere invariably represented only partial and often quite local publics, which generally conformed only poorly to Habermas's ideals of inclusiveness, transparency and formal equality. Moreover, by the first half of the twentieth century, these exclusions and inequalities were tending to become more rather than less marked, as institutions were appropriated and privatized by particular interest groups intent on self-advancement and the pursuit of social influence. *Pace* Habermas's view of the decline of the bourgeois public sphere in this period, however, it is not necessary to invoke the impact of state welfare provision on public autonomy to explain this process of privatization. On the contrary, we can in many cases attribute it simply to the internal dynamics of the institutions involved, and especially to the exploitation of structural inequalities by those in positions of relative power or influence. Voluntarism, in other words, is no guarantor of conformity to Habermasian ideals of publicness. It remains to ask whether it is a necessary condition for such conformity.

The state and the public sphere

Habermas's view of voluntarism as a precondition for the formation of an authentic public sphere is particularly evident in his insistence that such a sphere must necessarily be constituted at a clear remove from the sphere of public authority embodied in the state. This premise is fundamental to his account of the emergence and dissolution of the bourgeois public sphere: it was the emancipation of the bourgeoisie from identification with the agencies and institutions of the state that made authentic public opinion possible, and it was the re-infiltration of public authorities into the private sphere that undermined it. As we have seen, however, the institutions of the voluntary public sphere fell far short of Habermas's ideals of inclusiveness and the suspension of relations of domination and subordination. Meanwhile, empirical historical research is beginning to indicate that, during the late eighteenth and early nineteenth centuries at least, sections of the institutional machinery of the state may have provided at least as effective a site – and in many cases a more socially inclusive one – for the formation of public opinion, and for the representation of that opinion to government itself, as did voluntary institutions.[31]

This view is supported by several of the contributors to the present volume. Deborah Brunton, for instance, explores the role of local government as a site of public engagement with the work of the state in her chapter on the administration of public health and sanitary issues in mid-nineteenth-century Scotland. Brunton shows that local sanitary authorities were subject to intense lobbying by a remarkably wide public, for instance over proposals to construct public privies or to cleanse insanitary spaces, while their actions and powers were continually exposed to close public scrutiny and negotiation. The highly inclusive nature of these negotiations was facilitated by the integration of the local sanitary state into civil society more generally: officials on the relevant local government bodies were drawn from a wide spectrum of the citizenry, and elected by an even wider franchise. The boundary between state and civil society was thus not sharp or distinct but blurred and permeable. But whereas Habermas presumes that such interpenetration of state and society was inimical to critical reflection and debate, Brunton shows that, on the contrary, ready access to the state machinery made possible a vigorous public culture not just of critical discourse but also of direct representation and action. The local sanitary authorities were public institutions, not just in the sense that they were part of the machinery of public authority, but in the sense that they provided an institutional locus around which a wide public of householders, tenants and other private persons could articulate their needs and interests. Moreover, the effectiveness of this direct engagement with the state stands in marked contrast to the limited impact that literary public discourse made on local processes of public decision-making. The popular press provided a site for private citizens, philanthropic organizations and state officials to register their interest in sanitary matters, but this did not necessarily lead to reasoned debate, still less to the articulation of a settled public opinion over particular issues. Rather, the actual business of local decision-making was worked out pragmatically, at the level of the sanitary authorities, through the much more socially inclusive processes of direct representation, consultation and negotiation.[32]

This would not remain the case for long, however. By the mid-nineteenth century, local authorities were already acquiring new kinds of powers that tended to limit the extent of public participation in matters of sanitary regulation. Habermas notes that, from around this time, certain kinds of private dispute, which hitherto had been mediated through the pursuit of civil suits in the courts and settled by appeal to universal legal principles, now instead became the business of statutory agencies armed with specific and piecemeal regulatory powers.[33] Christopher Hamlin investigates an instance of just such a shift in his chapter for the present volume. Hamlin takes a detailed look at the mid-nineteenth-century expansion of statutory controls over environmental nuisances, especially dung, and shows how local government agencies, run by public health experts with categorical and specific powers to define and act against nuisances, increasingly displaced private litigation under common law as a means of policing and regulating the shared environment. To an extent, Hamlin's explanation of this shift is in accordance with that proposed by Habermas. Habermas attributes the growth of statutory authority to public demands for the state to intervene in order to mitigate the ill effects of structural inequalities in economic and legal power between corporate capital on the one hand and bourgeois and working-class interests on the other.[34] Hamlin agrees that this was certainly part of the story. With the growth of large-scale industry capable of inflicting widespread damage on the environment, private litigation by individual householders proved an ineffectual means of protecting bourgeois standards of environmental amenity. Consequently the bourgeoisie were generally in agreement that statutory agencies should be empowered to undertake that role on their behalf.

But Hamlin argues that there is another and equally important side to the story. New statutory powers to regulate nuisances were motivated less by a need to prevent corporate despoliation of the environment than by a concern to protect householders from annoyance caused by their immediate neighbours. Earlier in the nineteenth century, private litigation under the common law of nuisances had proved adequate to this task. But with the increasing density of population resulting from urbanization, and the increasingly complex network of relationships that this entailed between neighbours, private litigation proved too unwieldy to be practicable. The transfer of regulatory powers to the local authorities provided a convenient administrative solution to the problem. Significantly, it was also a solution that tended to favour the interests of the bourgeoisie over those of the proletariat. What the bourgeois householder deemed a nuisance – dung, for instance, or the smell of a pig – a poor man might regard as property or an unavoidable consequence of his trade. Such issues would once have been negotiable before the courts on a case-by-case basis, but the new statutes were categorical: a nuisance was a nuisance, whatever the circumstances. In effect, the accumulation of statutory powers by the local authorities represented a closure of the state around bourgeois standards of amenity, to the exclusion of the interests of the poor.[35] The state did not simply intervene to bolster the functional integrity of the capitalist system against structural distortions, as Habermas supposes. Rather, key institutions of local government were effectively appropriated by the bourgeoisie as a means of disciplining and domesticating their working-class neighbours, in a way that was remarkably similar to their use of philanthropic institutions of the voluntary public sphere.

It should of course be stressed that central government could not simply assume new statutory powers against the concerted wishes of those over whom such powers were to be exercised. Logie Barrow makes this clear in his chapter on the failure of the Vaccination Acts. Passed in the 1850s and 1860s, these Acts made it an offence for parents to refuse to vaccinate their children, while providing a free public vaccination service for those who could not afford to have the operation performed privately. These measures were widely approved by central and local government experts, but met with sustained resistance from large sections of the public. This was partly because parents were unwilling to expose their children to what many of them considered a risky operation. But their hostility was greatly exacerbated by the fact that public vaccination was provided under the auspices of the Poor Law. Despite being officially declared non-pauperizing, public vaccination was consequently stigmatized by association with the destitution services, while the notorious parsimony of the Poor Law Guardians ensured that public vaccinees received what was widely seen to be a second-rate service. In effect, the conditions under which public vaccination was delivered served to underline the exclusion of the poor from the ranks of the bourgeois public. Moreover, the central authorities insisted that public vaccination should be conducted solely in designated stations to facilitate official scrutiny and supervision. Working-class parents saw this as a further assault on their rights. Above all, they resented having to take their infants and children to the station to wait for treatment and inspection among other potentially infectious cases. As a result, many parents preferred to face a fine or imprisonment than submit to such discriminatory, degrading and dangerous treatment. Faced with the sheer administrative difficulty of enforcing compulsory vaccination, the government was eventually forced to admit that the situation was unworkable, and strict compulsion ceased in 1898. The failure of the Vaccination Acts thus makes clear the extent to which public pressure may be brought to bear on government, not just through the articulation of public opinion, but also through the cumulative power of concerted individual actions.

Conversely, public opinion alone, no matter how rationally formulated, did not automatically move the central state to action, as Bill Luckin shows in his chapter on the literary and parliamentary debates that grew up around the dramatic problem of London fog during the mid- to late nineteenth century. These debates, as Luckin shows, are notable for the extent to which they conformed to Habermas's ideals of authentic public discourse. Thus they involved a diverse public, and were conducted in an inclusive and relatively non-technical language that emphasized the moral costs of degeneration and urban decline as well as the social and economic costs resulting from damage to the public health. Equally notable is the fact that they took place at a time when, according to Habermas, the bourgeois public sphere was being undermined by the impact of state interventionism. But perhaps the most notable thing about them, in this regard, is that they were to a great extent facilitated by government itself, through the establishment of a House of Lords select committee that heard both lay and expert evidence and which published various recommendations for addressing the problem by limiting smoke emissions. None of this was to any avail, however. Despite invoking such clear expressions of public opinion, Parliament declined the opportunity to establish new forms of statutory control over private smoke production. This was partly due to a concern to protect householders from incurring further costs. But equally important was the continuing commitment in Parliament to self-government through the local authorities – a commitment that was in fact little more than a tacit acknowledgement of the distribution of regulatory power between central and local government: even when central legislation was passed to control the production of industrial smoke in cities, it went largely unenforced by local magistrates. As a result, little was done to address the fog problem, and matters only improved when the severity of the London fogs spontaneously declined in the early twentieth century. In this instance, then, public opinion, though clearly and forcefully articulated, was simply out of step with the concerns and activities of the state machinery, and government felt little compulsion to act on it.

The intrusion of the state into private life, and especially into private matters of health and medicine, would become far more aggressive and extensive from the early twentieth century onwards. A key factor in this process, as the chapter by Steve Sturdy reveals, was the decision to improve the health of the population by providing better access to good-quality personal medical care. One of the most widely debated schemes for effecting such improvement was put forward in

1909 by Beatrice Webb, assisted by a group of leading local authority public health officials, as part of the Minority Report of the Royal Commission on the Poor Laws. The Minority Report recommended the establishment of a universal state medical service, to be run by the local government health authorities. Part of Webb's intention in recommending such a service was to increase public involvement with the local authorities themselves. The creation of a state medical service would not only lead to better treatment of disease, she argued, but would also encourage the public to play an active role in the direction and administration of their own medical services through the democratic institutions of local government. Webb's hopes were frustrated when the government opted instead for a state-subsidized system of National Health Insurance (NHI), which came into operation in 1913. But this scheme, too, was seen by its proponents as a way of revitalizing the public sphere as much as providing better health care. In the case of NHI, however, the locus of public activity was not to be the local authorities, but rather the friendly societies, the largely worker-run provident associations that already provided a large proportion of working-class medical care, and which it was now assumed would take responsibility for providing treatment under NHI.

In the event, these hopes too proved unfounded. Private insurance corporations demanded and secured permission to participate in the national insurance scheme, and with their highly efficient systems of administration and marketing they quickly came to dominate the running of the scheme. Those friendly societies that did well under NHI were the ones that most closely resembled the commercial companies in scale and administrative culture, and which least embodied the ethos of mutualism and self-government that had commended the societies to the advocates of state welfare. In effect, the government had created a state-assisted system of corporate medical care that, far from providing a new institutional focus for public life, simply removed medical provision still further from public control.

Government initiatives in the remainder of the first half of the twentieth century did little to improve the public accountability of the medical services. Though the creation of the NHS in 1948 led to the nationalization of the hospital services, their administration did not become the business of local government, but rather of unelected and largely autonomous regional hospital authorities dominated by elite medical practitioners and hospital managers. Meanwhile general practitioner care, though now made universally available, continued to be organized on a contractual basis between central government and what were in effect independent private practitioners. As a result, the enormous expansion of state involvement in the provision of health services did little to facilitate active involvement of the public in the planning or supervision of those services. The public remained little more than consumers – albeit enthusiastic ones – of health care.

That is not to say that the architects of the early NHS were hostile to public involvement in the provision and oversight of medical services, but rather that they placed greater emphasis on the need to strike a deal with the medical profession and the hospitals.[36] Indeed, politicians and policy makers were initially quite willing to facilitate public discussion of those areas of medical practice that proved to be controversial. Abortion was a case in point, as Naomi Pfeffer argues in the final chapter of the present volume. One of the main concerns behind the passage of the 1967 Medical Termination of Pregnancy Act, as Pfeffer shows, was to make abortions more readily available under the NHS, and thereby to reduce the number of abortions being conducted in private clinics. Underlying this move was a widely felt conviction that the practice of abortions for private profit was disreputable and contrary to the public interest. NHS practice, by contrast, was understood to be disinterested, transparent and publicly accountable. Indeed, the 1967 Act sought to enhance such accountability by establishing a system of gathering and publishing figures on abortions performed under the NHS. Eight years later, the appointment of the Lane Committee of Enquiry provided an opportunity for both pro- and anti-abortion lobbies to present their case to government. Pro-choice activists, in particular, were able to use the newly available government statistics to highlight geographical inequalities of provision, leading to improved facilities in under-provided regions. By such means, Pfeffer argues, the welfare state maintained at least a measure of commitment to public involvement in the development of the health services.

The situation changed markedly during the 1980s and 1990s, however. During this period, as Pfeffer shows, the development of *in vitro* fertilization (IVF) techniques precipitated intense public debates that were in many ways continuous with earlier debates over abortion. But with the appointment of a pro-business Conservative government in 1979, public doubts about the morality of private provision of controversial treatments were over-ridden by more positive evaluations of private practice and the pursuit of profit. As a result, IVF services developed along largely private and entrepreneurial lines. Moreover, the government declined to interfere in the developing market by establishing a similar system of monitoring and regulation to that which had been set up for abortion. Consequently, it was left to the IVF industry itself to establish a system of self-regulation under the so-called Voluntary Licensing Agency, chiefly as a means of promoting public confidence in the practice. Significantly, voluntary self-regulation did not involve the publication of commercially sensitive information about numbers of treatments or success rates. The collection and publication of data was improved somewhat in 1990 with the establishment of a new government-appointed body, the Human Fertilization and Embryology Authority, with a statutory responsibility for licensing and monitoring IVF clinics. But beyond ensuring certain minimum standards of provision, the Authority assumed that regulation of practice would take place primarily through the market, and confined itself to publishing data on success rates and other performance indicators that would supposedly enable customers to make an informed choice.

This amounts to repudiation by the state of anything more than a residual commitment to representing the public interest in the provision of medical services. In the absence of statutory opportunities for public mobilization, public agency has been largely reduced to the sum of individual consumer choices in the medical marketplace. Meanwhile, the state has defined its own role as guardian of the public interest principally in terms of ensuring a minimal level of provision, while leaving decisions about the form of such provision largely to doctors and managers.[37] If anything, this has fuelled mounting public disquiet about the organization and direction of health care, expressed both in the media and in the courts. It remains to be seen whether such activity will lead to concerted public action to reclaim responsibility for health care provision.

That is not to say, as Habermas would have us do, that state intervention in the provision of health care is necessarily incompatible with the formulation and pursuit of an authentic public interest. As the various chapters in this part make clear, state institutions could provide highly effective sites for the mobilization of public opinion and public action. Indeed, in some cases statutory agencies have proved to be more inclusive and more transparent than many voluntary public institutions, particularly where this was underpinned by a commitment to realizing universal rights of citizenship and entitlement. On the other hand, statutory institutions have also proved to be just as liable as voluntary associations to appropriation by much narrower bourgeois publics and by private corporate interests. If statutory provision of health care is not intrinsically inimical to the realization of an authentic public sphere, then, it is equally no guarantee of such a realization.

Conclusions

Taken together, the chapters of the present volume begin to sketch out a narrative of the transformation of the public sphere in Britain over the past four centuries. But they depart from the overall tendency of much recent scholarship in this area by not focusing on the changing forms and communities of public discourse, but rather on the various medical institutions, both voluntary and state-related, that have participated in the constitution of the public sphere during this period. In broad outline, this narrative mirrors Habermas's account of the emergence and growth of the bourgeois public sphere during the early modern period, and its subsequent dissolution and decline during the later nineteenth and twentieth centuries. But it also diverges from Habermas in important ways.

Thus, rather than presupposing the existence of a single bourgeois public sphere, we acknowledge from the start the many different kinds of medical publics that emerged from the seventeenth century onwards. Voluntary and philanthropic institutions were prominent sites for the formation of such publics, particularly during the eighteenth and nineteenth centuries. Such institutions were predominantly middle class in their make-up, and generally shared an interest in promoting bourgeois forms of life and conduct, particularly among the urban poor. But the same institutions also commonly served more specific, local and sectional interests – the interests of women doctors, for instance, or of particular political and religious groups. Mechanisms of exclusion and domination were thus built into medical charities from the start. Consequently, it is hardly surprising to find that, in the twentieth century, those institutions tended to close ranks against the influence of an economically empowered working class, to ensure that control of their activities remained firmly in the hands of a relatively narrow stratum of the lay and medical elite.

The story of the publics that developed around the institutions of local government follows a somewhat different trajectory. Initially, at least, the local state provided a locus of vigorous public activity involving a relatively wide cross-section of the population, particularly in matters relating to public health. Nevertheless, here too it would appear that, in the course of the nineteenth century, the bourgeoisie were able to secure a degree of influence over such institutions that enabled them increasingly to marginalize if not entirely exclude the interests of the proletariat. Moreover, as central government subsequently took steps to meet growing public demand for provision of improved medical services, it tended to by-pass local government and to work instead with private corporations and with an increasingly privatized voluntary sector. Decisions to work in this way appear to have been a matter of political compromise in the first half of the twentieth century, as government found itself caught between the demands of the electorate and those of corporate medical business. But by the 1980s the links between central government and business were increasingly being consolidated, and little space remained for direct public involvement in medical affairs.

The narrative we develop in this volume, then, is not one of the decay of a once-unified public sphere of rational discourse and opinion formation. Nor need we rely, as does Habermas, on generalized structural-functional assumptions about the collapse of critical-rational bourgeois discourse under the clamour of sectional interests and the growth of the mass media. Rather, the story we tell is of the closure and privatization of voluntary organizations, of the bourgeois appropriation and marginalization of local government as sites for the formation and mobilization of local publics, and of the growth of corporate forms of central government that chose to work through private rather than public agencies of medical provision. In effect, many of the most important medical institutions, both voluntary and statutory, to have developed during the eighteenth and nineteenth centuries have since been removed from the public into the private sphere, while the various publics that were originally involved in directing the work of those institutions have been marginalized and excluded. The result has not simply been a decline in public influence over state policy. Medical institutions also had an important role to play in the self-governance of the publics who constituted them and whom they served. With the privatization of those institutions, the opportunities for self-governance have been correspondingly impoverished, while the publics who once directed them have in large part been reduced to the status of consumers of corporate health care.

As our insistence on the mechanisms of exclusion and dominance that characterized eighteenth- and nineteenth-century medical institutions should make clear, however, public institutions never approximated to the kind of universalism that Habermas identifies as one of the ideals of the bourgeois public sphere. Public institutions, be they voluntary or statutory, always tended to serve the interests of particular sections of the population over others. Consequently, we should not conclude that the privatization of those institutions necessarily represents the deformation of some idealized universal public sphere. Rather, we should see it simply as the failure of certain more-or-less inclusive sites of collective self-representation and action. Nor, by the same token, is there any a priori reason for assuming that similar institutions cannot once again be created through the common interests and activities of particular publics. On the contrary, once we start to regard the public sphere in this more pragmatic light, as constituted through specific institutional formations, we also recover the possibility that that sphere might once again be revitalized through appropriate forms of collective action.

It remains to be seen how far this might actually be possible in practice. In the medical field, for instance, we cannot escape the fact that the growth of large-scale and predominantly private institutions of medical provision, and the massive material, human and organizational resources that they command, has resulted in a disproportionate expansion of their economic and political power relative to that wielded by more locally constituted publics. Nevertheless, there is no need to indulge in the fatalism that comes from thinking that the public has been reduced to a passive mass of consumers, or in laments for the decline of idealized forms of public discourse. On the contrary, we should be encouraged by the extent to which local publics continue to form and to engage in collective social and political action, both by bringing direct pressure to bear on government and by asserting what they regard as their rights as consumers of commodities and services.[38] The field of medicine offers a rich illustration of the continuing significance of collective mobilization around matters of public concern, from direct-action organizations demanding public release of drugs against human immunodeficiency virus (HIV) to calls by aggrieved parents for restrictions on the post-mortem removal of their children's organs.[39] Such movements do not depend for their impact solely on rational debate, or even on more emotive forms of discourse. They also engage in collective action of various kinds – in the courts, on the streets and in the medical marketplace – that is co-ordinated through a wide range of more-or-less formal institutions. We may not be in a position to predict the long-term consequences of such movements with any confidence. But we impoverish our understanding of the public and its functions if we confine ourselves to thinking solely in terms of discourse, and thereby neglect the role of institutionalized action in the constitution of the public sphere.

Notes

1 J. Habermas, *The Structural Transformation of the Public Sphere: An Inquiry into a Category of Bourgeois Society*, trans. T. Burger with the assistance of F. Lawrence, Cambridge: Polity Press, 1989. See also Habermas, 'The public sphere: an encyclopedia article (1964)', *New German Critique*, 1974, vol. 1, no. 3, pp. 49–55, for a summary statement of the argument.
2 Habermas, *Structural Transformation*, p. 36.
3 Habermas's early critique of existing forms of liberal democracy culminated in his essay *Legitimation Crisis*, trans. T. McCarthy, London: Heinemann, 1976. We can

perhaps relate this tendency in his work to wider mid-twentieth-century sociological anxieties about the feasibility and consequences of mass democracy, and especially about the impact of the mass media on the formation of public opinion. See, for instance, J. Dewey, *The Public and its Problems*, Chicago: Gateway, 1946, orig. pub. 1927; C. Wright Mills, *The Power Elite*, New York: Oxford University Press, 1954, esp. ch. 13: 'The mass society'; idem, 'Mass media and public opinion', in I.L. Horowitz (ed.), *Power, Politics and People*, New York: Oxford University Press, 1970, pp. 577–98; H. Arendt, *The Human Condition*, Chicago: University of Chicago Press, 1958; R. Sennett, *The Fall of Public Man*, Cambridge: Cambridge University Press, 1977.

4 See, for instance, P. Dahlgren, *Television and the Public Sphere: Citizenship, Democracy, and the Media*, London: Sage, 1995; D.C. Hallin, *We Keep America on Top of the World: Television Journalism and the Public Sphere*, London: Routledge, 1995; M.E. Price, *Television: The Public Sphere and National Identity*, Oxford: Oxford University Press, 1995.

5 For a critical review of this literature, see C. Calhoun, 'Civil society and the public sphere', *Public Culture*, 1993, vol. 5, pp. 267–80.

6 Habermas, *Structural Transformation*, pp. 84–6.

7 For influential summary statements of this view, see M. Ryan, 'Gender and public access: women's politics in nineteenth-century America', and G. Eley, 'Nations, publics, and political cultures', both in C. Calhoun (ed.), *Habermas and the Public Sphere*, Cambridge, MA: MIT Press, 1992, pp. 258–88 and 289–339 respectively. See also J.B. Landes, *Women and the Public Sphere in the Age of the French Revolution*, Ithaca, NY: Cornell University Press, 1988; L.F. Cody, 'The politics of reproduction: from midwives' alternative public sphere to the public spectacle of man-midwifery', *Eighteenth-Century Studies*, 1999, vol. 32, pp. 477–95.

8 For instance M.P. Ryan, *Women in Public: Between Banners and Ballots, 1825–1880*, Baltimore: Johns Hopkins University Press, 1990.

9 J. Plotz, 'Crowd power: chartism, Carlyle, and the Victorian public sphere', *Representations*, 2000, vol. 70, pp. 87–114; J.L. Brooke, 'Reason and passion in the public sphere: Habermas and the cultural historians', *Journal of Interdisciplinary History*, 1998, vol. 29, pp. 43–67.

10 N. Fraser, 'Rethinking the public sphere: a contribution to the critique of actually existing democracy', *Social Text*, 1990, vol. 25/26, pp. 56–80.

11 See for instance N. Fraser, 'What's critical about critical theory? The case of Habermas and gender', in Fraser, *Unruly Practices: Power, Discourse and Gender in Contemporary Social Theory*, Cambridge: Polity Press, 1989, pp. 113–43. Fraser is responding in this article not just to Habermas's account of the public sphere as developed in *Structural Transformation*, but also to the more highly theorized account of discursive politics that he subsequently develops in his *The Theory of Communicative Action*, vol. 1: *Reason and the Rationalization of Society*, London: Heinemann, 1984, and vol. 2: *Lifeworld and System*, Cambridge: Polity, 1987. Habermas discusses his misgivings about the power of identity-based publics to contribute to the formation of a genuinely inclusive public sphere in vol. 2: *Lifeworld and System*, pp. 391–6. For a cogent reply, see Michael Warner, 'The mass public and the mass subject', in Calhoun (ed.), *Habermas and the Public Sphere*, pp. 377–401.

12 In an insightful critique of recent scholarship in this area, Harold Mah suggests that this results from a continuing political commitment, previously developed especially by feminist and labour historians, to attribute social agency to marginal and especially minority groups: Mah, 'Phantasies of the public sphere: rethinking the Habermas of historians', *Journal of Modern History*, 2000, vol. 72, pp. 153–82, at pp. 160–4.

13 Eley, 'Nations, publics', p. 306.

14 Fraser, 'Rethinking the public sphere', p. 27.

15 Thus for instance Nancy Fraser: 'To interact discursively as a member of a public...is to disseminate one's discourse into ever widening arenas...however limited a public

may be in its empirical manifestation at any given time, its members understand themselves as part of a potentially wider public.' Fraser, 'Rethinking the public sphere', p. 67.

16 Whether or not discussion and negotiation between contending publics can ever result in the formation of a univocal body of public opinion or even of common interest, particularly in the absence of agreed standards of rationality for the resolution of disagreement, remains a matter of debate. Agnes Ku, for example, builds on Benedict Anderson's notion of 'imagined community' to suggest how local publics might come to identify themselves as part of a larger and more inclusive public. A.S. Ku, 'Revisiting the notion of "public" in Habermas's theory – towards a theory of politics of public credibility', *Sociological Theory*, 2000, vol. 18, pp. 216–40, at p. 229. For a more critical evaluation of the contradictions inherent in any such imagined public, see Mah, 'Phantasies of the public sphere'.

17 Thus M. Emirbayer and M. Sheller, 'Publics in history', *Theory and Society*, 1999, vol. 28, pp. 145–97, define publics as 'open-ended flows of communication that enable socially distant interlocutors to bridge social-network positions...in pursuit of influence over areas of common concern' (p. 156).

18 Habermas, *Structural Transformation*, pp. 31–43. For a particularly sophisticated and satisfying history of the institutionalization of new forms of public discourse during the early modern period, see M. Warner, *The Letters of the Republic: Publication and the Public Sphere in Eighteenth-Century America*, Cambridge, MA: Harvard University Press, 1990, which endeavours to elucidate the full 'cultural meaning of printedness' (p. xi).

19 As does P. Langford, *Public Life and the Propertied Englishman, 1689–1798: The Ford Lectures Delivered in the University of Oxford, 1990*, Oxford: Clarendon Press, 1991.

20 It is worth noting here the existence of an important body of literature on the history of the public sphere that we largely neglect in the present volume (the chapters by Christopher Hamlin and Bill Luckin are honourable exceptions), namely that concerned with the public constitution and dissemination of medical and other forms of scientific knowledge and expertise. For an introduction to this literature, which includes some of the most challenging and innovative writing on the history of the public sphere to date, see C.W.J. Withers, 'Towards a history of geography in the public sphere', *History of Science*, 1998, vol. 36, pp. 45–78; T. Broman, 'The Habermasian public sphere and "science *in* the Enlightenment"', ibid., pp. 123–50.

21 Early feminist histories of women's exclusion from the public sphere are a case in point. See for instance J. Siltanen and M. Stanworth (eds), *Women and the Public Sphere: A Critique of Sociology and Politics*, London: Hutchinson, 1984; L. Davidoff and C. Hall, *Family Fortunes: Men and Women of the English Middle Class, 1780–1850*, London: Routledge, 1992.

22 Such, at least, is my reading of his discussion of 'audience-related privacy', its representation in the emerging literary form of the novel, and its relation to the literature of political critique: *Structural Transformation*, pp. 43–56.

23 Historians have recently identified a number of other areas of public political discourse that likewise prefigured elements of the bourgeois public sphere in advance of the privatization of bourgeois domesticity. See for instance P. Lake and M. Questier, 'Puritans, papists, and the "public sphere" in early modern England: the Edmund Campion affair in context', *Journal of Modern History*, 2000, vol. 72, pp. 587–627; S. Pincus, '"Coffee politicians does create": coffeehouses and Restoration political culture', *Journal of Modern History*, 1995, vol. 67, pp. 807–34; D. Zaret, 'Petitions and the "invention" of public opinion in the English Revolution', *American Journal of Sociology*, 1996, vol. 101, pp. 1497–555; H.R. French, 'Social status, localism and the "middle sort of people" in England 1620–1750', *Past and Present*, 2000, no. 166, pp. 66–99.

24 E. Langland, *Nobody's Angels: Middle-Class Women and Domestic Ideology in Victorian Culture*, Ithaca, NY: Cornell University Press, 1995. And see D. Riley, *Am I That Name?'*

Feminism and the Category of 'Women' in History, Basingstoke: Macmillan, 1988, ch. 3: "'The social", "woman", and sociological feminism', for a discussion of the designation of feminized spaces of personal morality in civil society more generally.

25 N. Armstrong, *Desire and Domestic Fiction: A Political History of the Novel*, Oxford: Oxford University Press, 1987. In the present volume, Pelling makes a similar point about public and private space when she notes that, for all its public display of transparency and inclusiveness, the early College of Physicians of London also conducted the most sensitive aspects of its business behind closed doors, thereby exerting a degree of disciplinary control over its members and licensees.

26 See also F.K. Prochaska, *Women and Philanthropy in Nineteenth-Century England*, Oxford: Clarendon Press, 1980.

27 On the centrality of universal law to the conception of the bourgeois public sphere, see Habermas, *Structural Transformation*, pp. 73–9. See also M.R. Somers, 'Citizenship and the place of the public sphere: law, community, and political culture in the transition to democracy', *American Sociological Review*, 1993, vol. 58, pp. 587–620. In *The Theory of Communicative Action*, Habermas goes on to identify 'juridification' as one of the main means by which elements of the lifeworld are rationalized and reutilized by the bureaucratic machinery of the state: vol. 2, *Lifeworld and System*, pp. 356f.

28 Langford, *Public Life and the Propertied Englishman*; R.J. Morris, 'Voluntary societies and British urban elites, 1780–1850: an analysis', *Historical Journal*, 1983, vol. 26, pp. 95–118.

29 R. Porter, 'The gift relation: philanthropy and provincial hospitals in eighteenth-century England', in L. Granshaw and R. Porter (eds), *The Hospital in History*, London: Routledge, 1989, pp. 149–78; A. Borsay, '"Persons of honour and reputation": the voluntary hospital in an age of corruption', *Medical History*, 1991, vol. 35, pp. 281–94; A. Wilson, 'The politics of medical improvement in early Hanoverian London', in A. Cunningham and R.K. French (eds), *The Medical Enlightenment of the Eighteenth Century*, Cambridge: Cambridge University Press, 1990, pp. 4–39.

30 See especially Porter, 'The gift relation'. For a contrary view of hospital committees as sites for renegotiating rather than reconciling religious and social differences, see M.E. Fissell, *Patients, Power and the Poor in Eighteenth-Century Bristol*, Cambridge: Cambridge University Press, 1991.

31 See in particular J. Vernon, *Politics and the People: A Study in English Political Culture, c. 1815–1867*, Cambridge: Cambridge University Press, 1995. Lake and Questier, 'Puritans, papists and the "public sphere"', emphasize the role of the state in promoting public discourse as early as the late sixteenth century. More generally, recent work on the 'mixed economy of welfare' has demonstrated how difficult it is to draw any clear demarcation between statutory and voluntary agencies throughout the nineteenth century. See, for instance, G.B.A.M. Finlayson, *Citizen, State and Social Welfare in Britain 1830–1990*, Oxford: Clarendon Press, 1994.

32 Calhoun, 'Civil society and the public sphere', and Mah, 'Phantasies of the public sphere', both suggest that this kind of direct involvement with the state should not be regarded as part of the bourgeois public sphere, which characterizes itself solely in terms of rational debate, but rather as persistent elements of older forms of public life. It is not clear what historiographical purpose is served by such strictures, however, other than to bolster the presumption that the bourgeois public sphere is necessarily constituted at a remove from the state.

33 Habermas, *Structural Transformation*, pp. 178–80.

34 Ibid., pp. 141–51.

35 Cf. Vernon, *Politics and the People*, who argues that a similar closure took place around the political functions of the local state.

36 C. Webster, *The National Health Service: A Political History*, Oxford: Oxford University Press, 1998.

37 R. Klein, *The New Politics of the National Health Service*, 4th edition, Harlow: Prentice Hall, 2001.

38 The notion of consumption as a form of collective action is particularly germane here. With his insistence on the discursive nature of the public sphere, Habermas tends to regard consumption in terms of essentially private 'acts of individuated reception': *Structural Transformation*, p. 161. However, historians and sociologists alike have recently demonstrated the extent to which markets operate as institutions in their own right, in which consumption is profoundly informed by collective concerns about identity and social status. For an analysis of the institutional nature of the economic relations of markets in general, see M. Granovetter, 'Economic action and social structure: the problem of embeddedness', *American Journal of Sociology*, 1985, vol. 91, pp. 481–510. A.O. Hirschman, *The Passions and the Interests: Political Arguments for Capitalism before its Triumph*, Princeton, NJ: Princeton University Press, 1977, examines the circumstances under which the pursuit of wealth came to be valued as the normative basis for the maintenance of social order through the market. A similar perspective informs H.C. Clark, 'Commerce, the virtues, and the public sphere in early seventeenth-century France', *French Historical Studies*, 1998, vol. 21, pp. 415–40. Research into the growth of bourgeois consumption of a range of commodities, including medical care, during the eighteenth and early nineteenth centuries has made clear that consumer choice was not simply a matter of individual preference, and that patterns of consumption need to be regarded as informal public institutions, collectively negotiated and maintained through the establishment and policing of generally accepted norms of bourgeois conduct and identity. See for instance R.L. Spang, *The Invention of the Restaurant: Paris and Modern Gastronomic Culture*, Cambridge, MA: Harvard University Press, 2000, and especially C. Jones, 'The great chain of buying: medical advertisement, the bourgeois public sphere, and the origins of the French Revolution', *American Historical Review*, 1996, vol. 101, pp. 13–40. In the context of the present volume, we can extend this analysis to understand the growth of working-class resistance to compulsory vaccination during the second half of the nineteenth century, for instance, or incremental changes in the way that individual divorce suits were brought before the courts during the first quarter of the twentieth, as examples of similarly informal publics constituted and co-ordinated around issues of common interest. Likewise, the notion of a 'citizenship of entitlement' among the consumers of publicly funded medical services may be seen, in this light, as a vital element in the formation of a collective public identity.

39 On acquired immunodeficiency syndrome (AIDS) activism, see S. Epstein, *Impure Science: AIDS, Activism, and the Politics of Knowledge*, Berkeley: University of California Press, 1996.

Part I

Public–private interactions

1 Public and private dilemmas

The College of Physicians in early modern London

Margaret Pelling

We have only to conjure up such epithets as 'public health', 'private practice' and 'secret remedies' to begin to realize how intimate is the relationship between medicine and concepts of privacy and the public. Moreover, medicine, with its apparently unique ethical responsibilities focusing on human survival on the one hand, and confidentiality and the human mind and body on the other, seems to have a major influence on the value attached to these concepts. As this chapter will try to illustrate, value and meaning are interdependent. A shift in values causes one or the other concept to become better defined. In what follows, the aim is to use an early modern case study to reveal the decidedly ambivalent antecedents of what professionalized societies in general, and Habermas in particular, take for granted as being valued positively. The subject of the case study is a small, isolated, homosocial medical institution in London, the College of Physicians, in the period before the English civil wars. My concern is with something like a 'history of interiority' for a select group of highly educated males as expressed in an account of themselves – the College's Annals – which was at least semi-public. The College's attempts at defining both itself, and its opponents, in the wider world of London medicine involved a complex of meanings for public and private in which we can perhaps see the germs of the modern stress on privacy, itself an aspect of the hegemony of the middle class.

We can also discern in the College something like the literate, self-regulating detachment that Habermas idealized as essential to the authentic public sphere. However, this too calls for close inspection, and, as a result, proves to be a peculiarly constructed phenomenon indicative as much of weakness as of strength. If the College achieved detachment, it was as a side-effect of dependency. Further, the medical role itself can be shown to entail status and gender disadvantages that are intrinsic to the style and content of the physician's connection with the political process, and to his influence on the demarcation of the public and private realms. Privacy in the relationship between patient and practitioner emerges as contingent, compromised and at odds with the contemporary ideal in which the relationship was one necessarily involving other people. In general, the case study of the London physicians demonstrates how the closest possible proximity to the project of professionalization – and, it may be argued, a prominent role in defining it – can nonetheless be associated with a movement not from the proto-private towards the proto-public, as Habermas postulated, but of something like its opposite.

Privacy and individualism

In terms of basic demarcations, the early modern period contrasts with our own. Our own era appears convinced that the private realm is now of greater interest than the public. The latter concept is, at best, in the process of redefinition. Modern opinion has disengaged itself fairly thoroughly from such concepts as public service and public life; scrutiny in the public interest is only valued if it is individualistic. For many, the significance of 'public' is in its meaning for the individual, and what duties the individual is owed by the state, including such liberal preoccupations as freedom of information and whether a 'right to privacy' can safely be the subject of legislation. In the context of medical services, analysis is dominated by the single instance, or the definitive personal experience. Any deviation within the patient–practitioner relationship from the ideals of privacy and personal autonomy is resisted and deplored, even in the context of calls for greater accountability. In an article published in 1989 on 'unconscious aspects of health and the public sphere', Karl Figlio reflected current opinion by characterizing 'public' as a bland word, desexualized and lacking in energy, which did not even have the status of being the polar opposite of 'private'. 'Health', he claimed, was itself a public word, and both 'health' and 'public' stood apart by providing 'reservoirs of non-conflictual phantasy'. The complacency so attributed may be an aspect of the 'culture of contentment', although Figlio does not say so. 'Disease', on the other hand, was personal.[1] Recent calls for an insurance-based system to replace the National Health Service (NHS) reinforce these impressions. It is less clear how far this analysis can be reconciled with the revival of public health concerns and public health historiography.[2] An illustration of recent shifts is the renaming of the linear descendant of the first British department of social medicine, founded by a Nuffield benefaction in Oxford in 1942. What in the 1970s was a department of 'community medicine' is now one of public health within a division of public health and primary care. It might be argued, however, that such changes reflect in a purely pragmatic way the return of infectious diseases as a subject of professional concern, and, with that, some of the freight of meaning of earlier decades, rather than a new phase of redefinition. In spite of the trend towards globalism, it would be difficult to argue that the notion of public health has regained anything like the currency and substance it enjoyed in this country before the Second World War.[3]

Many discussions are content to take the distinction between public and private as a dichotomy firmly founded in nineteenth-century individualism. The contrast can be effectively deployed without matters of definition being of great concern.[4] Here, however, an emphasis on intimacy, subjectivity and 'the home' can obscure the privacy of economic relations that is an essential aspect of the Victorian distinction.[5] This aspect of privacy connotes a rejection of the state's right to interfere. Medievalist and early modernist historiography, for its part, has given us a schema for the relationship between public and private in society at large that corresponds with the decline of feudalism, the impact of the Reformation and the increased prevalence – or perhaps intensity – of the values of the middling sort. In this schema, the main feature is not so much the decline of the public as the growing importance of the private, particularly as expressed by the professional classes and the urban bourgeoisie. For post-Revolutionary England, stress is also laid on the private gentleman, living modestly on his own land and of influence mainly in his own locality. Here again, issues of definition are not thought essential to discussions that focus on the contrast between private life and the rise and fall of party politics. In this context, privacy can become synonymous with the contemplative life, involving contrasts between the country and the town, and between 'enthusiasm' and 'retirement' in politics and religion.[6] However, our current interest in subjectivity has encouraged the discovery of the private even in periods, like the Middle Ages, in which the concept was previously thought inapplicable because, under feudalism, the public and the private were deliberately conflated in the interests of the ruling class. That is, where the dichotomy between public and private is challenged for earlier periods, it is the private world that is currently attracting the interest. As an inverted reflection of this, resistance has been offered by feminist historians, who have qualified, or even abandoned, the notion of separate spheres, at least as a period-specific, comparative development in which the private realm contained the feminine, and was defined by its feminine characteristics. Instead, the trend is towards a redefinition of the public that includes female agency. For many historians, however, the distinction between public (male) and private (female) remains both evident and serviceable.[7]

Early modern public spheres: the British case

The sociologists, for example Norbert Elias, and the sociologist-philosophers, like Habermas, who problematize the distinction between public and private for historians, focus on the conjunction of absolutism and enlightenment in eighteenth-century continental Europe. Within this framework, the English versions of absolutism under the Tudors and Charles I are inconveniently early, particularly for Habermas's adoption of England as the 'model case' of the emergence of a bourgeois public sphere. Much recent scholarship has reiterated the deliberate self-consciousness of humanist intellectuals in this period, and the shared activism of the reading and writing in which they engaged.[8] However, it is difficult not to conclude that, although disappointment could breed detachment, the predominant intention of these figures was employment for themselves and their ideas in the service of the state. Moreover, although humanists were mutually supportive, constructed epistolary communities and more or less invented prosopography, this period in England almost entirely lacked the structures of sociability, the informal clubs, salons, societies and other semi-private gatherings that provide the focus for Habermas's notion of the authentic public sphere and its detached criticism of the activities of the state. Similarly lacking before the mid-seventeenth century are the published, allegedly independent organs of opinion such as news-sheets and journals. Although recent historiography has criticized Habermas's chronology in terms of the development of a public sphere in England in the 1640s or even earlier, partici-pants, including writers and readers of the early newspapers, are seen as politically engaged rather than detached. For Habermas, civic society was forced into existence as a corollary of a depersonalized state power.[9] Authority in Tudor and early Stuart England was certainly becoming more centralized, but it was not yet depersonalized, nor was it represented by standing armies or a faceless bureaucracy. Hindle describes this society as one in which 'governmental and judicial resources were unprofessional and relatively shallow'.[10] Perhaps most importantly, religious affiliation in the earlier period has to be seen as an initi-ating and organizing principle for intellectual activity, and as a factor more likely to influence 'detachment' than any secular motive.

Habermas did see the British case as, in outline, the model for development, and mid-seventeenth-century England as producing a sense of 'the public' in advance of eighteenth-century France or Germany. British historians have however been primarily concerned with whether the civil wars and the Commonwealth were necessary to bring about a participation in politics and structures of authority by those below the level of the ruling elite. This version of the public sphere does have a private dimension, as well as a local one, but it implies participation in government, not detachment from it. Critiques of Habermas in these terms, such as that of Goodman, therefore focus on nation-alisms to which his formulations have appeared more applicable, such as that of eighteenth-century France.[11] This chapter follows suit in that it is not primarily concerned to find Habermas wanting as an analyst of England before the 1690s. Rather, it looks at relevant forms of interiority that appear to have projected themselves into future periods, and examines their ambivalence. Habermas himself implicitly singled out English interiority, attributing consid-erable significance to the Protestant Reformation as a factor in the evolution of privacy. Thus, England's bourgeois revolutions were prompted in part at least by issues of freedom of conscience. Religiously and politically, English people in the seventeenth century are seen as achieving the right to think differently in private from what might be demanded of them in public.[12] Private devotions, as opposed to the whited sepulchres of the Pharisees, had always had a value in Christian theology, but this was naturally accentuated when intermediaries between God and the individual soul were removed. The early seventeenth century was still exploring the dangers for the individual and the body politic of a century of religious change in which an individual's allegiances might be very different from those he or she appeared to espouse. Hence a degree of paranoia and resort to covert operations in which physicians and other medical practitioners played an active and sometimes central role. As is well known, Elizabethan and Jacobean literature and satire are much preoccupied by sincerity, by both the uses and abuses of techniques of persuasion, of self-presentation in person and in print, and by the differences between appearances and reality.[13] As one reflection of this, the College of Physicians in 1599 felt obliged to communicate in English rather than its own language of Latin, to make evident the 'truth, honesty and sincerity' of its proceedings.[14]

Recent revisionism notwithstanding, in this period, by contrast with the present, it was 'public' that was the defining category, and 'private' that was the residual. This is not to deny that 'private' had already acquired many of the shades of meaning familiar today. Rather, the balance of usage was fairly evidently in a particular direction, which, not surprisingly, bore a direct relationship to masculine authority and male experience. In academic discourse, for example, woman could be defined as a 'species privata'. Women were allowed to work as sextons in London in the eighteenth century because this office was regarded as both private and menial.[15] Privacy signified mainly a form of deprivation, or even bereavement, referring to areas of life that lacked contact with, or were cut off from, the world of authority. Hence private traders, or private soldiers, were those who lacked an office or public position or clear allegiance. A private man was not entitled to forgive wrongs that contravened the public laws. Even towns could be described as 'only private places' if they were not a seat of government. This usage was evidently related to classical sources, images of republican Rome, and especially to notions of the appropriate political role, defined as public, of the adult male. Privacy at home was defined not by domesticity in the modern sense but by property rights, an aspect that is echoed, but greatly expanded, in nineteenth-century usage.[16] As with the Roman paterfamilias, the political and public responsibilities of every married male began with his role as head of a household. Some early modern usages do suggest privileged rather than deprived aspects of privacy, but this is mainly by way of reference to privileged access to a public person who counted as a source of authority. Thus Francis Bacon attributed his falling out with his patron the Earl of Essex to a 'discontinuance of private-ness'.[17]

In this pattern of usage, in which the advantage lay with 'public' and with the male gender, there was obviously potential for overlap between, or conflation of, the private and the feminine, and this is evident in contemporary references to secrecy, conspiracy and subversion. Again, the religious element is important, if not definitive. Suspicion attached to practices like private baptism, or sacraments in private houses. If, as some historians argue, the great common denominator of this period in English society was anti-popery, this has considerable significance for notions of privacy. Such a mentality inevitably placed a positive value on public manifestations of loyalty, visible signs of an ordered society, and oversight by neighbours. Hypocrisy was feared and suspected – it was not yet institutionalized, or reinvented as a virtue conducive to stability and social harmony.[18]

The anomalousness of collegiate physicians

How does the case study of the physicians illuminate this context? The answer has to be, not so much by typifying it, as in contrast with it. This anomalousness of physicians has many different facets. First, in their own persons, the physicians did not behave like citizens. Instead of becoming heads of households in their twenties, they deferred marriage and, although often originating in large families, were frequently childless themselves. I have argued elsewhere that these patterns were one reflection of attempts to compensate for the gender and status disadvantages arising out of the proximity of the physician's work to the residual, private, female realm.[19] This disengagement from household responsibilities (in the early modern sense) was apparently matched by a disinclination for office, or even responsibility, at the parish level. Physicians sought various kinds of exemption as both a mark of privilege and a saving of expense, but the side-effect of their avoiding such duties as watch and ward, and musters, was to minimize their participation in the ramifying structures of male authority. Nor was their undoubted concern for status allied to a willingness to take higher office, as councilmen, aldermen, mayors or justices of the peace. That issues of eligibility arise in such contexts is in itself a measure of the self-imposed isolation of physicians. It is true that physicians not infrequently stood as members of Parliament; this however was an occasional role, less directly representative of authority than it was later to become, and more symptomatic of clientage.

The low visibility of physicians in normal times was not compensated for by any prominent part in public health emergencies, such as plague epidemics. Rather, both individually and institutionally, physicians were absent when popular appreciation of their presence would have been greatest. Contemporaries were disinclined to give much credit to their claims to be serving the state by ensuring the survival (well away from the usual locations associated with government) of members of the elite. In this context, as in many others, a collegiate physician appeared as a servant within a patronage relationship, but without the recognized, semi-public political influence exerted by such servants as secretaries, brokers or factors. Physicians had privileged access to the bodies and even the minds of their elite patients, but although they could make economic gains, they were largely unable to make public use of this knowledge, which contemporaries tended to equate with the forms of access more commonly available to women. This is not to conclude that physicians suffered from complete emasculation in terms of their public role. However, it is notable that the form of masculinity most often attributed to them was purely sexual, and limited in its force by being linked to a high degree of association with women and an unfair degree of access to private spaces in the household. Gowing and others have suggested that it was women whose reputations were constructed in predominantly sexual terms, and that, where this is the case, it can be construed as an aspect of gender disadvantage.[20]

Collegiate physicians displayed the same characteristics institutionally as they did individually. They aimed at a sober richness in dress, rather than instant recognition, and their buildings lacked presence, although ambition in this respect was held back by financial constraints. Unlike the freemen of companies and City dignitaries, they were hesitant about appearing in public as a body, and their feasts were semi-private, when they took place at all. Physicians were in any case absent from London for stretches of the ceremonial year, especially in summer. The College officebearers, especially the Censors (four in number), were expected to go forth in formal dress to conduct searches of apothecaries' shops, but this open declaration of a form of public responsibility was sporadically made and seems never to have become a recognized ritual.[21] Rather, the College's institutional life was defined and dominated by its interrogations of irregular practitioners, which took place behind closed doors. It was intended, however, that the outcomes of these confrontations, if satisfactory, should become a matter of public record. For the College this was signified by the creation of a semi-public text, just as their appeal was constantly to written statutes, or to the sacred texts of Galen, available in print, but not in English.

The College's contacts with other regulatory or ruling bodies in the City were frequently unsatisfactory; more importantly, they were tenuous. The City companies were bound ultimately by Parliament; the College was answerable to the monarch and the court of Chancery.[22] The co-operation of City officials was necessary for the College's censorial activity to be successful, but the College's lack of integration in City life made it an unwilling suppliant rather than an equal partner. Its relationship even with its own parish, St Martin Ludgate, seems to have been minimal. It is not that the College was different in kind from the corporations regulating the crafts and trades. Rather, it did not behave in the same way, or take on the same responsibilities. Just as physicians lacked credibility as heads of household, so the College's participation in the upbringing of young male citizens was confined to examinations (designed to be exclusive rather than inclusive), the sporadic inspection of apothecaries' apprentices, and occasional lectures. There were other major differences. Companies, or individual freemen, made their presence felt by setting up schools, founding almshouses or supporting members and their widows in old age. The College, again partly for financial reasons, failed to carry out the philanthropic functions to which many historians attribute the stability of early modern English society. Since the effects of philanthropy are not seen as dependent upon its scale, the College's failure to do anything at all represents a significant abdication from the public role that might have been expected of it. In short (and more contentiously), the College appears to have eschewed both patriarchy and paternalism. It did however, as we shall see, participate to some degree in patronage relationships.

As defined by its statutes subsequent to its foundation, the College closely resembled one of the types of collegiate medical organization present in Italian cities from the thirteenth century, although it also seems structurally to have borne a close relationship to the humanist foundation (1517) of Corpus Christi College in Oxford.[23] It was not of course the only anomalous body in London. It shared characteristics with two other pre-Reformation foundations, the College of Arms, chartered by Richard III in 1484, and Doctors' Commons, founded for the civil lawyers in 1511, a few years before the inauguration of the College of Physicians in 1518.[24] In the Jacobean period, the civil lawyers practised in the ecclesiastical courts of the Archbishop of Canterbury, the High Court of Admiralty and the High Court of Chivalry. The last adjudicated on gentle status and the right to bear arms, and consequently overlapped with the concerns of the heralds. Neither the Heralds' College nor Doctors' Commons was a teaching body. Each is generally described as a small professional elite; each existed to defend the claims of different forms of recondite knowledge; each, like the Physicians' College, saw itself as entitled to regulate its specialism throughout the country – not on an administrative basis, but when it so wished. The heralds, like the physicians, earned their living by taking fees. Also like collegiate physicians, heralds faced a challenge from 'unlicensed practitioners' – painter-stainers and other artisans – and attempted to exercise a kind of summary jurisdiction over these and other offenders behind closed doors. All three groupings were closer to the crown (including its dependencies the Privy Council and the equity courts, such as Chancery) as a source of authority than to the City or to Parliament. It is arguable that by 1600 the College of Physicians' brand of humanism was more that of the court than the civic humanism associated with its foundation.[25] All three bodies appeared in the Jacobean period to enjoy a degree of prestige and the monopoly of a kind of intellectual capital of high value but limited currency.[26] Each of the three bodies, over the course of the seventeenth century, saw its intellectual capital devalued or taken out of circulation. For the physicians, this kind of investment in Galenism was replaced by the new science inaugurated by its Fellows Harvey and Gilbert. The significance of the utilitarian phase of the 'new science' with which collegiate physicians sought to replace Galenism has been much debated, but was short-lived; as far as the College was concerned, the new forms of knowledge were intended to be widely respected but not to form the basis of a new inclusive intellectual community.[27]

'Public' and 'private' in collegiate practice

If we turn to the different ways in which collegiate physicians themselves recorded their sense of public and private, we find a complexity that can be referred to the College's own problems of status. First, the College was divided within itself between public and private, on hierarchical grounds. The quarterly comitia, at which all the members were expected to be present, were seen as 'public' meetings; these were in contrast to the occasionally 'private' meetings of officebearers, and the meetings of the most senior members, the President and Elects, which were private by definition. Thus the process of becoming an Elect, which could involve examination by the President, could only be witnessed by other Elects. Such privacy was designed to signify privilege and to protect reputations, a concern that was played out at lower levels of the hierarchy. Of the four examinations for admission as a Candidate, the prelude to becoming a Fellow, it was the fourth, that most likely to reflect credit on all sides, which was most often conducted at one of the 'public' meetings. Less objectionable irregulars or borderline examinees were offered the inducement, or the consolation, of being questioned at a private meeting, or off the record, just as proceedings against those categorized as intransigent or ignorant were written down and could be shown to outsiders. For those unwilling to accept the College's authority, it was desirable as well as an added penalty to require them to make a submission in public.[28] Similarly, the College sought to induce conformity in the apothecaries drawn under its supervision by suggesting that poor-quality drugs could be destroyed privately, rather than for all to see.[29] The College itself could be represented as a private arena, which irregulars could be expected to prefer to the public arena of the law courts. That both sides could prefer to be out of the public eye is signified in the relatively neutral offer by the refugee clergyman-physician William Delaune in 1582 to submit evidence for public or private trial.[30] These arrangements have an obvious connection with aspects of male honour concerned with loss of face.[31] They also, however, had a tendency to undermine public participation in and consent to regulatory practices.

Some of the College's usages were undoubtedly similar to those traditional in the trades and crafts. Thus, it was the duty of members to protect the 'secrets' of the craft, while, at the same time, 'private' negotiations by members acting on an individual basis, especially when they were not officebearers, could be deplored as likely not to conduce to the common good.[32] Similarly, both private and public practice by those not members of the craft could be condemned. Those who practised in secret, or claimed secrecy for their remedies, were taking an unfair advantage in which secrecy was a shadow for ignorance and falsehood.[33] It was equally reprehensible to flout the College's authority by publicly proclaiming a right to practise, or making 'public declarations of wonderful things', although it was a little easier for the College to carry conviction (if not to convict) where this was the case.[34] Other forms of privacy observable in the Annals connect with areas of exercise of trades and crafts within the household that were traditionally, although not invariably, exempted from company control. These include working by family members for the benefit of the family, and work done as a privileged servant or retainer of a royal or noble household. Patrons, collegiate physicians and irregular practitioners all made strategic reference to this version of private practice. Thus the Earl of Essex justified the actions of his protégé Leonard Poe in terms of his 'privat practising upon his freendes'.[35] Richard Berry's confrontation with the College was in terms of his practising only 'in private houses or for the sake of charity'. Berry was then a Bachelor of Medicine (MB) and licentiate in medicine of Oxford University of several years' standing; later, as a Doctor of Medicine (MD) of Padua, he was suspected of popery.[36] Berry and others like him cannot have been unaware that the College was at its most compromised in seeking to repress practitioners who enjoyed the patronage and protection of members of the ruling class. In many respects, such practitioners were the collegiate physicians' closest competitors; at the same time, the risks of trying to suppress them were higher than in any other context, and the chances of being able to do so correspondingly small. This apparent notion of private life as exempt from intrusion was a concept forced upon the College by expediency, but one that was also defined by privilege.

'Citizen' or contractual medicine: an alternative relationship

The real difficulty for the College lay in the fact that it was this version of the relationship between patient and practitioner that was nearest to its ideal. The alternative, which I have called contractual or 'citizen' medicine, offered a contrasting, public framework and a degree of equity between patient and practitioner.[37] The contract system, which was similar to that prevailing in other areas of trade, consisted of an agreement, usually verbal, between the two parties, defining the patient's condition and a feasible outcome. Very often part of the price of the contract was paid in advance, and the remainder on completion of the cure. In the event of dissatisfaction, either side could pursue the other by informal and by legal means, as in a debt case. It was naturally important that such a contract be witnessed; it was also desirable for there to be witnesses to the practitioner's proceedings during the cure, and the patient's response to treatment. Thus it was actually detrimental for the patient–practitioner relationship to be private in the modern sense. Contractual medicine was not marginal. Versions of it can be located in European urban settings that range widely both geographically and chronologically. It had the capacity to be flexible, and varied according to context. Like any other system it could be distorted or abused, and instances of this kind can give the impression that it belonged only to the least reputable sectors of medicine. Similarly, cases surviving in legal records can mislead the historian into concluding that 'patient satisfaction' was less in surgery than in physic. Instead, such cases should be seen as routine, and interpreted more positively as evidence of a degree of accountability, expressed in the public realm as well as in that private to the craft.

It should not be assumed that contractual medicine had a distorting effect in requiring patient–practitioner relations to be public. Rather, medical practice in the early modern period still belonged in shops and shared spaces, and it was exceptional rather than otherwise for a patient to be private with his or her practitioner. More plausibly seen as distorting, in fact, are the personal relations that could be enjoyed by a patient and his or her attendant who closeted themselves together in order to share secrets, conversation or intellectual interests. Most pervasive however in the many accounts of practice in the Annals is the notion of privacy as discreditable, which also points to practice in public as normative. In the urban setting, consulting a practitioner in private was closely associated with suspicion of venereal disease, which patients would hesitate to disclose both on the grounds of reputation, and the consequences of being known to be infectious. The disease was protean in character, and so ubiquitous had it (or the fear of it) become in the metropolitan environment that a very wide range of conditions can be found in contracts and other forms of relationship into which a new twist of secrecy had been introduced.[38]

Contractual medicine belongs to a context in which practitioners were both varied and numerous. It implied a process of bargaining between patient and practitioner that depended to some extent on shared knowledge, and active definition by the patient of his or her state of health. These are features usually attributed to medicine as dominated by patronage. By contrast, contractual medicine entailed a degree of equality between patient and practitioner irrespective of differences in social status or level of formal education. It also offered forms of accountability and redress that were commonplace in early modern society and similarly operational across a wide social spectrum.[39] If the practitioner in question belonged to a company, the seniors of the craft had rights of supervision over the transaction, especially in dangerous cases. The company provided the first formal port of call in cases of breakdown of contract when one or the other party was considering a resort to law. Contractual medicine should not be idealized. However, it is necessary for it to be restored to its appropriate place in the medical systems of early modern England, which most recent historiography has defined as unregulated on the basis of the inadequacy of forms of regulation specific to medicine.

Not surprisingly, contractual medicine was at its most effective when integrated with the forms of control over standards that were exerted by the companies. In such contexts, it provides an example of the public regulation of economic relationships still characteristic of the earlier period and either underestimated or misinterpreted by later commentators, including Habermas, who saw the twentieth century as the period in which private matters had become the concern of the state. However, contractual medicine was not dependent on the existence or the continued survival of the companies in their traditional form. Nor was it wholly public in its characteristics. Its congruence with economic transactions in general meant that medical contracts had the potential to be classified as belonging, like private property, to the realms that classical economics defined as *laissez faire*. The existence of contractual medicine is still traceable in legal sources in the eighteenth century, when the companies had lost much of their public character, and it may have survived into the nineteenth.[40] However, it was by then vestigial, and likely to be found only in fringe areas of medicine. Among the reasons for its decline must be counted the College of Physicians, and, even more so, the criteria of professionalization that the College was instrumental in establishing for all aspirants to status in medicine.

There is no doubt that physicians in the medieval and early modern periods involved themselves in contracts with their patients, even though it is sometimes difficult to distinguish a true contract from action taken on the traditional advice to extract a fee from the patient in advance, when he or she was still grateful for the physician's care and attention. The London College was explicit, first in its partial acceptance of contractual medicine, and then in its rejection of it. Although physicians used contracts partly as a means of ensuring payment, they nonetheless condemned contractual medicine as covetous. Less clearly stated are their other grounds of objection. Contractual medicine materialized the relationship between patient and practitioner. It defined outcomes and included time constraints. It was predicated on considerable autonomy for the patient, and constrained the autonomy of the practitioner. For reasons connected with both status and gender, physicians wished to distance themselves from most of their patients, and to establish a disembodied mode of practice in which they would be paid purely for their advice, regardless of outcome. Contractual medicine involved economic transactions of the most tangible kind; physicians by contrast sought to identify with orders of society who lived on the equivalent of unearned income. In contractual medicine, treatment could not begin until the patient and the practitioner had agreed on a diagnosis. For the physician, his skill in prognosis was his pre-eminent asset and often the main service for which he was paid.

Privacy and detachment

This is not to argue that the physician's ideal was a form of practice that involved his sitting at home or (later) in a coffee-shop and being paid by proxy for advice given to patients whom he never saw. Rather, the latter was the form of practice adopted by physicians in the absence of the ideal patient–practitioner relationship as they saw it. Ironically, this inferior pattern of practice, the result of various species of avoidance, was also a form of socializing given a positive value by historians as an aspect of the authentic public sphere.[41] By contrast, the physician's ideal, as already suggested, included many features of a privileged, essentially private form of communication within a patronage relationship. This form of relationship dominates the historiography for the transition in medicine from traditional to modern society, but without full analysis of its origins, recognition of its ideal status or, most importantly, awareness of rival forms. There are obvious ways in which it was preferable for physician and elite patient to be alone together. If others were present, these would either be of higher status than the physician, or they would be servants with whom the physician would not wish to be identified. Moreover, although physicians traditionally advised each other on how best to deal with those about the sick, there was little certain gain for the physician in having witnesses to his attempts to establish his authority over an elite patient. There were no structures of accountability in this relationship other than the personal (as broadly interpreted to include clientage). The ideal would include the longer-term relationship in which the patient's dependence upon the physician increased to the extent that other practitioners were excluded. However, it can be assumed that privacy was the sought-after exception rather than the norm of actual practice even of collegiate physicians at this period. They were more likely to achieve private relations while treating those nearer to them in social status, but this would be very much second-best. It is the latter relationship that subsequently became the norm, and then the location for the definition of professionalization in terms of such qualities as trust.

Inside its own space, and in the account it tried to give of itself to the outside world, the Jacobean College certainly pursued an ideal of rational discourse in which extravagance of any kind was stigmatized as improper, unbalanced or simply foreign. Moreover, the College was commendably persistent in opposing its discourse to the more personal wielding of power by members of the elite. Having judged a practitioner as ignorant by its own criteria, the College was very rarely persuaded to think otherwise, whatever other compromises it might make. However, its favoured discourse was not founded upon debate, but on the truths already defined in Galenic texts. Further, as a 'community of equals' the College was hierarchically organized and extremely small. Although a proportion of those who challenged its authority became members, the College's practices were so exclusionary as to disbar many whose educational and intellectual profiles should have entitled them to a share in its proceedings. It is hard to see any sense in which the College recognized 'parity of citizenship' with those in the outside world. Collectively as well as individually, collegiate physicians isolated themselves from civic consciousness and instead spent anxious care on their ambivalent relationship with the ruling class.[42] There are certainly ways in which the College could be seen as consisting of men groping towards that image of the private, responsible individual, located in the urban environment but detached from the political process, which underlies Habermas's concept of the authentic public sphere. At the same time, the College's isolation in the contemporary context, its hybrid nature between estate and class, and its detachment from male structures and processes of authority of the modernizing variety placed severe limits on the match between its view of itself, and its role in the public world. The 'privacy' of its relationships was only bourgeois by default.

Acknowledgements

I am grateful to the audience at the Edinburgh Public Sphere conference for their responses, and in particular to Steve Sturdy for bibliographical information and perceptive comments on my text.

Notes

1 K. Figlio, 'Unconscious aspects of health and the public sphere', in B. Richards (ed.), *Crises of the Self: Further Essays on Psychoanalysis and Politics*, London: Free Association Press, 1989, pp. 85–6, 90.

2 As well as reviving the claims of agency and improvement, recent historiography has also stressed gender, and cultural interpretations. See D. Porter, *Health, Civilisation and the State: A History of Public Health from Ancient to Modern Times*, London and New York: Routledge, 1999; *idem* (ed.), *The History of Public Health and the Modern State*, Amsterdam: Rodopi, 1994; A. Bashford and C. Hooker (eds), *Contagion: Historical and Cultural Studies*, London and New York: Routledge, 2001.

3 D. Porter, 'Changing disciplines: John Ryle and the making of social medicine in Britain in the 1940s', *History of Science*, 1992, vol. 30, pp. 137–64; *idem*, 'The decline of social medicine in Britain in the 1960s', in *idem* (ed.), *Social Medicine and Medical Sociology in the Twentieth Century*, Amsterdam and Atlanta: Rodopi, 1997, pp. 97–119; C. Webster, 'Medicine', in B. Harrison (ed.), *The History of the University of Oxford*, vol. 8: *The Twentieth Century*, Oxford: Clarendon Press, 1994, pp. 331–2; J. Lewis, *What Price Community Medicine? The Philosophy, Practice and Politics of Public Health since 1919*, Brighton: Wheatsheaf, 1986, esp. pp. 35–44.

4 See for example J. Harris, *Private Lives, Public Spirit: A Social History of Britain 1870–1914*, Oxford: Oxford University Press, 1993.

5 For one relevant critique, see A. Mitzman, 'Privacy no more: historians in search of nineteenth century intimacy', *Journal of Social History*, 1991, vol. 24, pp. 359–70.

6 See for example I. Coltman, *Private Men and Public Causes: Philosophy and Politics in the English Civil War*, London: Faber & Faber, 1962; H.R. French, 'Social status, localism

and the "middle sort of people" in England 1620–1750', *Past and Present*, 2000, no. 166, pp. 66–99; B. Vickers, 'Public and private life in seventeenth-century England: the Mackenzie-Evelyn debate', in Vickers (ed.), *Arbeit, Musse, Meditation*, Zürich: Centre for Renaissance Studies, 1985, pp. 257–78; P. Langford, *Public Life and the Propertied Englishman 1689–1798*, Oxford: Clarendon Press, 1991.

7 Cf. for example C. Pateman, 'Feminist critiques of the public/private dichotomy', in Pateman, *The Disorder of Women: Democracy, Feminism and Political Theory*, Cambridge: Polity Press, 1989, pp. 118–40; A. Vickery, 'Golden age to separate spheres? A review of the categories and chronology of English women's history', *Historical Journal*, 1993, vol. 36, pp. 383–414; M.E. Wiesner, 'Nuns, wives and mothers: women and the Reformation in Germany', in S. Marshall (ed.), *Women in Reformation and Counter-Reformation Europe: Public and Private Worlds*, Bloomington and Indianapolis: Indiana University Press, 1989, pp. 8–28; B. Capp, 'Separate domains? Women and authority in early modern England', in P. Griffiths, A. Fox and S. Hindle (eds), *The Experience of Authority in Early Modern England*, Basingstoke: Macmillan, 1996, pp. 117–45.

8 Cf. L. Jardine and A. Grafton, '"Studied for action": how Gabriel Harvey read his Livy', *Past and Present*, 1990, no. 129, pp. 30–78; A. Fox, 'Custom, memory and the authority of writing', in Griffiths, Fox and Hindle, *Experience of Authority*, pp. 89–116; A. Stewart, *Close Readers: Humanism and Sodomy in Early Modern England*, Princeton, NJ: Princeton University Press, 1997; K. Sharpe, *Reading Revolutions: The Politics of Reading in Early Modern England*, New Haven and London: Yale University Press, 2000; J. Raymond, 'The newspaper, public opinion, and the public sphere in the seventeenth century', in Raymond (ed.), *News, Newspapers and Society in Early Modern Britain*, Portland, OR: Frank Cass, 1999, esp. pp. 124, 131–2.

9 J. Barry, 'A historical postscript', in D. Castiglione and L. Sharpe (eds), *Shifting the Boundaries: Transformation of the Languages of Public and Private in the Eighteenth Century*, Exeter: Exeter University Press, 1995, p. 223; Raymond, 'The newspaper, public opinion and the public sphere', pp. 110, 114, 128; J. Habermas, *The Structural Transformation of the Public Sphere*, trans. T. Burger, Cambridge: Polity Press, 1989, p. 19.

10 See P. Clark, *British Clubs and Societies 1580–1800: The Origins of an Associational World*, Oxford: Clarendon Press, 2000; Barry, 'Historical postscript', pp. 228–30; Raymond, *News, Newspapers and Society*; S. Hindle, 'The keeping of the public peace', in Griffiths, Fox and Hindle, *Experience of Authority*, p. 236.

11 See for example Hindle, 'Public peace', p. 238; D. Goodman, 'Public sphere and private life: towards a synthesis of current historiographical approaches to the old regime', *History and Theory*, 1992, vol. 31, pp. 1–20.

12 Habermas, *Structural Transformation*, pp. 11–12, 57ff., 90–1.

13 See for example J.M. Archer, *Sovereignty and Intelligence: Spying and Court Culture in the English Renaissance*, Stanford, CA: Stanford University Press, 1993; P. Zagorin, *Ways of Lying: Dissimulation, Persecution and Conformity in Early Modern Europe*, Cambridge, MA: Harvard University Press, 1990. On the involvement of medical practitioners, see M. Pelling, 'Appearance and reality: barber-surgeons, the body and disease', in A.L. Beier and R. Finlay (eds), *London 1500–1700: The Making of the Metropolis*, London and New York: Longman, 1986, pp. 82–112; M. Pelling, 'Compromised by gender: the role of the male medical practitioner in early modern England', in H. Marland and M. Pelling (eds), *The Task of Healing: Medicine, Religion and Gender in England and the Netherlands 1450–1800*, Rotterdam: Erasmus, 1996, pp. 101–33; M. Pelling, *The College of Physicians and Irregular Practitioners in Early Modern London* (Oxford University Press, in press).

14 London, Royal College of Physicians, Annals, 11 January 1599, p. 120. Page references are to the transcript/translation of the Annals. I am grateful to the President and Fellows of the College for permission to quote from their records.

15 I. Maclean, *The Renaissance Notion of Woman*, Cambridge: Cambridge University Press, 1980, pp. 3, 44–5; S. Mendelson and P. Crawford, *Women in Early Modern England*, Oxford: Clarendon Press, 1998, pp. 57–8.

16 See *Oxford English Dictionary*; R. Williams, *Keywords: A Vocabulary of Culture and Society*, London: Croom Helm/Fontana, 1976, pp. 203–4 (the keyword being 'private'); R. Shoemaker, *Prosecution and Punishment: Petty Crime and the Law in London and Rural Middlesex, c. 1660–1725*, Cambridge: Cambridge University Press, 1991, p. 88; cf. Habermas, *Structural Transformation*, pp. 5, 11, 74ff. Brewer argues that 'privacy' remained the residual category even into the nineteenth century: J. Brewer, 'This, that and the other: public, social and private in the seventeenth and eighteenth centuries', in Castiglione and Sharpe, *Shifting the Boundaries*, esp. pp. 8–9.

17 Quoted in L. Jardine and A. Stewart, *Hostage to Fortune: The Troubled Life of Francis Bacon 1561–1626*, London: Phoenix, 1999, p. 211. See also L.A. Pollock, 'Living on the stage of the world: the concept of privacy among the elite of early modern England', in A. Wilson (ed.), *Rethinking Social History*, Manchester and New York: Manchester University Press, 1993, pp. 78–96.

18 For some reflections see Pelling, 'Compromised by gender'; Langford, *Public Life*.

19 These points are more fully developed in M. Pelling, 'The women of the family? Speculation around early modern British physicians', *Social History of Medicine*, 1995, vol. 8, pp. 383–401; *idem*, 'Compromised by gender'. For what follows on physicians, see also *College of Physicians*. Officebearing by physicians will be the subject of a separate essay. Not surprisingly, Habermas's is not a gendered account, except in terms of such concepts as patriarchy: see A.J. La Vopa, 'Conceiving a public: ideas and society in eighteenth-century Europe', *Journal of Modern History*, 1992, vol. 64, pp. 112–15.

20 L. Gowing, *Domestic Dangers: Women, Work and Sex in Early Modern London*, Oxford: Clarendon Press, 1996; cf. A. Shepard, 'Manhood, credit, and patriarchy in early modern England c. 1580–1640', *Past and Present*, 2000, no. 167, pp. 75–106.

21 Although cf. P. Wallis, 'Medicines for London: the trade and regulation of London apothecaries c. 1610–c. 1670', Oxford University DPhil thesis, forthcoming.

22 G. Clark, *A History of the Royal College of Physicians of London*, 2 vols, Oxford: Clarendon Press, 1964–6, vol. 1, p. 61.

23 C. Webster, 'Thomas Linacre and the foundation of the College of Physicians', in F.R. Maddison, M. Pelling and C. Webster (eds), *Linacre Studies*, Oxford: Clarendon Press, 1977, pp. 214–19.

24 Clark, *College*, vol. 1, pp. 27, 61–3; H. Cook, 'Against common right and reason: the College of Physicians versus Dr Thomas Bonham', *American Journal of Legal History*, 1985, vol. 29, pp. 303–5.

25 See Webster, 'Thomas Linacre'; H. Kearney, *Scholars and Gentlemen: Universities and Society in Pre-Industrial Britain 1500–1700*, London: Faber & Faber, 1970, pp. 34–5, endorsing a distinction first made by Baron.

26 See G.D. Squibb, *The High Court of Chivalry: A Study of the Civil Law in England*, Oxford: Clarendon Press, 1959; *idem*, *Doctors' Commons: A History of the College of Advocates and Doctors of Law*, Oxford: Clarendon Press, 1977; B. Levack, *The Civil Lawyers in England 1603–1641: A Political Study*, Oxford: Clarendon Press, 1973; W. Prest, *The Rise of the Barristers: A Social History of the English Bar 1590–1640*, Oxford: Oxford University Press, 1986; A.R. Wagner, *Heralds of England: A History of the Office and College of Arms*, London: HMSO, 1967. There were of course differences: the heralds, for example, were notoriously quarrelsome, especially in the 1590s, their expertise was less clearly defined and their College was residential, housing even their wives and children.

27 These issues are inseparable from that of the College's religious and political allegiances, which have been extensively debated. Cf. Clark, *College*; W. Pagel, *William Harvey's Biological Ideas: Selected Aspects and Historical Background*, Basle: Karger, 1967; C. Webster, 'The College of Physicians: "Solomon's House" in Commonwealth England', *Bulletin of the History of Medicine*, 1967, vol. 41, pp. 393–412; C. Webster

(ed.), *The Intellectual Revolution of the Seventeenth Century*, London and Boston: Routledge & Kegan Paul, 1974; L. Sharp, 'The Royal College of Physicians and Interregnum politics', *Medical History*, 1975, vol. 19, pp. 107–28; C. Webster, *The Great Instauration: Science, Medicine and Reform 1626–1660*, London: Duckworth, 1975; C. Webster, 'William Harvey and the crisis of medicine in Jacobean England', in J. Bylebyl (ed.), *William Harvey and His Age*, Baltimore and London: Johns Hopkins University Press, 1979, pp. 1–27; R.G. Frank, *Harvey and the Oxford Physiologists: A Study of Scientific Ideas*, Berkeley: University of California Press, 1980; W.J. Birken, 'The Royal College of Physicians of London and its support of the Parliamentary cause in the English Civil War', *Journal of British Studies*, 1983, vol. 23, pp. 47–62; H.J. Cook, *The Decline of the Old Medical Regime in Stuart London*, Ithaca and London: Cornell University Press, 1986; and most recently, H.J. Cook, 'Institutional structures and personal belief in the London College of Physicians', in O.P. Grell and A. Cunningham (eds), *Religio Medici: Medicine and Religion in Seventeenth-Century England*, Aldershot: Scolar Press, 1996, pp. 91–114.

28 See for example Annals, 22 November 1610, p. 26; 1 September 1620, p. 140; 22 December 1609, p. 18.

29 Annals, 12 November 1619, pp. 131–2.

30 Annals, 22 December 1582, p. 16.

31 See E.A. Foyster, *Manhood in Early Modern England: Honour, Sex and Marriage*, London and New York: Longman, 1999, pp. 7ff.; Shepard, 'Manhood, credit and patriarchy', esp. pp. 102ff.

32 Annals, 1556/7, p. 27; 26 March 1621, p. 140.

33 Annals, 3 December 1596, p. 104; 20 March 1618, p. 109; 5 July 1623, p. 171; 11 July 1623, p. 172.

34 Annals, 2 June 1609, p. 9; 3 May 1616, p. 83; 5 July 1616, p. 86.

35 Annals, 30 June 1590, p. 67.

36 Annals, [blank] October 1618, p. 117; 29 March 1626, p. 202. In his will, proved 1652, Berry described himself as 'doctor in physic', leaving bequests to a brother, nephews and a natural daughter: PRO, PROB 11/217 (138 Grey).

37 See Pelling (trans. G. van Heteren), 'Een eerlijke overeenkomst? Contractrelaties tussen patienten en medisch practici in het vroegmoderne Londen', *Gezondheid: Theorie in Praktijk*, 1996, vol. 4, pp. 6–15; Pelling, *College of Physicians*. On contractual medicine see also G. Pomata, *Contracting a Cure: Patients, Healers and the Law in Early Modern Bologna*, Baltimore: Johns Hopkins University Press, 1998.

38 See Pelling, *College of Physicians*. For an instance, see Annals, 30 September 1586, p. 44. Cf. Brewer, 'This, that and the other', p. 9.

39 See esp. I. Archer, *The Pursuit of Stability: Social Relations in Elizabethan London*, Cambridge: Cambridge University Press, 1991; Shoemaker, *Prosecution and Punishment*; C. Muldrew, *The Economy of Obligation: The Culture of Credit and Social Relations in Early Modern England*, Basingstoke: Macmillan, 1998; C. Brooks, *Lawyers, Litigation and English Society since 1450*, London: Hambledon, 1998.

40 See C. Crawford, 'Patients' rights and the law of contract in eighteenth-century England', *Social History of Medicine*, 2000, vol. 13, pp. 381–410.

41 Habermas, *Structural Transformation*, p. 59; S.B. Dobranski, '"Where men of differing judgements croud": Milton and the culture of the coffee houses', *The Seventeenth Century*, 1994, vol. 9, pp. 35–56; Raymond, 'The newspaper, public opinion and the public sphere'; J.J. Keevil, 'Coffee house cures', *Journal of the History of Medicine*, 1954, vol. 9, pp. 191–5.

42 There are suggestive parallels here with La Vopa's discussion of 'service elites', exclusionary practices and 'literary authority' in the eighteenth century: La Vopa, 'Conceiving a public'.

2 Producing the public

Public medicine in private spaces

Pamela K. Gilbert

'"Having a room of one's own" is a desire, but also a control.'

Gilles Deleuze[1]

In the nineteenth century, public medicine, especially sanitary science, was first conceived as a way of containing the spread of disease. The public that it served was, early in the century, elite and bourgeois, and, later, composed of largely bourgeois and bourgeois-aspirant citizens; the portion of the population upon whom it was practised was generally outside this 'public'. Initially, this second population was perceived as a permanently marginal group to be contained and managed. By the 1850s and 1860s, though, this target group was to be brought within the pale if possible, and this necessitated a different approach to public medicine: holistic and prophylactic rather than specific and ameliorative. Historians have begun to understand public health in the light of narratives of what Foucault called 'governmentalities,' or the system of knowledges and practices used within the liberal state to produce a consenting liberal subject.[2] I would like to contribute to this project by showing how a specific aspect of the mid-century public health movement, housing reform, was interwoven with other moral discourses and practices. Matters of physical health in housing were connected to notions of appropriate domesticity, both of which were believed to contribute to the formation of the nascent citizen.

Public medicine, as it evolved out of the sanitary movement, initially meant state-supported health intervention, practised on behalf of a public formed of individual private citizens in whose service the state laboured and to whom it was accountable. My concern in this chapter is with the way that private citizens active in the bourgeois public sphere of literature and politics – in particular the literature and politics of public health and housing reform – brought that public understanding to bear on the domestic habits and practices of the poor. I explore this issue specifically in terms of what recent theorists and historians have called 'the social', a term that has assumed a wide and sometimes contradictory range of meanings in the current literature.[3] Here, I will use it to denote mid-nineteenth-century bourgeois practices that mediated between the shifting boundaries of public and private, in order to safeguard and produce that very split, in the service of the emerging liberal conception of citizenship. It is the hazy demarcation of the social as a buffer zone between public and private that underwrote efforts to discipline the lives of the poor. Put another way, it is this formulation that enabled so many for so long to see poverty, filth-related epidemic disease and so forth as 'social problems' to be handled through an extension of actions in the private and social spheres rather than primarily as public, political or state-economic issues requiring far-reaching government intervention. The citizen was to be produced in the domestic sphere and through the social to eventually participate in the public sphere; paradoxically, although the domestic was discursively 'cordoned off' from the public, its relation to the public sphere necessitated a great deal of practical 'leakage' between them that the social came, uneasily, to contain. With this in mind, in examining the relation of public medicine to the social, we can interrogate the notion of a bourgeois 'public sphere' and see how it depends on forms of panoptic oversight of the so-called private to secure the conditions of its possibility.

Public, private and domestic

By the mid-nineteenth century, as is well known, 'private' had come to refer to two areas: the domestic (what Habermas calls the intimate sphere)[4] and the economic rights of private property. These are closely related: just as the nuclear family is held in this period to be the basic unit of society and to mirror appropriate models of authority (benevolent paternalism), so is the economic freedom of the head of household to be exercised in the interest of the family, and hence in the interest of the community that is figured as an aggregate of families.[5] Obviously, this model could be and was contested at the time; still, it remained the dominant model in popular understandings of political economy, and reflected the liberal formula that only an atomized, economically independent *private* individual could or would properly participate as a citizen in the public sphere of a liberal polity. These distinctions between public and private, and within the private, the domestic and economic, though important, were quite tenuous.[6] State or public economics were believed to depend on appropriate private economics, yet there was to be no state intervention into the economics of the private sphere. Habermas clarifies:

> The sphere of the market we call 'private'; the sphere of the family, as the core of the private sphere, we call the 'intimate sphere'. The latter was believed to be independent of the former, whereas in truth it was profoundly caught up in the requirements of the market.[7]

In the same way, the separation between public and private economics could be defended because appropriate economic behaviour was seen to be 'natural' and therefore did not need to be legislated; in practice however, many did not enact these 'natural' economic behaviours, such as placing a high priority on spending for certain kinds of domestic improvements or saving for the schooling of offspring, and the presence or absence of such behaviours came in part to demarcate those who could be good citizens and those who were considered defective material unready for citizenship unless retrained.

The criteria for such inclusion were largely shaped by ideals of economic and social behaviour within the home. Habermas observes that the subjectivity explored and celebrated within the public sphere was one shaped by the nuclear family. I would add that this was the nuclear family experienced in a certain way: within a particular practice of domestic space with carefully mediated levels of publicity and seclusion, both within and from the immediate family. This demanded multiple rooms and a certain amount of space devoted to the *enactment and display of privacy*. As Elizabeth Langland points out, privacy itself had to be displayed, open to inspection; bourgeois privacy, as an index of respectability, was also the visible representation of having *nothing to hide*.[8] Hence, perhaps, the ever increasing differentiation of levels of privacy in the upper middle-class home, as we see in Robert Kerr's contemporary model of the gentleman's house: the absolute distinction between public and private, family and guests, and then again between inside and outside, allowed for a 'social life' supposedly divorced from business and politics, but in reality deeply embedded within them.[9] Langland states:

> The [bourgeois country] house metaphorically and metonymically stood for power and one's moral entitlement to that power. Because it operated most effectively through its continual visibility, it was thus open...and even its most intimate spaces could be penetrated with impunity...at the center of that visible structure stood the lady of the house, whose motions were precisely regulated by etiquette...that put her continually on display. The maintenance of wealth and power demanding continual visibility; continual visibility justifying the penetration of even private spaces; and private space gendered feminine so that the woman who is most protected by the architecture is also most exposed by it.[10]

The much vaunted privacy of the upper middle-class family was precisely the setting for semi-public rituals of visiting, dinners, at-homes and so forth, conducted and overseen largely by women, which provided the vital stage upon which respectability might be displayed, power consolidated, alliances forged, courtships conducted.[11] This display of privacy, as an extension of domesticity, was enacted within an intermediate public of social peers and near peers within which intimate–public processes (like friendly business) were conducted, and which was conceived as representative of the larger public realm. Although levels of social life were defined by exclusions, the social as a whole modelled inclusiveness and visibility.

This display of private life, and its surveillance and approval by a society of peers, was a key element in policing and enforcement of bourgeois norms that were taken to constitute universal and natural standards of behaviour and value. Observation of such standards of social (and related economic and political) practices is connected to a notion of citizenship that posits adherence to a 'natural' standard of conduct and values. Citizenship itself was conceived as membership in a social body offering participation in the public sphere through the franchise, and in a public national culture through consumption. Increasingly, by the 1860s, citizenship was counterposed against local identities, especially class, which were seen as threatening the coherence of the social body. Monitoring and assurance of properly private forms of life promoted public well-being. The lower working classes, however, just outside the borders of the social body, just beneath the minimal economic requirements for the franchise, were worrisome precisely because they did not seem to practise a private form of domesticity: doing paid work in their domestic space, sharing sleeping quarters with non-family members or with those of the opposite sex, etc. In response, public medicine now developed as a means of promoting proper privacy. Social experts pushing for house-to-house visitation and intervention found themselves in the peculiar position of arguing that working-class privacy must be penetrated because it did not exist, or that proper privacy could only be learnt under supervision. Middle-class women, the centre of the domestic and social, must take working-class women under their tutelage, to enable them in turn to produce the social in their own domestic space.

The social

Denise Riley has argued that the social is gendered feminine from the moment of its construction, not only in its intimate and familial concerns, but also in its articulation of an emotional and moral standard for perception.[12] She notes also that the feminization of the social distances it from the political arena. Poovey in turn observes that 'Because the metaphor of the social body highlighted intimate bodily processes and championed the feminized epistemology of sympathy, its proponents inadvertently reinforced women's claims to be naturally suited to work which could be seen as an extension of domestic offices'.[13] It is worth paying attention to where the 'feminized epistemology of sympathy' was being constructed and found its authority. Nancy Armstrong has analysed the claims of this authority at length in *Desire and Domestic Fiction.* She argues that by figuring men 'no longer [as innately] political creatures so much as they were products of desire and producers of domestic life', novels positioned women as individuals to be valued for their innate qualities of mind, cultivated by moral education given them in girlhood.[14] These qualities were in turn, in adult women, to be directed at managing male desire and inculcating sympathy, and ultimately shaping in the domestic sphere the masculine psychology that would lead to right political action in the public sphere. Although this development was key to the construction of separate (gendered) spheres, she avers, it apparently depoliticizes the feminine and sentiment.[15] Habermas sees the public sphere, comprised of both political and literary discourse, as seamlessly intertwined, although he observes that individuals had differing levels of access to these two arenas of subject formation:

The circles of persons who made up the two forms of public were not even completely congruent. Women and dependents were factually and legally excluded from the political public sphere, whereas [they]...took a more active part in the literary public sphere....Yet...in the self understanding of public opinion, the public sphere appeared as one and indivisible.[16]

But we know that the areas of public discourse were not perceived as homogenous, but clearly demarcated in elaborate, if unstable, hierarchies. Literary discourse, especially Habermas's privileged form, the novel, was seen as inferior, suspect, feminine and requiring careful discipline and surveillance throughout this period.[17]

Poovey makes the same move with the social that Habermas makes with the public: Poovey appears to see the whole social domain as essentially homogenous instead of stratified in its own right (for example, as I will argue below, between analysis and intervention). Certainly, the moral authority of feminine sympathy and management of desire came at the cost of any site of direct political address for women. Interestingly, then, the domain of the social that became a site of public address for women social workers had to do with precisely sexuality, household management and sympathy – putatively non-economic, apolitical, feminine concerns, mobilized in the service of a particular economic and political model. Private persons as 'human beings pure and simple' were to be formed within and by domestic attachments, under the primary authority of the mother; it is this maternal figure who is the harbinger and ruler of the social. Thus, the social mediated between the public and private, but in a very particular way, in that the social prepared potential citizens for public life, but essentially involved the regulation of what was perceived as private: in the case which I will discuss below, it involved middle-class intervention in the domestic practices, individual economic practices (especially those related to domesticity, such as saving for furniture and rental) and the bodily practices of those deemed to have an insufficient sense of proper domestic privacy. Poovey seems to imply that the understanding of the social as 'work that could be seen as an extension of domestic offices' was a sort of accidental by-product of the construction of the social 'in the image of the economic'; in fact, this femininity is quite central to the construction of the social as mediator between public and private identities.

The social as a field of practices (in addition to knowledge), like the 'two forms' of public sphere identified by Habermas, was also stratified. In order to transform social information into policy through the expert biopolitical knowledges of social control, that information was abstracted through statistics. Thus, the construction of the social at the legislative level required, as Poovey notes, a certain abstraction.[18] However, biopolitical knowledges moved in two directions – the gathering of information, and the putting of that information into practice through intervention, where abstract knowledges must be, at least in part, reparticularized. This stratification is what enables the use of the social as a field of regulatory and disciplinary practices ('social work') separate from the public sphere. Poovey connects the construction of the social with a privileging of abstraction; she then argues that women like Ellen Ranyard, who began the 'Bible women' movement, were able to use the feminization of the social against abstraction and in the service of a more richly individualized understanding and intervention.[19] However, this personal connection was based on what was thought to be (abstractly enough) a more or less universal feminine aptitude for personalizing and relating on a maternal basis (one might think of Romney Leigh's indictment of women as 'hard to general suffering').[20] This was what made women such good social workers, the logic ran – and such bad politicians. Therefore, social work, although indeed generally feminized, had two aspects, analysis and intervention, each of which worked on a real and metaphorical level in a polarized gender relationship: observation, analysis and finally legislation by male administrators, often sanitarians; and individual intervention by female and (feminized) male district visitors, clergy and paid sanitary police. When tutelary intervention became the norm, it was almost entirely practised at mid-century by women and clergy – the 'private', voluntary sector. The feminization of the social worked to separate social problems effectively from political discourse and action, in part by casting them as susceptible to maternal correction through proper socialization: women and clergy operated in the tutelary role of socializing children and men for proper participation in the social and eventually public spheres; while social problems were cast as the problems of childlike working-class individuals who had not been properly mothered and so were unable to properly mother others. Although I agree with Poovey that individuals exploited and resisted the construction of the social to a number of ends, and that for middle-class women it was a realm that provided particularly empowering possibilities for identity construction, I think we have to be careful about 'romanticizing resistance'. The power of the social enabled liberal feminism eventually to make many of the moves it did; it also created some of the conditions that necessitated those moves in the first place (and often operated at the expense of less powerful groups).[21]

Housing and public health

The social problems of hygiene, defined in response to epidemic disease, by the 1850s were no longer specified as problems solely of nuisance removal but of the people who lived in 'problem' environments. Moral health and physical health cannot be separated in this era: in the 1830s it was thought that cholera struck populations that were immoral and excessive in their habits, and by the 1850s it was still largely believed that unsanitary environments were as much a result, if not more, of the habits of those who lived within them as of infrastructure or economics. By the 1860s, the moral problems of citizenship and inclusion in the social body were defined very much as problems of hygienic self-discipline of individual bodies through moral education, i.e. socialization, which in turn was dependent upon providing an environment that would promote moral and cleanly habits. In short, public medicine cannot be separated in this period from housing or from moral education. The housing movement itself, although legislatively concerned with sanitation – the destruction of slums, the repair of drains, the construction of new housing up to a certain code – was just as concerned at the level of intervention with the inculcation of domesticity and the performance of privacy, particularly among the lower working classes.

In the housing movement, social operations took two peculiar forms: the first was the insistence on multiple rooms for poor families. The second, borrowed directly from the sanitary movement's methods of disease/nuisance control, was house-to-house visitation in order to inculcate appropriate habits and values. The insistence on multiple rooms peaked in the 1850s and early 1860s. As philanthropic efforts shifted from the artisan to the very poor casual labourer, however, the 'three room dogma' began to be challenged by highly visible figures such as the famed architect Kerr, who in 1866–7 proposed his plan of one-room tenements for the very poor, scandalizing his auditors.[22] Although most historians attribute this to a newly realistic attitude towards expenditure, I would argue that it might also be related to the understanding, following the second Reform Bill, that renters at this level would not be eligible for citizenship until they had acquired not only the physical surroundings, but the *desires* and habits associated with domesticity as practised in multiple rooms – practices that privileged privacy, individualism and bourgeois consumption habits. Enough social experiments had placed poor tenants in multiple rooms for social workers to begin to understand that these practices would not just spontaneously emerge given the necessary but not sufficient condition of more space.

The nineteenth century saw the creation of suburbs, the middle-class country house and, in the urban space, the emergence of architecture reflecting an ever more carefully differentiated culture of privacy. Daunton summarizes overall changes in architecture and the practice of urban space as follows:

> The dwelling became more enclosed and private, whilst the external space became 'waste' space or connective tissue which was to be traversed rather than used....Space that was not encapsulated within the private sphere of the individual unit became totally public, and hence open to view and regulation.[23]

Slum clearance and building laws over the mid-century gradually abolished the communal, semi-private space of the court in favour of the wholly public space of the street. Within private spaces, increased distance between bodies and segregation of rooms became a key concern.

Medical science had begun to insist in the 1840s on the importance of clean air, and the dangerous nature of air 'vitiated' by previous breathing. By the 1860s, many doctors determined the healthiness of a building primarily in terms of the number of cubic feet of air per person. An underlying concern, however, in terms of 'overcrowding' was not space, but its uses.[24] Descriptions of persons 'of all sexes' huddled together in one room usually implicitly, and often explicitly, define incest as an inevitable result of such crowding.[25]

'Talk of morality!' says Dr. Bickersteth, in a lecture…'amongst people who herd – men, women, and children – together, with no regard of age or sex, in one narrow, confined apartment! You might as well talk of cleanliness in a sty, or of limpid purity in the contents of a cesspool…the first token of moral life is an attempt to migrate, as though by instinct of self-preservation, to some purer scene.'[26]

The model housing built in the 1840s and 1850s all featured the priority given to room separation, and many reformers were horrified when, despite the avail-ability of a second room, the poor preferred to 'pig together' in one room. Certainly, it is probable that many of the poor could not afford second rooms, and when they had them, they could not heat or light them. However, it is also quite possible that many, accustomed to a way of life in which little waking time was actually spent confined to that room, and accustomed to different standards of physical distance, really did find the multi-room lodging oppressive – unneces-sary, uncomfortable and difficult to maintain.

When housing those too poor to afford the new model housing, however, such questions did not arise. Economic necessity alone was sufficient to limit the space that could be provided to this class, especially in the face of the dictum that there should be no subsidizing to 'pauperize' tenants, and the demand for a 5 per cent return. Before the mid-1850s, no one had seriously attempted to house the very poor, and so this inevitability had been, to some extent, ignored. And despite the fact that most poor people lived in one-room tenements (Daunton cites a 1854 report on the cholera in Newcastle that places the proportion of householders in overcrowded single rooms at approximately half),[27] suggestions that the poor should be offered or encouraged to take single rooms generated storms of controversy.[28]

Octavia Hill: domesticating the poor

Octavia Hill provides a subject of unique interest because of her commitment to housing precisely this class. A model for modern social work, her project included not only housing the very poor, but also intimately managing and counselling them. Her work dramatizes the operation of the social, its opportunities for middle-class women and also some of the limits of those opportunities. Although Hill believed in the necessity of multiple rooms, pragmatism, she believed, dictated that reformers begin with single rooms and then foster desire for more space. 'Good sized single rooms should be built…thousands of small poor families…want only one large room, who indeed prefer it to two small ones.' She adds:

Near to these single rooms, but separable from them, smaller ones should be built which could be let with them, whenever wages, or the standard of comfort, rose. There are many tenants who can be induced by a little gentle pressure and encouragement to spend a rather larger proportion than they now do in rent.[29]

Hill never ordered her tenants to do anything other than pay the rent on time. Her goal was to 'befriend and persuade', using her considerable cultural and moral authority (backed, not incidentally, by her status as landlady) to mobilize consent. Hill is the perfect exponent of the social; the coercion at the back of social practices is rarely seen as coercion because those practices appear as the result of natural desire – even if bad environment has so thwarted nature that it requires a little coaxing to re-emerge. Hill rather proudly relates an instance of 'gentle pressure and encouragement':

> They [her tenants] are easily governed by firmness, which they respect much. I have always made a point of carefully recognizing their own rights; but if a strong conviction is clearly expressed, they readily adopt it....One tenant – a silent, strong, uncringing woman, living with her seven children and her husband in one room – was certain 'there were many things she could get for the children to eat that would do them more good than another room'. I was perfectly silent. A half-pleading, half-asserting voice said: 'Don't you see I'm right, miss?' 'No,' I said; 'indeed I do not. I have been brought up to know the value of abundant good air; but of course you must do as you think best – only I am sorry.' Not a word more passed; but in a few weeks a second room was again to let, and the woman volunteered: 'She thought she'd better strive to get the rent; good air was very important, wasn't it?'[30]

We can easily see why Beatrice Webb and Henrietta Barnett criticized Hill for her arrogance and 'hypocritical' cordiality to the poor;[31] from a present-day perspective the emphasis on space over food seems particularly inhumane. But Hill did not differ signally from other housing reformers on this point; indeed, what was different about her approach was the personalized relationship she insisted on with her tenants and – paradoxically – the amount of 'freedom' the tenants had to make their own decisions. Hill's model of intervention – which became the dominant model for social work – used domesticity and a maternalist ideal to situate its cultural authority and its careful negotiation between the social and the public, between the need to centralize authority and fit into governmental and public policy structures on the one hand and the need to maintain autonomous and private status on the other.

Friendly visiting saw itself as tutelage by example – as Hill put it 'living side by side with people, til all that one believes becomes clear to them'.[32] Hill in particular did not merely see herself, as so many before her did, as establishing a small community of support for some poor. She saw herself as 'governing' the desires of the poor in order to transform them, and as teaching those who were outside of the social body to behave in a manner that must bring them within it.[33]

> That the spiritual elevation of a large class depended to a considerable extent on sanitary reform was, I considered, proved; but I was equally certain that sanitary improvement itself depended upon education work among grown-up people....I further believed that any lady who would help

them to obtain things, the need of which they felt themselves, and would sympathize with them in their desire for such, would soon find them eager to learn her view of what was best for them; that whether this was so or not, her duty was to keep alive their own best hopes and intentions...governing more than...helping.[34]

The visitor's authority depends on two things equally: her status as a lady, and her sympathy with tenants' needs. On the one hand, she is a social and economic authority figure (and exerts direct authority as landlady, in Hill's case); on the other, she is a private individual, in a relationship of equality and what Poovey would call 'structural equivalence' with her tenant. It is particularly important that it be a 'lady', not a 'gentleman' – the lady's moral authority is based in the private and the social, on her domestic identity. The striking thing in reading Hill is not her casual assertion of the authority of her position as 'governor' of her tenants, which is frequently present, but her equally frequent insistence on her relationship as friend and equal – her denial that she exerts any authority save that of reason and example. In her belief in a government by consent that masks any reference to her power, in her separation of the social (her friendships) from the economic (Hill was unyielding in her rule that anyone who didn't pay rent on time would be turned out), and finally in her belief that the separation of the economic from the social was mutually supportive with her moral goals for her tenants' behaviour, Hill embodies the precise contradictions and ideals of liberal government in the period.

Hill's method depended on relations of intimacy with her tenants: 'My people are numbered, not merely counted, but known, man, woman, and child....Think of what this mere fact of *being known* is to the poor!'[35] The choice of words here, I think, is particularly opportune. The investigative side of the social is the side that 'counts' the poor, abstracting them into specific information; Hill's method does not oppose this, but supplements it – the poor who are counted by sanitary authorities are 'numbered' by her in the biblical sense. There is a practical aspect, of course: being 'known' means that the very poor have some access to the cultural capital of the workings of the social in a higher economic class – they can get references for jobs, and take advantage of networking. But more to the point, being known, as individuals, by someone who 'matters' de-massifies the poor as unreasoning atoms of a large unreasoning mass and reconstructs the person in the image of individualism – there is someone there with a unique and valuable subjectivity to 'know'. It also means that Hill can 'know' them because they are not the Other – their desires are 'known' because they are similar to hers as part of the same social body. She and her tenants are structural equivalents because they both belong to families that are 'natural' and therefore identical in structure and operation:

> I have heard...girls...talk rather enviously of those who can give their time wholly to such work; but have they ever thought how much is lost by such entire dedication? – or, rather, how much is gained by her who is not only a visitor of the poor, but a member of a family with other duties? It is the

families, the homes of the poor, that need to be influenced. Is she not the most sympathetic, most powerful, who nursed her own mother through her long illness...who obeyed so perfectly the father's command when it was hardest? Better still if she be wife and mother herself, and can enter into the responsibilities of a head of a household, understands her joys and cares, knows what heroic patience it needs to keep gentle when the nerves are unhinged and the children noisy. Depend upon it, if we thought of the poor primarily as husbands, wives, sons and daughters, members of households, as we are ourselves, instead of contemplating them as a different class, we should recognize better how the house training and high ideal of home duty was our best preparation for work among them....What, in comparison with these gains is the regularity of the life of the weary worker, whose life tends to make her deal with people en masse, who gains little fresh springs from other thoughts and scenes? For what is it that we look forward to as our people gradually improve? Not surely to dealing with them as a class at all, any more than we should tell ourselves off to labour for the middle classes, or aristocratic class, or shop-keeping class. Our ideal must be to promote the happy mutual intercourse of neighbours.[36]

Several important points can be made about this interesting statement. The first is Hill's belief that the moral authority of middle-class women derives from the similarities of their lives to the lives of the poor in the universals of sickness, nursing, patriarchal domestic structure, etc. (Obviously, this elides the real differences between homes with servants and adequate food and water, and those that have none, to name only one example.) The statement that the 'most sympathetic' is 'most powerful' deflects attention from coercive aspects of power and grounds power in equivalence, which is explicitly counterpoised to class; in fact the goal of this exercise in sympathy is to erase class, not by improving the person's economic situation, although that may be part of the process, but by erasing the significance of economic difference. But perhaps most interesting of all is Hill's suspiciousness of professional social workers. Despite the fact that Hill did much to create an institutional context and method for social work, and that students of social work came from the continent and North America to study her method, Hill opposed the professionalization of social work to the end of her life.[37] Her reaction to Jane Addams's Hull House style of intervention, in which a community of women live domestically within the neighbourhood in which they are working, is that these 'Homes' are false – they are not really replicative of patriarchal nuclear families, and, worse, they make work with the poor a substitute for, rather than an extension of, home duties.

[W]e want very much more the influence that emanates not from a 'Home', but from 'homes'....I hope for...men and women coming out from bright, good, simple homes, to see, teach, and learn from the poor; returning to gather fresh strength from home warmth and love, and seeing in their own homes something of the spirit which should pervade all.[38]

Yet, despite her desire that visitors should not professionalize, Hill worked hard
to establish structured relationships between voluntary visitors and statutory
bodies like the Poor Law Guardians in a centralized structure of authority. She
was committed to structures that mediated between, but did not erase, the strati-
fications of the social between policy analysis and implementation discussed
above.[39] Firmly believing, as many Victorians did, that charity was often pauper-
izing and that too often aid was dispensed in ways that harmed, rather than
helping recipients to achieve independence, Hill believed that all charities should
work together through a centralized agency, the Charity Organization Society,
and, in turn, work with institutional bodies like the Guardians, to co-ordinate aid
and share information so recipients could be tracked and managed in the light of
their personal histories. She proposed an elaborate tri-level system involving the
visitors, whose job it was to know the poor thoroughly and decide when and
what kind of help should be given or withheld, an intermediary female super-
visor with some knowledge of the Poor Law and the workings of government, to
whom these women would report and from whom they would take direction,
and who in turn would report to the male administrators of local Church and
government bodies, as well as charity boards. The advantages of this system
were, she argued, that a more accurate sense of needs could be determined,
since the poor were unreliable and inarticulate about their own needs; that
follow-up could be performed within the context of the 'friendship' of the visitor
without being resented (indeed the function of the visitor was explicitly, as a
'friend', to 'persuade' recipients to accept the Board's often unpalatable advice),
and that all efforts could be brought to bear on bringing the poor within the
social body rather than providing counter-productive short-term melioration.
Why then, in this elaborate and highly formal system, is it important to maintain
the 'front line' of workers as non-professionals – that is, as fully private individuals? Again, it is based on the notion of sympathy and equivalence. Hill
explains:

> The Relief Committee…have before them not only the valuable informa-
> tion of the Charity Organization Society, gathered, sifted and examined by
> their paid officer and representative committee, but also the detailed
> account of a volunteer, who brings to bear on the case a fresher and more
> personal sympathy than a paid agent ordinarily possesses, who has much
> more patience to listen to, and probably more patience to elicit the little
> facts upon which so much may depend. Anyone will appreciate this who has
> had the experience of the difficulty of obtaining the evidence of uneducated
> people, women more especially; they are nervously confused, they cannot
> understand what are the real points of the case, nor state them clearly.[40]

Hill's insistence on equality with her tenants has often been dismissed as disingenuous, most famously by Beatrice Webb. However, most observers miss the
point of Hill's sense of community with her tenants. It is not that Hill thought of
her tenants as social equals; she didn't. It was that she believed them to be poten-

tial participants in the social body and public sphere – citizens, whose *interests* (narrowly defined) counted equally with her own. It is this that is reflected in her insistence on the oneness of national community and in her emphasis on both the necessity and the danger of local community. Local community is good, but activism should begin in one's own neighbourhood because one had to conceive of community as a group of individuals with whom one's relationships were personal – one's own social sphere. But that was only valuable in so far as, like one's own family, it enabled one to sympathetically understand and claim solidarity with other families, other communities. To the extent that it was used as a marker of identity, such as class, it became dangerous. Local identities that are not connected to a larger sense of community actually cause community to degenerate. She exhorts her colleagues:

> [R]emember well your duties; and, never forgetting the near ones to home and neighbourhood,…remember also that when Europe is sacrificed to England, England to your own town, your own town to your parish, your parish to your family, the step is easy to sacrifice your family to yourself.[41]

Hill sees her 'raw' tenants as riven by local identity. But most of all, an inadequate sense of family responsibilities and relationships keep poor people from having possibilities of sympathy for one another in Hill's view – community is made possible by the structural equivalence that begins with one's sense of identity within a family role. In response, Hill took on the role of mother, happy when her tenants shelved their differences to please her or because they felt that their quarrels hurt her – as, according to her, they often did. Hill provided classes at some of her tenements; upon bringing women together for classes, sewing and cleaning, Hill remarks:

> [A] neighbourly feeling is called out among the women as they sit together on the same bench, lend one another cotton or needles.…The babies are a great bond of union.…That a consciousness of corporate life is developed in them is shown by the not infrequent use of the expression 'One of us'.[42]

What is striking about this moment is that Hill utterly fails to remark on any of the other bonds of community to which historians of the working classes have alluded and which are so evident in the communal uses of stair, courts and the like; nor does she regard the common experience of shared labour habits or economic struggle as legitimate sources of communal feeling. Her triumphant citation of the common phrase 'one of us' may indicate that this phrase was rarely used by her tenants; it more likely indicates that it was rarely used in a manner that Hill recognized as meaningful. For Hill, meaningful corporate life is organized apolitically, through sympathy rooted in the structural equivalence of roles in the patriarchal, heteronormative nuclear family.

Ultimately, of course, the Victorian model of the social as profoundly separate from government could no longer withstand the pressure of its centrality to the aims of government itself, and social work became professionalized – both the ultimate success and failure of Hill's ideal. Hill's troubled response to professionalization (and institutionalization) illustrates both the discursive and ideological barriers between public and private, state and social, and the absolute permeability of those boundaries in practice, the messy inadequacy of these terms as separate categories of cultural or civil life. Hill was active from the 1860s through to the end of the century; she never swerved from her firm commitment to voluntarism. Only in private, individual relationships, paradoxically, could the aims of nation be bodied forth and realized: in 1883, she still believed that:

> The people's homes are bad, partly because they are badly built and arranged; they are tenfold worse because the tenants' habits and lives are what they are. Transplant them tomorrow to healthy and commodious homes and they would pollute and destroy them. There needs...a reformatory work which will demand the loving zeal of individuals which cannot be had for money, and cannot be legislated for by Parliament. The heart of the English nation will provide it – individual, reverent, firm, and wise. It may and should be organized, but cannot be created.[43]

Nationhood depends both on individuality and the sense of community called forth by voluntarism; professionalizing and legislating social work would destroy that bond of sympathy between individual private persons upon which both Habermas's public sphere and the social are based, and upon which citizenship and civil consent are founded. Economic aid can be given by the masculinized professional, but only from a position of privacy can the domestic feminine intervene in and produce in turn the fragile privacy of the newly socialized poor. And only then may the poor emerge into and through the social into the social body itself as bearers of a public and proudly English identity.

Notes

1 G. Deleuze, 'Foreword' to J. Donzelot, *The Policing of Families*, trans. R. Hurley, New York: Pantheon, 1979, p. xvii.
2 M. Foucault, 'Governmentality', in G. Burchell, C. Gordon and P. Miller (eds), *The Foucault Effect: Studies in Governmentality*, Chicago: University of Chicago Press, 1991, pp. 87–104.
3 See, for example, M. Poovey, *Making a Social Body: British Cultural Formation 1830–1864*, Chicago: University of Chicago Press, 1995; D. Riley, *'Am I that Name?' Feminism and the Category of 'Women' in History*, London: Macmillan, 1988; G. Procacci, 'Social economy and the government of poverty', in Burchell *et al.* (eds), *The Foucault Effect*, pp. 151–68.
4 J. Habermas, *The Structural Transformation of the Public Sphere*, trans. T. Burger with F. Lawrence, Cambridge, MA: MIT Press, 1991.
5 As Pitkin observes, 'utilitarianism not only favored the representation of persons, but made interest an increasingly personal concept': H.F. Pitkin, 'Representation', in T. Ball, J. Farr and R.L. Hanson (eds), *Political Innovation and Conceptual Change*, Cambridge: Cambridge University Press, 1989, pp. 132–54, at p. 145.

6 It is important to remember that Habermas chronicles the history of an ideal (though he himself sometimes appears to forget that), not an actual cultural structure. The distinction between the public and private spheres, which imaginatively structured social and political life in this period, was widely admitted and probably nowhere coherently practised. (Amanda Vickery has famously charted the follies of too literal interpretations of this division. See A. Vickery, 'Golden Age to separate spheres? A review of the categories and chronology of English women's history', *The Historical Journal*, 1993, vol. 36, pp. 383–418.) Also, the fantasy of an ideal public sphere is, throughout Habermas, shadowed by its less savoury but more interesting twin, the development of public opinion in an increasingly literate and powerful populace, to which the public sphere of Habermas's coffee houses bears the relation of the good citizen to the unreasoning mass of the mob. Although public opinion is not inherently and necessarily a degraded form of public communication, Habermas suggests that it can only realize its proper form under conditions that have not and do not exist.

7 Habermas, *Structural Transformation*, pp. 55–6.

8 E. Langland, 'Enclosure acts: framing women's bodies in Braddon's *Lady Audley's Secret*', in M. Tromp, P. Gilbert and A. Haynie (eds), *Beyond Sensation: Mary Elizabeth Braddon in Context*, New York: SUNY Press, 1999, pp. 3–16.

9 R. Kerr, 'On the problem of providing dwellings for the poor in towns', lecture delivered before the Royal Institute of British Architects, on Monday, 3 December 1866, RIBA *Journal of Proceedings*, 1866–7, pp. 37–47.

10 This increasingly important tension between visibility and invisibility – or publicity and privacy – is exploited in the 1960s by sensation novels, in which the middle-class home veils a dark secret.

11 Elizabeth Langland's *Nobody's Angels* gives a fine overview of the complex nature of these social practices: E. Langland, *Nobody's Angels: Middle-Class Women and Domestic Ideology in Victorian Culture*, Ithaca: Cornell University Press, 1995.

12 Riley, *'Am I that Name?'*.

13 Poovey, *Making a Social Body*, p. 43.

14 Armstrong, *Desire and Domestic Fiction*, p. 4.

15 Ibid., p. 10.

16 Habermas, *Structural Transformation*, pp. 55–6.

17 It might be useful here to think in terms of Nancy Fraser's concept of multiple publics in multiple relationships to the dominant one, with varying degrees of 'strength' (i.e. performative power), whose discourse interacts with the hegemonic public in various ways: supporting, modifying, opposing and, in the case I cite, supplementing. N. Fraser, 'Rethinking the public sphere: a contribution to the critique of actually existing democracy', *Social Text*, 1990, vol. 8–9, pp. 56–80.

18 Poovey, *Making a Social Body*.

19 Ibid., p. 27.

20 E. Barrett-Browning, *Aurora Leigh*, Chicago: Academy Chicago Publishers, 1979, pp. 43–4.

21 Also pertinent here is F.K. Prochaska's very useful *Women and Philanthropy in Nineteenth-Century England*, Oxford: Clarendon Press, 1980. Prochaska makes the point that women's philanthropic activities prepared them over the course of the century for eventual entry into the public sphere, especially the campaign for women's suffrage, towards the end of the period – a point with which I basically concur. Here, however, I am interested in clarifying this complex trajectory, which necessitates understanding the relationship between public, private and social, on which Prochaska does not elaborate. This relationship, however, is crucial to understanding why, in Prochaska's view, women like Octavia Hill were, as a contemporary critic charged, too interested in the social, and not in what Prochaska calls 'theory' (p. 133) – i.e. issues such as politics and political economy. Prochaska attributes the lack of such interest to a 'pragmatic, unanalytic mentality encouraged in the other spheres of their lives',

which discouraged them from being interested in abstract concepts (p. 134). On the contrary, I would say that Hill, for example, had a rather comprehensive theory about the organization of the social body and its relationship to nation; it is the explicit connection of that to political economy and politics that she regards as outside the appropriate feminine sphere of the social, and, indeed, antithetical to it. It is impossible to understand this disconnection without understanding the vexed relationship of the social to the mid-Victorian public sphere.

22 Kerr, 'On the problem of providing dwellings'.
23 M.J. Daunton, *House and Home in the Victorian City: Working Class Housing 1850–1914*, London: Edward Arnold, 1983, p. 12.
24 As Rodger points out, 'It was not simply the physical structures themselves which undermined decency and the family unit – there were many examples of generously proportioned and well maintained terrace housing and tenement flats – it was the congestion with which they were associated': R. Rodger, *Housing in Urban Britain 1780–1914: Class, Capitalism and Construction*, London: Macmillan, 1989, pp. 40–1.
25 For one of the more explicit references to incest, see E. Chadwick, *Report on the Sanitary Condition of the Labouring Population of Great Britain (1842)*, ed. with an introduction by M.W. Flinn, Edinburgh: Edinburgh University Press, 1965, p. 193.
26 Quoted in G. Godwin, FRS, *Town Swamps and Social Bridges. The Sequel to a Glance at the Homes of the Thousands*, London: Routledge, Warnes and Routledge, 1859, p. 21.
27 In Daunton, *House and Home*, p. 16.
28 Charles Gatliff argued as early as 1854 that working-class families did not generally need or use three rooms, but he was unheeded (J.N. Tarn, *Working Class Housing in 19th Century Britain*, London: Lund Humphries, 1971, p. 11) – and even Gatliff insisted on separate sculleries and lavatories for each tenement. Kerr's 1866 proposal to provide one-room housing was met with incredulity, despite the fact that he was only suggesting it for households without children at home, or headed by single women: Kerr, 'On the problem of providing dwellings'.
29 O. Hill, *Homes of the London Poor, Octavia Hill; and, The Bitter Cry of Outcast London…, Andrew Mearns*, London: Frank Cass and Co, Ltd, 1970 [1883], p. 15.
30 Hill, *Homes*, p. 21.
31 N. Boyd, *Three Victorian Women who Changed Their World: Josephine Butler, Octavia Hill, Florence Nightingale*, Oxford: Oxford University Press, 1982, p. 134.
32 J. Lewis, 'Presidential address: family provision of health and welfare in the mixed economy of care in the late nineteenth and twentieth centuries', *Social History of Medicine*, 1995, vol. 8, pp. 1–16, at pp. 6–7.
33 In France, this role is made explicit much earlier. As early as 1820, in Gerando's manual for visitors of the poor, the philanthropist is admonished to investigate the lives of the recipients closely: '*Morality was systematically linked to the economic factor*, involving a continuous surveillance of the family' (J. Donzelot, *The Policing of Families*, p. 69). In other words, morality was measured in large part by the subject's willingness to engage in economic behaviours (saving, consuming) that supported bourgeois domestic values – using wage rises to spend more on rent, for example.
34 Hill, *Homes*, pp. 17–18.
35 Hill, *Homes*, pp. 34–5.
36 O. Hill, *Our Common Land and Other Short Essays*, London: Macmillan, 1877, pp. 24–7.
37 Boyd remarks of Hill's system that 'The ideal manager combines two principles: she is to participate as "a volunteer", that is "a spontaneous undertaker of tasks"…and she is to be trained as a "professional", a worker whose knowledge of science, sociology and economics enables her to reconcile the care of individual tenants with the needs of the community.…In later life, Octavia Hill expressed reservations about the…increasing tendency of workers to specialize.…Emphasis must remain on "*knowing* people with whom you work" not on exercising skills.…The professional

status of the visitors might be considered to make them superior to their clients, yet as volunteers they can be equals.' Boyd, *Three Victorian Women*, pp. 53–4.

38 Hill, *Homes*, p. 66.
39 This trend continues. Most social workers in the United States are female, especially social workers involved with family issues (as opposed to parole officers). Hoover *et al.* point out that 'the number of programs utilizing [prophylactic] home visiting as a strategy for delivering services has rapidly expanded' in the 1990s (p. 17), and identify the key goals of home visiting as role modelling and providing 'social support' by 'developing a trusting relationship': T.D. Hoover, F. Johnson, C. Wells, C. Graham and M. Biddleman, *A Guest in my Home*, published through the collaborative efforts of the Family and Community Health, and Children and Families Program Office; the Ounce of Prevention Fund of Florida; and the Bureau of Student Services and Exceptional Education, Florida Department of Education, 1996, p. 18. This volume, which instructs home visitors, admonishes them to 'Keep the home a home', noting that 'Home should be where families can retreat from other influences or pressures of the outside world' (p. 51). This rather Victorian distinction between domestic and public spheres not only emphasizes a discontinuity between private and public, but fails to acknowledge that traumatic incidents are very likely to occur within the domestic sphere – indeed, for children and women more likely to occur within that sphere than outside it. In England and Wales, the casework model of social work predominates (M. Payne, 'United Kingdom', in N.S. Mayadas, T.D. Watts and D. Elliott (eds), *International Handbook on Social Work Theory and Practice*, Westport, CT: Greenwood Press, 1997, pp. 161–83, especially p. 172), despite a tradition of theoretical emphasis among many social workers on structural inequalities (p. 178). In the United States, the trend has been even more heavily individualist (L. Leighninger and J. Midgley, 'United States of America', in Mayadas *et al.* (eds), *International Handbook*, pp. 9–28, especially pp. 11, 23); although recent discussions have focused on issues of social justice, these almost always translate in practice into an emphasis on avoiding harmful stereotypes and respecting cultural difference in working with individual 'clients'; the predominant mode of intervention is psychotherapeutic. Union organization, for example, is considered political activism, not social work.
40 Hill, *Homes*, p. 58.
41 Hill, *Our Common Land*, pp. 172–3.
42 Hill, *Homes*, p. 28.
43 Hill, *Homes*, p. 10.

3 'Should the doctor tell?'

Medical secrecy in early twentieth-century Britain

Andrew A.G. Morrice

For those with the modern habit of looking back to Hippocrates to find an ancient root for current medical concerns, the confidentiality clause of the Hippocratic Oath appears to provide a satisfying case in point.[1] The undertaking that 'whatever I see or hear, professionally or privately, which ought not to be divulged, I will keep secret and tell no one'[2] appears to endorse the view that the privacy of the medical encounter has a long history of being given special status. This was certainly the view of many Edwardian doctors, but it should not be taken for granted. Societies exist in which such a conception of a healing encounter as private and secretive would be both suspect and nonsensical.[3] Equally, a closer look at early twentieth-century medical opinion brings out a view of the privacy of medical work that differs in important senses from contemporary thinking.

The view that the clinical encounter was essentially a private, often domestic affair, occurring between people in an ongoing relationship of care and compliance, can be traced in writings about doctors' behaviour and moral standards at least as far back as the eighteenth century.[4] By the late Victorian and Edwardian period it was well entrenched in discourses on medical ethics. However, the same period saw new pressures on doctors to co-operate in the public processes of the state, calling into question the assumptions and values inherent in the injunction to maintain secrets.[5]

This chapter examines a set of controversies dealt with by the British Medical Association (BMA) and its Central Ethical Committee (CEC). The period 1914–24 saw an escalating dispute between the BMA and the judiciary over the issue of disclosure of clinical information to the authorities and courts of law. The doctors who took the lead in this debate wanted to defend the right of doctors to reveal only what their patients had consented to have divulged. They argued that doctors should have complete 'privilege' to prevent this principle being over-ridden in the courts. Lawyers argued that this would undermine legal processes including doctors' ability to defend themselves in malpractice cases. But the doctors who fought for professional secrecy and privilege saw it as a matter of honour: a defence of an 'ancient', 'sacred' and 'traditional' moral code.[6] This appeal to tradition was important on two counts. First, tradition itself was seen as a crucial underpinning and authorizing principle in medical behaviour. Second, Hippocrates' stock was already high with some doctors in the 1920s, the corpus being seen by many as a source of authority, revitalization and reorientation of a medicine lost in science and the tightening embrace of the state.[7]

The primary issue at stake was the conflict between public pressures that urged doctors to reveal information about their patients, and the need perceived by doctors for medical secrets to be preserved in order for the medical profession to retain both its usefulness and status. Most of these discussions were prompted by the increasing use that agencies of the state, including the judiciary, wished to make of information held by doctors about their patients. Since these wrangles usually involved matters such as sex outside marriage and venereal disease (VD) they were highly emotionally charged debates in which the public and private faces of medicine related in complex ways. For some protagonists in these debates over the extent to which medical knowledge of patients should remain a private matter, Hippocrates appeared a particularly 'big gun' that could be usefully trained on their opponents. Few noted that Hippocratic statements on confidentiality amounted to little more than an injunction against gossip, or that a great deal rode on the judgement as to what ought or ought not be divulged.[8] Neither did they appear to see what the social historian would assume, that despite the perennial inclusion of confidentiality in codes of medical conduct and ethical traditions, the way in which the issue was framed shifted in different times and contexts. The fact that doctors at the time used the term 'secrecy' rather than 'confidentiality' indicates that their conception was different from, and in many cases more absolute than, the one in current use.

The BMA and medical ethics

The BMA provides historians of medicine with an exceptionally informative window on the concerns of the medical profession in Britain during the nineteenth and twentieth centuries.[9] By the period in question the Association represented the vast majority of the working profession in Britain, and had evolved an extremely effective structure that allowed grassroots medical opinion to guide its policy while also allowing its leaders and secretariat to exert remarkable disciplinary influence over its members. The Association's aim to 'maintain the honour and interest of the medical profession' was essentially a public function carried out on behalf of its private members, who contributed financially and committed themselves personally to support this work. In other words, the Association was a mechanism by which doctors could collectively exert influence over public affairs to further the collective and public status of medicine as well as their private interests as practitioners.[10]

The Association was formed in 1832 by provincial medical men seeking to reform and energize a profession that was still defined and regulated by languishing collegiate oligarchies in the British capitals, particularly London. Among the issues on which the Association's founders felt that they could take a lead was medical ethics, as they understood the term. But the middle years of the nineteenth century were characterized by failure to produce any code for the profession at all. This was a marked contrast to the American Medical Association, which had produced a formal code as part of its foundation process.[11] Written and unwritten rules did exist in the United Kingdom, but they appear to have been the hallmark of particular localities where the profession was organized into associations or societies. Jukes de Styrap, a member of the BMA, took it on himself to add to one such local rule list – that of his own Shropshire branch – by compiling locally used conventions, rules and comments from correspondents deemed able to give guidance on medical conduct.[12] This work appeared in four editions from 1865, but was never intended to be adopted by the Association.[13] In fact de Styrap's *Code of Medical Ethics* reads more like a collection of exhortations and suggestions, and, particularly in its later editions as the original formulations and suggestions attracted comment, like a discussion on the problems in producing such a set of rules.

By 1933, however, the Association had 'gone from strength to strength' as perhaps the most successful professional body of its times, and it was often 'credited with powers it d[id] not in fact possess'.[14] This degree of success and influence was in large part a result of the reorganization of the Association in 1902, prompted by the medico-legal crisis over contract practice arrangements,[15] which created a dynamic democratic and disciplinary structure that has since remained essentially unchanged. Included in the BMA's new constitution of 1902 was a network of local, area and central ethical committees. In contrast to other organizations dealing with doctors' conduct, the Association was required to debate and decide its policies with reference to its members. This allowed for issues considered to involve medical ethics to be debated and resolved upon, and occasionally codified in a way that sought to balance the needs of practitioners with their professional ideals. As a result, the Association attempted to influence the General Medical Council (GMC), the statutory body overseeing medical practitioners, and worked closely with professional defence bodies, particularly the Medical Defence Union (MDU), to secure codification of particular disciplinary offences by the GMC from 1905 onwards.[16] Meanwhile Robert Saundby, the founding chairman of the BMA's CEC, was furthering debate by publishing and updating his own proposals for a formal code of medical ethics.[17]

An initial survey of 'medical ethics' between the turn of the nineteenth century (when Thomas Percival chose the phrase as the title for his codification of professional behaviour)[18] and the mid-twentieth century would show that it was concerned largely with doctors' behaviour towards other practitioners. Thus arrangements for conferring over cases without threatening the original doctor (consultation ethics) featured strongly, along with matters of propriety, mutual respect for medical brethren and the avoidance of disputes. The 'opprobrium' often caused by doctors' behaviour towards each other both in private and in public was felt not only to be un-Christian, but to damage the 'usefulness' of the profession.[19] In other words, by influencing the interactions between practitioners both in the domestic and public spheres, medical ethics was considered to be a method of raising the stock of medicine with the public as well as with individual patients. Later in the nineteenth century relationships with unorthodox healers and the strict avoidance of anything that might be construed as advertising had become prominent issues.[20] Again, the aim here was to present a unified public display of inconspicuousness in order to prevent unseemly competition and to promote a public image of medical men as gentlemen rather than tradesmen. By the turn of the century the relationship of doctors to lay organized medical services, whether mutual self-help organizations or commercial enterprises, joined the list of major concerns.

While discussions of confidentiality can be found in works on doctors' conduct throughout this period, they were never the authors' defining or overriding concern and were never prominent. Nevertheless it is useful to examine these discussions in order to make sense of the early twentieth-century debates on the subject. Charles Hawthorne, writing in the 1930s, put it thus:

> frankness on the part of the patient and silence on the part of the doctor are essential conditions of medical practice. Clearly it would be a most dishonourable action for a doctor to reveal what he learns of a patient's affairs in the secrecy of a professional interview, and a talkative doctor, if one can be imagined, would be a social nuisance and a mischief maker.[21]

This description frames beautifully the problems that could be generated by routine breaches of confidentiality. Aitchison Robertson, a teacher of medical jurisprudence in Edinburgh, struck a similar note, but with more emphasis on the private healing relationship, when he wrote that 'to anyone of true gentlemanly feeling the giving away of a confidence is repellent'. For him secrecy was 'the first commandment of medical ethics' and one of the foundations of the 'very close and intimate relationship between doctor and patient.'[22]

These quotes highlight the perceived need for the patient to be entirely truthful, which was felt to be essential if an accurate history was to be taken and appropriate treatment provided. This was in turn predicated on the patient's faith in the doctor's secrecy. Less obvious but no less important were the potentially ruinous social effects of disclosure. Both writers appealed to honour and gentility to maintain trust in the doctor–patient relationship, and to prevent scandals which would harm not only patients but doctors themselves. The words 'scandal' and 'ruin' are appropriate. Debates about the ethics of secrecy were in almost every instance triggered by matters involving extra-marital sex. Doctors were often involved with its after-effects. Unwanted pregnancies were often aborted, either by lay abortionists or, less commonly, by doctors. Most nonmedical abortions were performed clumsily and doctors often treated patients damaged in this way. Unwanted pregnancies were also concealed, and the baby given away or abandoned. In the latter situation, or where a bungled abortion resulted in a woman's death, the police often sought medical information. VD contracted by one partner within either an established or proposed marriage was another important source of secrets, since medical evidence of VD could be used to object to a marriage or to prove 'matrimonial causes' for divorce.[23]

Discussions of secrecy and sexuality were of course deeply nuanced and inflected by considerations of gender and class. The gender of the parties could crucially influence the behaviour of (almost invariably) male doctors. Moreover, medical ethics was primarily concerned with private practice (notwithstanding the fact that the original impetus for Percival's code was the need to avoid disputes within the new public institution of the hospital), and was thus mainly concerned with those classes of society that could afford to pay a doctor. Within this private setting, however, it was generally agreed that the doctor enjoyed considerable discretion over how far to maintain strict secrecy. Writing in the late nineteenth century, de Styrap continued to emphasize the importance of secrecy, but he also set out many ordinary circumstances that justified the breaking of secrecy, albeit tactfully, 'to a near and prudent relative'. These included 'a case of threatening insanity, or of pertinacious concealment of pregnancy after seduction'.[24] For de Styrap, prudent *private* disclosure could be consistent with the overarching and paternalistic medical virtue of doing what was in the patient's best interests – a virtue or consideration that was implied in most writings on medical conduct during this period. In effect, it was generally assumed that the gentlemanly private practitioner was a trustworthy judge of what was best for his patients, and a skilled navigator of the network of private obligations and relationships within which he operated.

Public disclosure, for instance in the courts, was a very different matter, and could be seriously damaging to the patient where it involved potentially scandalous information. Nonetheless, before the early twentieth century it seems to have been regarded as a relatively unproblematic issue. Given the popularity of Hippocrates and the convenience of the confidentiality clause in the oath it is striking that Percival, the putative 'father of medical ethics', was able to write on tact, confidentiality and the duty to give evidence in court without reference to the supposed 'father of medicine'. Percival's code stated that 'secrecy...when required by peculiar circumstances, should be strictly observed' and that confidences should be 'used with discretion and with the most scrupulous regard to fidelity and honour'.[25] However, giving evidence in court was something Percival saw as a duty to society – a public duty – and not to be shirked.[26] Strangely neither his discussion of the duty to testify nor the need for tact mention the case, heard in 1776, that set the legal precedent for the doctor's duty to testify in court. The Duchess of Kingston was tried for bigamy before the House of Lords, and the sergeant-surgeon to the King was asked to give evidence. He asked whether 'professional honour' would allow disclosure of information obtained as a medical attendant. The judge Lord Mansfield said that while voluntary disclosure was 'a breach of honour and...a great indiscretion...a surgeon has no privilege to avoid giving evidence in a Court of justice, but is bound by the law of the land to do it'.[27] It is not clear whether Lord Mansfield was breaking new ground with this judgment on confidentiality, but it seems unlikely since it was not seriously disputed during the nineteenth century. Indeed, the judiciary were well aware of the difficulties that public disclosure of medical secrets might pose for doctor and patient alike, to the extent that they would occasionally rule in favour of medical confidentially where this was pleaded – as de Styrap noted with evident satisfaction.[28]

This comfortable consensus was placed under increasing strain as public agencies began to invade the world of private medicine. As the nineteenth century advanced and medical ideas increasingly informed state provisions, powers and legislation, medical practice moved more and more out of the sphere of the private drawing room or bedroom and into the hospital, the clinic and the workplace. The most important instances of this were structures put in place for the notification and control of infectious diseases. Graham Mooney has demonstrated that doctors' concerns about the impact of notification and the involvement of Medical Officers of Health on both the honesty of patients and their respect for their usual doctor led many to resist notification arrangements.[29] The notification of tuberculosis and of neonatal gonorrhoeal eye infection were resisted, and only imperfectly acted on by doctors.[30] Medical attitudes to such things varied widely, however, with doctors involved in public health work being keener to support such procedures, while those in private practice were more likely to object to their application to specific patients. It was this latter class of practitioners, in particular, who would lead the charge against the growing use of medical evidence in the courts.

Abortion and the problem of medical secrecy in Edwardian Britain

The impression that secrecy was socially and legally endorsed was dramatically reinforced during the famous 1896 slander trial of William Playfair, an eminent London gynaecologist.[31] The case was brought by Playfair's niece, Linda Kitson, on whom he had conducted a dilatation and curettage of the womb. He identified some of the currettings as placental tissue, and since Kitson's husband had been away for well over a year Playfair assumed she had been up to 'hanky panky'. Playfair communicated this assumption to his wife, and this brought about Linda Kitson's financial ruin. Kitson sued, successfully portraying herself as a tragic victim, and the case resulted in the award of massive damages to the plaintiff, generating a great deal of alarm in medical circles. As Angus McLaren has pointed out, this affair turned on social class and gender issues. Thus although the circumstances were unusual, the litigant and defendant belonged to the class that most concerned doctors – their own. But McLaren's account of this affair also includes the assessment that the trial clarified the law on the issue of confidentiality. In fact, although doctors were left in no doubt that the sharing of medically obtained secrets with family members was risky, the judgment created far more confusion than clarity.[32]

Much of this confusion stemmed from tangential evidence and the judge's comments on it. In the course of the trial, medical witnesses had stated that they might consider informing the authorities of a woman suffering the after-effects of an illegal abortion – a question of *public* rather than private disclosure and hence quite dissimilar to the situation of William Playfair. The judge, evidently thinking of Linda Kitson's social ruin, commented that he 'doubted very much' if doctors 'would be justified' in informing the authorities in such circumstances, describing 'a thing like that' as 'a monstrous cruelty'. These comments were widely (and mistakenly) cited as a legal pronouncement on the issue of secrecy generally, and on the issue of informing the authorities about abortions in particular. The Royal College of Physicians of London sought the opinion of two barristers on the issue of informing the authorities in cases of suspected abortion. This report was leaked twice in the medical press although it was supposed to be *secretum collegii*.[33] Despite much detail about exactly how statements for evidence should be taken, readers in whose ears Justice Hawkins's words were still ringing could easily read the report as endorsing the view that even illegal abortions were to be regarded as absolute medical secrets.

Robert Saundby, writing on secrecy in 1907, described a disputed area, in which the legal profession and the courts loomed large. His formulation, balancing the obligations of doctors against the power of the courts, was that 'a medical practitioner is under an obligation to his patient to preserve his secrets, and in legal matters should, except with the patient's consent, answer questions only at the express direction of the judge'. Above all, a doctor should never volunteer sensitive information. Here we see a vital and apparently new idea: the need for consent to revelation. Saundby's contention was that it was 'ethically wrong' to volunteer information without it.[34] He also stated, however, that there might 'be cases where it was the obvious duty of the medical man to speak out', and gave the example of a wounded murderer seeking treatment. But in other respects, Saundby's views were strict. Commenting on the opinion obtained by the Royal College of Physicians after the Playfair trial, he stated that 'a medical man should not reveal facts which had come to his knowledge in the course of his professional duties' even where a criminal offence such as abortion was suspected.[35]

Abortion was of course widely practised in Edwardian Britain. And even when the operation was performed by an amateur abortionist, doctors were still often involved since abortees were frequently subject to severe sepsis and bleeding.[36] Doctors were potentially in a position to elicit information that could be used to prosecute abortionists, but frustrated the legal establishment and the Lord Chief Justice in particular by their reluctance to obtain or pass on this information. This reticence was often attributed to the Playfair trial.[37] However, Horace Avory, one of the lawyers who had advised the Royal College of Physicians in the aftermath of the trial, subsequently repudiated the commonly held view that the judge had endorsed the principle of secrecy. Avory himself went on to become a judge, and at Birmingham Assizes in December 1914 he heard a case that gave him an opportunity to give voice to the Lord Chief Justice's concerns, although publicly he appeared to speak entirely independently.[38] The Birmingham case concerned a woman who had sought medical help after an abortion carried out by a lay woman, and had died suddenly from infection and massive bleeding. Because no proper statement had been taken by her doctors Avory decided that a charge of murder could not be brought against the abortionist, and he commented that he could not doubt that it is the duty of the medical man to communicate with the police or with the authorities in order that [a statement be made]....The desire to preserve...confidence[s] must be subordinated to the duty [of] every good citizen to assist in the investigation of a serious crime.

He went on to state that his opinion of twenty years previously had been misinterpreted in Saundby's *Medical Ethics*. Contrary to Saundby's interpretation, he stated that his opinion had been clearly that it was in the public interest for doctors to inform in such circumstances. In retrospect it is clear that both men were drawing selectively on the document in question, but such an analysis was not undertaken at the time, and the matter proceeded to a full-blown dispute.

Within days the Director of Public Prosecutions wrote to the BMA asking that 'the inaccuracy in Dr. Saundby's book...be corrected' and Avory's views circulated to doctors.[39] However, the CEC felt that that doctors were justified 'in [their] own conscience' in withholding information because systematic informing would create so many scandals that it would lay the doctor open to suits for slander. The Committee also suggested that the public supported this approach. One striking feature of the correspondence is that the public prosecutor several times appealed to the BMA to avoid publicizing their disagreement. The fact that he was at pains to avoid any public discussion of the issue, and the fact that the BMA was prepared to publish details in their journal, would tend to support the supposition that the BMA was taking the more popular position.[40] The BMA Council passed a resolution that the state had 'no authority' to claim an obligation to inform, unless they legislated to protect doctors from slander charges such as those brought by Linda Kitson. Furthermore they endorsed a key statement on confidentiality drafted by the CEC. It stated that 'a medical practitioner should not under any circumstances disclose voluntarily, without the patient's consent, information which he has obtained from that patient in the exercise of his professional duties'.[41] At a subsequent meeting with the Lord Chief Justice specific 'circumstances' in which informing was justified were set out to representatives of the BMA.[42] These 'circumstances' were essentially a polite way of pointing out that doctors should inform in situations that could lead to prosecutions. When the list of circumstances was published in the *British Medical Journal*, however, they appeared alongside the Association's own conflicting resolution.[43]

The BMA evidently felt that public opinion (by which they would almost certainly have meant the opinion of the *Times*-reading classes) would support them in containing scandal by refusing to divulge details of abortions where there was any chance of such repercussions. The private nature of the medical encounter was upheld and seen as over-riding the public concern over illegal abortion. The fact that the detailed file on this question closes as this point, and the lack of any repeat of the dispute, suggests that on this occasion the BMA's view prevailed.

Venereal disease, divorce and medical secrecy

Another issue that was to provoke medical debate on the question of secrecy involved infection with a venereal disease. The issue figured so often in discussions of medical secrecy during the early twentieth century that it is worth denoting it 'the case of the syphilitic fiancé'. In its basic form it supposed a situation in which the doctor knew that his patient had VD and that marriage was proposed. The doctor's dilemma was a simple one: should he tell the bride-to-be, or perhaps her father, in order to protect the 'innocent' third party from infection? A common variation on the theme involved a venereal patient who was already married. One of the fascinating aspects to this trope is its basis in gender and class stereotype and in the double standard. It was never the bride-to-be who was imagined to suffer from VD, while in the married version it was always assumed that whichever partner presented to the doctor with VD was the one guilty of bringing the infection into the home (an assumption that now appears unsafe in the light of modern knowledge of the biology of some forms of urethritis). A conflict between gentlemanly gallantry and gentlemanly professionalism thus lay at the root of the dilemma.[44]

Writing in the years before the First World War, Saundby simply advised 'objecting to the marriage' in such cases, but did not say whether to breach confidentiality.[45] But this hypothetical dilemma would become more urgent when, just a few months after Avory made clear his views on doctors' responsibility to report cases of illegal abortion, the recently appointed Royal Commission on Venereal Disease consulted the BMA about secrecy in connection with the network of VD clinics that they proposed to establish. On the one hand, the Commissioners wanted to encourage attendance at the clinics by making all information obtained during treatment confidential. In this, it seems likely that they drew on the advice and evidence of medical practitioners, and allowed themselves to be persuaded that the promise of secrecy was a factor in bringing people to medical attention and treatment, and as such was of public benefit. But, on the other hand, the Commissioners' primary aim was not to treat VD but to prevent its spread. Consequently, they were keen that doctors should be allowed to warn partners and potential partners of VD patients. To this end, they recommended statutory changes to make such communications 'privileged'.[46] In other words they proposed to establish statutory instruments to protect doctors from slander suits when privately divulging information obtained in clinics that the Commission itself intended to be confidential.

The CEC regarded the proposed safeguard of privilege as deeply unsatisfactory. The Committee upheld the view that doctors owed a private duty of secrecy, and they were unwilling to accept any legislative measures that might be seen to sanction breach of that duty. Equally, however, the Committee were prepared to accept that they also had a public duty to prevent the spread of venereal disease. But they preferred to see that duty enshrined in statute, in the form of a compulsory responsibility to notify VD cases to the public health authorities, who would then be responsible for any further preventive measures including disclosure to those at risk of infection. The Commissioners' proposals for voluntary but privileged disclosure represented an unsatisfactory 'half-way house' between these two desirable principles, which left responsibility for private disclosure in the hands of the private practitioner. As such they were unacceptable to the CEC, who framed a clumsily worded resolution for the Annual Representative Meeting (ARM) stating that no privilege as outlined by the Royal Commission was called for.[47] At the ARM there was disagreement between those who felt the regulations should compel disclosure and those who were affronted by any suggestion that individual judgement was insufficient. This discussion was not helped by the opaque syntax of the draft resolution. Only one delegate was able to distinguish the issue of whether or not 'to tell' from the question of privilege, and in the confusion the motion was lost.[48] The clinics were put in place with non-statutory rules that stipulated confidentiality, but that failed to specify circumstances in which practitioners might be allowed or compelled to disclose information either to public bodies or to private individuals.

This system of non-statutory confidentiality appears to have worked satisfactorily during the war years. But the lack of clarity in the system became highly problematic not long after the war ended, when evidence of VD began to play an increasingly common role in divorce cases. Until the early years of the twentieth century divorce had been the preserve of the wealthy, and only a hundred years previously had actually required an individual Act of Parliament. The twentieth century was marked by a number of legislative changes that made divorce easier for first the middle and then the lower classes, and by a corresponding rise in the number of marriages ending in divorce. The period immediately after the First World War saw one such steep rise, which coincided with greater ease of access to divorce hearings in provincial Assize courts. It appears than no extra judicial time or other resources were made available to support this new workload until the 1940s and it came as an unwelcome addition to the circuit judge's routine.[49]

It was in this context that the non-statutory confidentiality of the VD clinic system was challenged in 1920. Justice McCardie, a hard-working judge with progressive views on divorce, contraception and abortion,[50] was presiding over a hearing for divorce on the grounds of adultery and cruelty, the proof being the passing of syphilis from husband to wife. McCardie ordered a Medical Officer from one of the wartime VD clinics to give evidence of the husband's condition. He ruled that, although secrecy was desirable, 'in a Court of Justice there were even higher considerations'.[51] The matter was debated by the CEC and a report prepared for the next meeting of the BMA Council. The CEC and the BMA solicitor acknowledged that many doctors and lay people felt that the partner had a right to be informed in the 'case of the syphilitic fiancé'. But they advised Council that they were nonetheless 'strongly against any relaxation of the immemorial tradition of the profession that the confidence of patient must be regarded as sacred'.[52]

The CEC subsequently put forward a resolution for the 1920 ARM which reiterated the principle that the doctor should not voluntarily breach secrecy without the patient's consent, and specifically so with reference to VD. But the discussions that took place around this resolution reflected not only the real moral dilemma involved – between the duty to protect the interests of individual patients on the one hand, and to protect the health of other individuals and of the public on the other – but also a continuing confusion between discreet private disclosure to an interested party and public disclosure in the courts. Consequently, when the Association's Solicitor spoke to the resolution at the ARM, his rhetorical question as to whether they would inform in 'the case of the syphilitic fiancé' was met with an uproar of yes's and no's. The issue was further confused by a discussion on the lack of medical 'privilege', which failed to distinguish between two different legal meanings of the term. The kind of privilege earlier proposed by the Royal Commission on Venereal Disease, and rejected on that occasion by the ARM, was the kind that *allows revelation* without fear of action for slander. But many at the present meeting of the ARM now evidently resented their lack of a very different kind of privilege, namely that enjoyed by lawyers, which would *allow them not to reveal* information about their clients in court of law without being held in contempt. The meeting became heated, with much harking back to the 'organization' of the 1900s and 1910s (a euphemism for what had been concerted boycotting of contract practice posts), and the first mention of the idea that the BMA's membership might be capable of establishing a new legal precedent on the question. The meeting was impressed by this argument that the profession could take a stand on the issue, and asked the CEC to consider to what extent the Association could support those who defied the Courts.[53]

The CEC's response was cautious. The Committee drafted a series of resolutions, subsequently endorsed by the Council, which upheld the view that court rulings and existing statutory requirements were reasonable and justifiable exceptions to the rule of professional secrecy, and that anyone defying court orders would do so 'entirely on his own responsibility'. The resolutions then went on to state that if any extension of these exceptions was proposed, the Association should resist by 'all lawful means', and should 'accord support...to any individual practitioner...assailed through such new encroachments'.[54] Before the draft resolutions could be considered by the 1921 ARM, however, two further judicial interventions early in that year ensured that the Meeting would be in no mood to accept the CEC's policies. The first of these cases was essentially a bad-tempered re-run of the one recently heard by McCardie.[55] But the second – again a divorce hearing – involved the revelation of confidential statutory information contained in a birth registration of a stillborn child to prove that the child was not the husband's.[56] This represented not just an over-ruling of a convention, but a formal abuse of the stillbirth notification statutes. The fact that the cases occurred within a few weeks of each other heightened medical reaction against breaches of secrecy more generally.

Consequently, by the time the ARM came to consider the CEC's recommendation that doctors should comply with court orders, the gathered representatives were disinclined to agree. The chairman of the CEC, Reginald Langdon-Down,[57] did his best to explain to the ARM that any other stance than that recommended by the Committee would be simply illegal, but stronger passions prevailed. To great applause one representative urged 'a much stronger attitude' since the judiciary were going to 'destroy [the] whole basis of confidence' between doctors and patients. Further cheers and applause met the comment that the ordinary layman was quite positive that his doctor should never under any circumstances tell anybody his private affairs. After a long and unbalanced debate in which Hippocrates and public opinion figured large, the meeting decided to support an *ad hoc* resolution that did not seek to overturn all statutory breaches of secrecy, but effectively drew a line in the sand. It stated:

> that the Association use all its power to support a member...who refuses to divulge, without the patient's consent, information obtained [during] his professional duties, except where it is already provided by Act of Parliament that he must do so.[58]

Langdon-Down later described this as intended to create a stir, so that defiant doctors 'will be hailed as martyrs by a grateful public and that a new custom will in due course be established according full privilege to a doctor'. Many within the BMA still thought of the organization as capable of using its disciplinary and fraternal functions to bring about concerted medical action, of a type more usually associated with militant trade unions.[59] The strategy had brought the Association into collision with the courts over the issue of boycotting low-paid appointments during the 1910s, and while most responsible members of the BMA secretariat had no wish to re-run their trial for conspiracy, slander and libel,[60] there were others who still had a taste for such action. The purpose of the ARM resolution was to set up a system whereby doctors could risk contempt of court because the BMA would arrange to maintain their practices during their prison sentences. Moreover, the supporters of the resolution assumed that the public (many of whom would have something in their private lives they wished to keep secret) would side with the doctors in taking this stance. By encouraging what they hoped would be widely publicized prosecutions for contempt of court, the protesters thus hoped to provoke public opinion and thereby secure a change in the law.

At the meeting Langdon-Down acted quickly, using a technicality to prevent the resolution from becoming BMA policy for a year. But clear battle lines had been drawn up within the Association, which would shortly find itself forced into a bruising confrontation with the legal profession.

Should the judge order the doctor to tell?

The moderate view can be found expressed in an eminently reasonable memorandum by Langdon-Down that he intended to be the starting point for discussion, but which his committee simply adopted as a report.[61] He pointed out that the BMA could not retain two resolutions – one implying exceptions to secrecy and the other rejecting any exceptions without consent. The principle could not be absolute, doctors' opinions on notification of disease showed how attitudes changed, and their tendency to assert contradictory responses in 'the case of the syphilitic fiancé' showed inconsistency of thought. There were many situations where duty and moral sense would over-ride secrecy: for example discovering a spy, a dangerous criminal, 'an epileptic driving a train' or 'a lunatic...at large'. He suggested that the judge was perhaps the best person to decide when secrecy should be breached, and that public awareness of the limitations of secrecy was the key to the problem. If the exceptions to secrecy were fully explained then people could not complain 'that we have acted dishonourably'. It would be better 'for our own self-respect...to warn the public clearly'.

The CEC proposed a clear set of exceptions to the rule of secrecy. These were: when obliged by an Act of Parliament or Order in Council; when ordered by a Court of Law; and where a practitioner's duty as a citizen over-rode his professional obligation, including where this was in the patient's best interest. A further resolution cancelled the troublesome undertaking of the previous ARM to support doctors who defied the courts, and pledged instead 'to sustain the principle of professional secrecy on the highest level consistent...with...the public interest'. To this end the BMA would, if appropriate, support any doctor who was treated 'harshly or unjustly...in the exercise of his professional duties to the highest public interest'.[62]

Leading the opposition to the CEC proposals was a small group of eminent and successful practitioners, including Lord Dawson,[63] E.B. Turner and Guy Dain,[64] who regarded the principle of secrecy as absolute, the doctor as the final moral arbiter and the law and the judiciary as reasonable targets for organized conscientious objection. These men disliked the CEC document so much that they took unprecedented steps to destroy it. Discussion was postponed to a special Council meeting, at which the report was referred back, not to the CEC itself, but to a 'special meeting' to be attended by Dawson, Dain, Turner and three other extremely senior members of Council.[65] In other words, the CEC were sat down with a group of heavyweights, and made to reconsider. One submission from a long-serving Council member argued that secrecy was 'a matter of *conscience*...of honour and honesty; of compassion and chivalry; of patriotism and altruism'.[66] Another felt that it was 'a moral issue, and must remain a matter for the individual conscience in every case'.[67] All felt that the doctor–patient relationship was more important than 'the disposal of litigation',[68] although one memorandum suggested that a distinction might be drawn between civil cases, such as divorce, and criminal charges such as murder.[69] This latter point is important: one of the aspects of the situation that appears to have riled doctors was the fact that divorce cases did not involve matters of high justice or dramatic criminal activity, just the rather sorry parading of personal misery through the public courts. It is striking that it was not decided to make more of this distinction in the proposed campaign for privilege.

At the meeting Lord Dawson proposed a motion calling for 'a measure of privilege' for doctors in Courts of Law 'above and beyond what is accorded to the ordinary witness'. After 'considerable discussion' this privilege was defined as preventing the revelation of any information without the patient's consent.

Moreover it was resolved to 'support in any possible way' cases of conscientious refusal to testify considered by the Council to be worthy of such support. Last, it was agreed 'that the Hippocratic Oath be published in the *Journal'*.[70]

Four days later the Association's solicitor wrote to Alfred Cox, the BMA Secretary, expressing his concern that the Association's stance could cause real problems with malpractice cases, in which doctors' evidence for the defence routinely broke professional secrecy. Cox, no mean medical unionist and the virtual father of organized medical solidarity, said he had 'never felt less comfortable over anything than I do over this'. He felt there was 'something rather fine' about the scenario envisaged by the hard-liners, but that their 'attitude rests on sentiment and tradition and it is no good trying to invest it with logical consistency'. [71]

The Secrecy Committee met again a few days later and considered a draft report obviously pasted together from the various memoranda submitted and including an 'appendix' by Langdon-Down that argued against the rest of the Report. Langdon Down disowned the report and resolutions when they were presented to a poorly attended meeting of the Council, which approved them by the narrow majority of sixteen votes to fourteen.[72] Lord Dawson and the others had achieved a complete reversal of policy within the space of a month. Despite the efforts of Langdon Down and other leading CEC members, the 1922 ARM adopted the resolutions framed by Dawson, which were intended to establish a new legal precedent to over-ride the Mansfield judgment of 1776.

One motivating factor in the elite hard-liners' stance on absolute secrecy was jealousy of the legal profession, and an inflated sense of their own public status. Thus the BMA was prepared to accept a statutory duty to notify the authorities of cases of infectious disease, for instance, since such a public duty was imposed by Parliament or the executive. Orders in court were a different matter. Dawson and his sympathizers resented the fact that a judge had the power to compel disclosure at his own discretion – often, it seemed, simply in order to secure a convenient and expeditious end to a petty case of divorce. This inter-professional jealousy became clear when the newly ennobled Lord Dawson gave an ill-advised speech at the Medico-Legal Society in early January 1922.[73] At the heart of Dawson's talk was a perfectly sensible proposal to imitate the distinction found in New Zealand law that allowed secrecy to be over-ridden in criminal cases only. But he ruined his case by declaring, in front of an audience of leading lawyers, that the Law was 'the spoilt child of the professions', and that the argument that medical evidence was required to ensure justice was a cover for judicial laziness. Speaking of the 'spirit of the English Law', which allowed lawyer–client communication absolute privilege, he then invoked the 'spirit of English Medicine' and asked: 'Can it be contended that one is more important than the other?' He spoke of the threat to the 'art' of the general practitioner, which relied entirely on the evidence of the patient's own history, and thus on their frankness. He spoke movingly about two 'hypothetical' cases, both of which involved sexual misdemeanours. Dawson may have intended to give the impression that these cases were based on his own patients, whom his audience would have known were often drawn from the social elite. Dawson asked, 'is the law to have the power to take advantage of [a] patient's illness and compel the doctor to disclosure?...If so all honour is at an end'.

This speech was not printed in the society's *Transactions* – indeed, it would have been completely out of place there – but it did appear in *The Lancet*, along with a summary of the ensuing discussion, which spilled over into a second meeting a week later. It is clear that most of those present felt this was an inter-professional dispute. One doctor spoke passionately in favour of Dawson's view, and looked forward to 'more doctors in Parliament'. Lord Riddell (who later published on secrecy) said that 'Doctors were always anxious to improve their status', while Lord Russell pointed out that 'Doctors were a numerous class and not all of them had [such] high ideals'. Others argued that individual doctors could not be relied on to act in the interests of public health. The society's President, in summing up, asked if doctors really wanted to be put into a position whereby their fee bought their silence, at the price of their honour and duty as citizens.[74]

This latter view was very much that held by Dr Francis Crookshank, who was not only Vice-President of the Society but also a member of the CEC, and who resigned from both bodies shortly after these events. His views are worth noting for their incisiveness. In a speech to a local BMA Branch that summer, he described the Medico-Legal Society meeting as a disaster, saying that 'a very bad impression was made on the distinguished lawyers then present when one medical man after another propounded various hypothetical and fantastic cases...revealing an extraordinary ignorance of the practice of our Courts...and the rules of evidence'.[75] The only cases of real hardship, he argued, were the two cases that had triggered the furore in the first place. The Hippocratic Oath contained no absolute injunction against anything other than gossiping, and nobody swore it in any case. The 'case of the syphilitic fiancé' was, he said, 'the favourite instance of the medical casuist...so often spoken of as likely to occur, yet which hardly ever does'. As for evidence or knowledge of crimes, 'the doctor who gives an absolutely binding pledge of secrecy...is a fool and a negligent fool, for whom there is no excuse'. Crookshank's disdain for many in the medical profession was clear. 'I can quite conceive', he said:

> that some gentlemen whose clientele is drawn from certain classes of society may feel the shoe to pinch them more frequently than it does others...the proportion of my own patients who are either criminal or immoral and who fear exposure in Court, is almost negligible.

For Crookshank, the duty to tell the truth in court was 'more urgent than the shadowy obligations said to be imposed by the so-called Oath of Hippocrates'. For him medicine had to be subordinate to public interests and abstract justice, for 'Public Health without public justice is mere brutality'.

Both Dawson and Crookshank addressed class issues in one way or another. For Dawson the threat to the social fabric through the avoidance of medical advice or the exposure of sordid secrets among the upper classes was prominent.

And just as he wished to keep the elite out of the cruel glare of public exposure, he wished to keep medical judgements about what should remain secret, if not above the law, then at least parallel to it. Crookshank, by contrast, appears to have regarded the social elite as degenerate and dispensable, and looked to the rule of law as the absolute guarantor of public welfare. These differing views of public polity informed radically different views about the extent to which the private sphere should be protected through medical confidentiality.

However, the most effective contribution to this debate had yet to come. Since Lord Birkenhead (Frederick E. Smith) had been Lord Chancellor between 1918 and 1922, his critique, entitled 'Should a doctor tell?' and published in a book of essays for general readership in 1922, was most significant.[76] Birkenhead combined his high office with well-practised skill in writing entertainingly for the public.[77] For him, the question was not one of 'professional partisanship' but 'of the broadest concern'. He started his argument by demolishing the legal grounds for absolute privilege in any profession including law. He admitted and affirmed that 'common sense and ordinary feelings of honour would prevent a doctor from gossiping'. However, he judged the arguments put forward for medical privilege to be 'discordant and loose'. This woolly medical thinking was exposed in cases where doctors had knowledge of crime. 'The doctor,' said Smith, 'assumes his tongue is tied, [and] that he must impale himself on the horns of a dilemma.' All that had resulted was that 'innumerable' crimes such as poisoning and abortion went unpunished. More damaging still, Birkenhead effectively charged doctors with complicity in child sexual abuse. To devastating rhetorical effect, he recounted the 'amazing' refusal of a medical laboratory worker to disclose VD test results that would have proved a child had been sexually assaulted. He asked, 'what kind of confidential relation has been set up between this elderly syphilitic violator of his own child and the laboratory staff to whom he is only known through a specimen...of his...blood?' Thus, he said, the argument was not between two professions, but between 'those who claimed' medical privilege in court 'and the parents of the children the law sought to protect'. He did not stop there, observing that 'doctors have no monopoly of medical practice' and asking, 'are the Christian Scientist healer, the herbalist, the quack, the bone setter, the chemist to be covered by the same doctrine as the doctor?' Modern life, he argued, depended on a 'web' of confidential relations. They could not all be absolute, without the complete collapse of legal redress in court. The privilege asked for by doctors would be 'retrograde...and [un]justified', and was opposed by all judges and barristers.

Conclusion

Not only would a dramatic courtroom showdown with extensive newspaper coverage have suited the hard-line camp in the BMA, it would also have satisfied some basic narrative imperatives in bringing this story to a conclusion. In reality the affair moved swiftly to an anti-climax. The BMA Council had already shown signs of realizing the weakness of their stance. The CEC still had to devise the detail of the scheme of resistance, but Council simply put the matter off several times. They adopted the CEC's suggested delaying tactic of seeking a united approach with the Royal Colleges, reporting that 'the task before the profession...may well be one of extreme difficulty'.[78] Birkenhead's book was cited as 'an indication of the opposition [we] may...encounter'. But it was not until 1924, when a member of the Association proposed to refuse to give evidence that he regarded as confidential, that the CEC for the first and last time considered a 'test case'. After a brief discussion, the member was advised to outline his reasons for not wishing to testify, and then obey the judge's orders.[79] A further attempt to push for privilege was made at the ARM in 1929, but the CEC used a wily bureaucratic manœuvre to ensure that it was never recorded as BMA policy.[80] Hope sprang eternal in some breasts however. In 1927 and 1937 the dermatologist MP for London University, Ernest Graham Little, introduced Private Members Bills to allow for medical privilege, but both were easily defeated by the deployment of Lord Birkenhead's arguments.[81]

Meanwhile the CEC continued to advise doctors on specific issues of secrecy. The cases, which involved all the usual stock-in-trade of medical secrecy – VD, marital cruelty and divorce, abandoned babies and the like – demonstrate how easily doctors could enmesh themselves in problems that they could have avoided by simply following the advice readily available in BMA handbooks and year-books.[82] Usually either the doctor, or in one instance an entire Division of the BMA,[83] was persuaded by more or less honourable sentiment that the principles of non-disclosure were best breached. But doctors' need for such guidance is hardly surprising in view of the conflicting opinions that continued to be aired. Thus Aitchison Robertson's influential textbook took a more liberal stance than the BMA, arguing on ethical grounds that exposure of the name of the aborted was justified by the conviction of the abortionist, that a patient dying after abortion ought to make a dying declaration and that, in 'the case of the syphilitic fiancé', the patient should be put off marrying or the father of the bride informed.[84] On the other hand, Hugh Woods, secretary of the Medical Protection Society, was prompted by fear of litigation to adopt a contrary stance. In a series of articles on secrecy that appeared in *The Lancet* in 1927 – subsequently published in a volume on medical conduct – Woods offered the strictest advice of any of the published discussions. 'Apart from legal compulsion,' he said, 'the obligation of secrecy is absolute.' It was clear that he would have preferred it to be absolutely absolute. When it came to the risk of being asked to give evidence his advice was not to let anyone, especially solicitors, know what you knew beforehand.[85]

This continuing divergence of opinion reflected deeper tensions and anxieties within the profession, as to how they should situate themselves in the context of the wider social and political changes that troubled Britain in the years around the First World War. Hitherto, doctors appear to have had little difficulty with issues of secrecy. In general confidentiality was preserved, since it served both the doctor, by promoting his trustworthiness, and his patients, who could consult without fear of private misdemeanours or mistakes becoming widely known. The public responsibilities and duties that doctors shared with all citizens – notably the duty to disclose information demanded in court by a judge – generated exceptions to this principle. Conflicts between these public pressures and the basic considerations of tact, delicacy and regard for the patient's reputation that underpinned notions of secrecy before the early twentieth century were either quietly resolved, or were not felt to merit ethical or political debate within the profession. Serious anxieties only emerged with the expansion of the state into matters of public health, when doctors also found themselves bound to disclose information about their patients to the requisite authorities. But it was only when medical evidence of sexual conduct began to assume a new prominence in the courts, particularly as a result of mounting concern over abortion and growing rates of divorce, that the dramatic but essentially futile reactions discussed in the present paper were elicited.

The hardening of medical opposition to disclosure during the first twenty-five years of the twentieth century represented a reaction against this growing tendency of the public authorities to intrude into private affairs, and to fears that such intrusion represented a threat to the prevailing social order. This is evident from the fact that the medical secrets at issue were almost always sexual. Doctors were being asked to expose private behaviour of a kind that was publicly deplored. Elite doctors like Lord Dawson, in particular, feared that such revelations would undermine public respect for the wealthy classes among whom they practised. In this as in several other areas of medico-political or ethical difficulty, they responded by invoking the Victorian ideal of the medical gentleman. Supposedly a man of private and independent moral and financial means, and of general and scientific learning, this ideal doctor served the public by deploying these gifts to relieve suffering and dispel disease, primarily in the context of the private domestic encounter. The medical ethics that doctors like Dawson espoused – the framework of ideals, rules and discipline that guided medical behaviour – aimed to promote this ideal at every turn, by ensuring the correct public and private demeanour of these gentlemen, both individually and collectively. Medical secrecy, in particular, served to delineate the boundary of a sacred and private space occupied by the patient and doctor, and closed to public scrutiny.

But there were also many for whom the need to prevent degeneration and disease from destabilizing society implied a more pragmatic approach to the information gleaned in the medical encounter. This view – which for some amounted to a promotion of the ideal of the scientific public officer to replace that of the Christian gentleman of science – was steadily gaining ground by the early twentieth century. It was seen not least in calls from public health doctors for the establishment of a state medical service to replace private practice.[86] In the light of such proposals, the Victorian values underlying much of medical ethics could be seen to support a reactionary position. Medical unwillingness to expose the venereal and the extra-maritally impregnated, in particular, could be seen as implying complicity with a deeply entrenched social hypocrisy. This point, whether consciously or unconsciously perceived, might also have fed into the marked reaction described in this chapter. Early twentieth-century medical ethics did much to promote the idea that a patient should primarily entrust their medical care to one doctor at a time, who then organized further specialist or consultant care, and to protect that almost matrimonial relationship in the marketplace. This was widely sensed and often viewed with suspicion or frustration; indeed, some observers portrayed the insistence on secrecy as little more than an attempt to bolster private practitioners' own interests in the medical marketplace. The publisher and lawyer Lord Riddell quipped that 'if medical advertising were permitted, I am sure that a sign reading "Dr. Blank is a regular oyster; he never talks about his patients" would be a valuable recommendation to the laity'.[87] A leading GP made a similar point, but without the irony, when he advised young doctors that 'silence is golden, and a reputation for being as close as wax about your patients…is a very valuable asset'.[88]

That is not to say that there were not still good practical reasons to urge secrecy. In the absence of compulsory treatment structures, delay in seeking treatment for whatever reason would stifle attempts to contain diseases that threatened the social fabric. But the same concern with public order led to the identification of many instances in which the doctor should tell, the least contentious of these being where the doctor had knowledge of criminal activity. The publicly responsible image that the profession wished to project thus did not imply a simple attitude to confidentiality, except for those who regarded the private sphere and private moral judgement as paramount. Debates about secrecy thus revolved, at one level, around how the profession could best use the private information they gleaned in the course of their practice to protect or promote the public good. Some prioritized the stability of the web of private relationships that constituted elite society, while others looked to more public and universal structures and measures of medical and social regulation.

The waters were further muddied by elite doctors' jealousy of the judiciary. Most doctors accepted that Parliament had the power to compel disclosure, in the public interest, of information known to doctors that would otherwise have remained secret. But in their discussions over secrecy they allowed themselves to become obsessed with the question of whether the judiciary too should have this power. Caught up in these tensions, many leading doctors failed to distinguish clearly between matters of private and public disclosure, between different meanings of privilege, and between civil and criminal cases. As a result, the BMA failed to provide a clear lead on the issue, and the profession gradually subsided into grudging compliance with the courts.

By the 1930s it appears the fight to enforce secrecy in the courts was largely forgotten, just as objections to notification had been swept aside. If the problem had been resolved in practice, however, it was at the expense of any higher consideration of principle. For one medical observer at least, commenting in 1937 on the swift rise in medical testimony for divorce, this could only cast a dishonourable light on the profession:

The present attitude of most doctors…seems to me despicable. They usually salve their conscience by uttering a formal protest, and then proceed to throw the patient to the wolves of the law. So long as the 'responsibility' is shifted to the judge, the realities of personal and professional honour seem to matter little.[89]

Acknowledgements

The author remains indebted to the Wellcome Trust for funding the research on which this chapter is based, which was undertaken in 1997–8 under a Medical Graduate Research Fellowship. This work would not have been possible without the teaching, support and inspiration of Bill Bynum, Roy Porter, Michael Neve, Christopher Lawrence, Chandak Sengoopta, Mark Harrison and many others involved in the former Wellcome Institute between 1987 and 2000. I am grateful to Steve Sturdy and Holger Maehle for their ongoing interest, support and patience in allowing me the opportunity to publish some of my findings.

Notes

1   B. Hurwitz and R. Richardson, 'Swearing to care: the resurgence in medical oaths', *British Medical Journal*, 1997, vol. 315, pp. 1671–4.
2   G.E.R. Lloyd (ed.), *Hippocratic Writings*, London: Blackwell, 1950, p. 67.
3   Isabel de Salis, private communication. De Salis's forthcoming PhD concerns spiritual healing practices in contemporary northern Malawi where healing ceremonies involve the whole community and only black magic or witchcraft would be carried out in secret. See also Margaret Pelling's chapter in the present volume for a discussion of the problematically public character of much medical consultation in early modern England.
4   T. Percival, *Medical Ethics; or a Code of Institutes and Precepts Adapted to the Professional Conduct of Physicians and Surgeons*, orig. pub. 1803, reprinted in C.D. Leake, *Percival's Medical Ethics*, Baltimore: William & Wilkins Co., 1927, pp. 61–205, at II.i.
5   G. Mooney, 'Public health versus private practice: the contested development of compulsory infectious disease notification in late-nineteenth century Britain', *Bulletin of the History of Medicine*, 1999, vol. 73, pp. 238–67.
6   J. de Styrap, *A Code of Medical Ethics: With Remarks on the Duties of Practitioners to their Patients, etc.*, London: J. & A. Churchill, 1878, preface; R. Saundby, *Medical Ethics: A Guide to Professional Conduct*, Bristol: John Wright, 1902, p. 2; W.G. Aitchison Robertson, *Medical Conduct and Practice, A Guide to the Ethics of Medicine*, London: A. & C. Black, 1921, p. 1.
7   C. Lawrence, 'Still incommunicable: clinical holists and medical knowledge in interwar Britain', in C. Lawrence and G. Weisz (eds), *Greater than the Parts: Holism in Biomedicine, 1920–1950*, New York: Oxford University Press, 1998, pp. 94–111, and S. Sturdy, 'Hippocrates and state medicine: George Newman outlines the founding policy of the Ministry of Health', in ibid., pp. 112–34.
8   G. Riddell (Lord Riddell), 'Should a doctor tell?', *John O'London's Weekly*, July 16 1927, vol. 17, pp. 441–3.
9   A. Morrice, '"Honour and interests": medical ethics in Britain, and the work of the British Medical Association's Central Ethical Committee, 1902–1939', University of London, MD thesis, 1999. Sequential minute books of all BMA committees, including the Council, the CEC and its sub-committee are held in the BMA Archive, Tavistock House, Tavistock Square, London. Invaluable correspondence, press

cuttings and other revealing ephemera on medical ethical issues dealt with by the CEC are also held in the Wellcome Library for the History and Understanding of Medicine, Contemporary Medical Archive Centre (CMAC), series SA/BMA/D.

10 P. Bartrip, *Themselves Writ Large: The British Medical Association, 1832–1966*, London: British Medical Journal, 1996.

11 R. Baker, 'Introduction', in *idem* (ed.), *The Codification of Medical Morality*, vol. 2: *Anglo-American Medical Ethics and Medical Jurisprudence in the Nineteenth Century*, Dordrecht, London: Kluwer Academic Publishers, 1995, pp. 1–22.

12 P. Bartrip, 'An introduction to Jukes Styrap's *A Code of Medical Ethics* (1878)', in Baker, (ed.), *Medical Morality*, vol. 2, pp. 145–8.

13 De Styrap, *A Code of Medical Ethics*, London: J. & A. Churchill, 1878; 2nd edn, London: J. & A. Churchill, 1886; 3rd edn, London: H.K. Lewis, 1890; 4th edn, London: H.K. Lewis, 1895.

14 A.M. Carr-Saunders and P.A. Wilson, *The Professions*, Oxford: Clarendon Press, 1933 (reissued London: Frank Cass & Co., 1964), pp. 90–1.

15 D.G. Green, *Working Class Patients and the Medical Establishment: Self Help in Britain from the Mid-Nineteenth Century to 1948*, Aldershot: Gower, 1985, pp. 21–98.

16 It was the lobbying of the MDU and then the BMA that wrung a series of 'Warning notices' from the reluctant GMC, which saw itself much more as a court than as an instructor or guide. R. Smith, 'The development of ethical guidance for medical practitioners by the General Medical Council', *Medical History*, 1993, vol. 37, pp. 56–67.

17 R. Saundby, *Medical Ethics*, Bristol: John Wright, 1902; 2nd edn, London: Charles Griffin, 1907.

18 Percival, *Medical Ethics*, 1st edn.

19 W.B. Kesteven, *Thoughts on Medical Ethics...From the London Medical Gazette*, London: private imprint, 1849, p. 3.

20 This is a central issue in de Styrap, *Medical Ethics*, 1st edn.

21 C.O. Hawthorne, 'General practice no. IV – medical ethics', *Practitioner*, 1936, vol. 137, pp. 646–56.

22 Robertson, *Medical Conduct and Practice*, p. 32.

23 Where a wife sought a divorce from her husband, she had to prove both infidelity and cruelty on his part, while a husband had only to prove that his wife had committed simple adultery. In both cases, however, venereal infection was deemed to constitute sufficient grounds. O.R. McGregor, *Divorce in England: A Centenary History*, London: Heinemann, 1957.

24 De Styrap, *Medical Ethics*, 3rd edn, pp. 39–40.

25 Percival, *Medical Ethics*, 1st edn, I.v.

26 Ibid., IV.xvi.

27 J. Glaister, *A Textbook of Medical Jurisprudence and Toxicology*, 3rd edn, Edinburgh, E. & S. Livingstone, 1915, p. 54.

28 De Styrap, *Medical Ethics*, 3rd edn, pp. 39–40.

29 Mooney, 'Public health versus private practice'.

30 *Lancet*, 1922, vol. 1, pp. 641–3.

31 A. McLaren, 'Privileged communications: medical confidentiality in late Victorian Britain', *Medical History*, 1993, vol. 37, pp. 129–47.

32 D.H. Kitchin, *Law for the Medical Practitioner*, London: Eyre & Spottiswoode, 1941, p. 54.

33 A.M. Cooke, *A History of the Royal College of Physicians of London*, vol. 3, Oxford: Clarendon Press, 1972, p. 980.

34 Saundby, *Medical Ethics*, 2nd edn, p. 111.

35 Ibid., p. 114.

36 B. Brookes, *Abortion in England*, London, New York: Croom Helm, 1988; J. Keown, *Abortion, Doctors and the Law*, Cambridge: Cambridge University Press, 1988.

37 Cooke, *A History of the Royal College of Physicians*, vol. 3, pp. 981–2.
38 *Lancet*, 1914, vol. 2, pp. 1430–1.
39 Sir Charles Matthews, letter of 14 December 1914, CMAC SA/BMA/D170.
40 Correspondence, December 1914, CMAC SA/BMA/D170.
41 BMA CEC minutes, 8 January 1915.
42 Hempson to Cox, 4 April 1915, CMAC SA/BMA/D170.
43 *British Medical Journal*, 1915, vol. 2, *Supplement*, 3 July 1915.
44 It may have been this fundamental moral tension that sustained medical fascination with 'the case of the syphilitic fiancé', since one commentator could state that the situation 'hardly ever' arose in practice. F.G. Crookshank, *Professional Secrecy*, London: Ballière, Tindall & Cox, 1922. On the other hand the problem actually seems rather likely to occur in the context of a state-run VD clinic.
45 Saundby, *Medical Ethics*, 2nd edn, pp. 68–9.
46 Agenda, BMA Council, 28 June 1915; Kitchin, *Law for the Medical Practitioner*, p. 282.
47 BMA CEC minutes, 28 May 1915.
48 *British Medical Journal*, 1916, vol 2, *Supplement*, 5 August 1916, p. 51.
49 McGregor, *Divorce in England*, pp. 1–36. This reform had been envisaged by the 1857 Matrimonial Causes Act, but the judiciary had managed to resist its implementation until 1920.
50 G. Pollock, *Mr. Justice McCardie*, London: John Lane, 1934.
51 *British Medical Journal*, 1920, vol. 1, pp. 102, 132.
52 Ibid.
53 *British Medical Journal*, 1920, vol. 2, *Supplement*, p. 10.
54 BMA Council minutes, 16 February 1921.
55 BMA CEC minutes, 17 June 1921.
56 BMA CEC minutes, 17 June 1921; BMA CEC subcommittee minutes 10 November 1921.
57 Reginald Langdon Langdon-Down (1866–1955) was a member of the CEC for four decades, and chairman 1919–26. He had a secure medical income from the mental home set up by his father in Teddington, and devoted enormous amounts of time and energy to the BMA, specifically in medical ethics, but never held high office. See obituary, *British Medical Journal*, 1955, vol. 1, p. 1433; *Medical Directory*, London: J. & A. Churchill, 1983–1955.
58 *British Medical Journal*, 1921, vol. 2, *Supplement*, 23 July 1921, p. 38.
59 Morrice, "Honours and interests", pp. 105–39.
60 *British Medical Journal*, 1918, vol. 2, *Supplement*, 26 October 1918, pp. 53–60.
61 Memorandum, BMA CEC sub-committee minutes, 10 November 1921.
62 BMA CEC sub-committee minutes, 19 December 1921.
63 Bertrand Dawson, Lord Dawson of Penn (1864–1945) was an eminent Royal Physician and medical politician, best known for his report of 1920 into the future of medical services. Dawson was President of the Royal Society of Medicine, 1928–30, of the BMA in 1932 and of the Royal College of Physicians, 1931–8, as well as serving on the Privy Council after 1929. See 'Dawson, Bertrand Edward, Viscount Dawson of Penn (1864–1945)', *Dictionary of National Biography (1864–1941)*, London: Oxford University Press, 1959, pp. 201–4; *The Times*, 8 and 10 March 1945; *British Medical Journal*, 1945, vol. 1 p. 389; *Lancet*, 1945, vol. 1, p. 353.
64 H. Guy Dain (c.1871–1966) was a very long-serving member of Council (resigning in 1960). He chaired the Representative Body between 1937 and 1943, and then became Chair of Council, and was thus in the forefront of the prolonged negotiations over the NHS. See obituaries in *The Lancet*, 1966, vol. 1, p. 607; *British Medical Journal*, 1966, vol. 1, pp. 616, 683, 868.
65 BMA Council minutes, 18 February 1922.
66 E.R. Fothergill, memorandum, BMA CEC Professional Secrecy Committee minutes, 31 March 1922.

67 Guy Dain, memorandum, BMA CEC Professional Secrecy Committee minutes, 31 March 1922.
68 The phrase is from Fothergill, memorandum.
69 Dain, memorandum.
70 BMA CEC Professional Secrecy Committee minutes, 31 March 1922.
71 Cox to Hempson, 6 April 1922, CMAC SA/BMA/D170.
72 BMA Council minutes, 26 April 1922.
73 B. Dawson, 'Professional secrecy', *Lancet*, 1922, vol. 1, p. 619.
74 *Lancet*, 1922, vol. 1, pp. 641–3.
75 Crookshank, *Professional Secrecy*.
76 F.E. Smith, *Points of View*, vol. 1, London: Hodder & Stoughton, 1922, pp. 36–74.
77 'Smith, Frederick Edwin, first Earl of Birkenhead (1872–1930)', *Dictionary of National Biography 1922–1930*, London: Oxford University Press, 1937, pp. 782–9.
78 BMA CEC minutes, 26 September 1922; and BMA Council minutes, 25 October 1922.
79 BMA CEC minutes, 18 November 1924.
80 BMA CEC sub-committee minutes, 20 December 1925.
81 *The Times*, 23 November 1927, col. 9a; *Hansard*, 5 February 1937, cols 1984–2013.
82 BMA CEC minutes, 16 April 1925, 16 January 1929, 6 May 1936, 22 December 1936.
83 Correspondence included in BMA CEC minutes, 15 January 1935.
84 Robertson, *Medical Conduct and Practice*, pp. 132–6.
85 H. Woods, 'Medical secrecy', in *The Conduct of Medical Practice, by the Editor of 'the Lancet' [S. Sprigge] and Expert Collaborators*, London: The Lancet, 1928, p. 79–81.
86 Such views, and their relationship to ideas of a new state-centred social order, are discussed in Steve Sturdy's chapter below.
87 G.A. Riddell (Lord Riddell), *Medico-Legal Problems*, London: H.K. Lewis, 1929, p. 442.
88 E.K. le Fleming, *An Introduction to General Practice*, London: Edward Arnold, 1936, p. 94.
89 H. Roberts, *Medical Modes and Morals*, London: Michael Joseph, 1937, p. 53.

Part II

Voluntary institutions and the public sphere

4 The Birmingham General Hospital and its public, 1765–79

Adrian Wilson

This chapter seeks to relate Habermas's concept of *bürgerliche Öffentlichkeit*, the 'bourgeois public sphere', to the voluntary hospitals of eighteenth-century England, and particularly to the origins of such hospitals. As a test case I shall use the Birmingham General Hospital, which is of particular interest because it was in effect founded twice: first and unsuccessfully in the 1760s, then again a decade later, when the Hospital was relaunched, this time with success. I shall conclude by asking what light this troubled history sheds upon Habermas's conception.

The premise of this study is a point emphasized in Steve Sturdy's introduction to the present volume: that the concept of the *bürgerliche Öffentlichkeit* needs to be refined so as to take on board the founding of institutions, over and above those (such as coffee houses and newspapers) which by definition belonged to that sphere as sites for what Habermas called 'rational-critical debate'. It is a truism, but one that bears repeating, that institutions did not arise, in this or any other setting, by 'spontaneous generation';[1] rather, their genesis needs to be seen in each case as a concrete initiative arising from a specific socio-political context. Thus the creation of any new institution within the 'public sphere' must reflect the very nature of that 'sphere'; and this point acquires special force in the setting of eighteenth-century Britain. For it was there, according to Habermas, that the *bürgerliche Öffentlichkeit* first came into being;[2] we also find there a remarkable array of new institutions; and many of these initiatives arose precisely within the 'public sphere'. In this context, therefore, the birth of new institutions ought to shed light on the birth, or at least the development, of the 'public sphere' itself.

The dominant component of the eighteenth-century British polity was England; and in this period England was especially rich in such novel institutions – assembly rooms, banks, debating societies, dispensaries, infirmaries, libraries, literary and philosophical societies, music festivals, newspapers, theatres and more. Although London of course played its part in this process,[3] the most striking feature of these developments was that they took place in dozens of provincial towns, from Lancaster to Norwich and from Exeter to Newcastle. Without doubt this 'urban renaissance', as Peter Borsay has dubbed it,[4] was closely bound up with what Habermas depicted as the development of the 'bourgeois public sphere'.[5] Consequently, the 'urban renaissance' presents a trea-sure-trove of initiatives through which to explore the emergence of the *bürgerliche Öffentlichkeit* in England.

With respect to medicine, the key such institutions were the voluntary hospi-tals and dispensaries – and especially the hospitals, for these preceded the dispensaries,[6] outnumbered them until the nineteenth century[7] and had a much more conspicuous public profile. Thus the topic of medicine and the 'public sphere' directs our attention to the foundation of these hospitals; and here we have an *embarras de richesse*, for by 1800 there were twenty-eight provincial infir-maries,[8] along with another dozen or so voluntary hospitals in London.[9] This raises the question as to how to make manageable such a plethora of exam-ples;[10] the strategy that I have chosen is to restrict attention to a single infirmary, treating this not in the mode of institutional biography (for that genre tends to treat the genesis of the given institution as a matter for celebration rather than explanation),[11] but rather within the framework of a local study that attempts to reconstruct the specific conjuncture in which that hospital was founded.[12]

The particular infirmary whose origins I shall be examining is the Birmingham General Hospital, which was first launched in 1765 but did not open until 1779. One reason for this choice is that the history of eighteenth-century Birmingham is unusually accessible, thanks to the existence of John Money's pioneering *Experience and Identity*.[13] The other consideration, mentioned already, is that the Birmingham General Hospital was founded not once but twice, which makes it easier to problematize such acts of foundation as I am seeking to do. It should be remarked that this hospital was not alone in failing initially, for the same had already happened in four other cases,[14] while at least three of those infirmaries that got off the ground at the first attempt had faced local opposition.[15] Thus, although no such individual infirmary can be taken as 'representative', the difficulties which the Birmingham General Hospital experi-enced were by no means unusual. And we shall see that the reasons for those difficulties, though highly specific in their local expression, were anchored in issues that obtained throughout the counties of England.

Before proceeding to this case study, let us recall the salient characteristics of the voluntary hospitals in general.[16] They originated in the eighteenth century: the first of them, the Westminster Infirmary, was established in 1719, and as we have seen, some forty such hospitals had been created by the end of the eighteenth century. The reason that they are called 'voluntary' is that they were financed by voluntary subscriptions (regular annual gifts) and benefactions (one-off donations). They were thus wholly dependent on the goodwill of their subscribers; and indeed in a very real sense they revolved around those subscribers.[17] For the subscribers not only funded the hospitals but also managed them (typically through an elected committee), and were therefore also called governors; it was these subscribers/governors who appointed the medical staff (commonly a salaried apothecary and rotas of honorary surgeons and physi-cians); and the subscribers had a considerable say as to the patients who were admitted, for although prospective patients were vetted by the medical staff, patients normally required a letter of personal recommendation from a subscriber in order to be considered for admission. These arrangements had specific medical consequences, for admissions were typically restricted to curable illnesses, which assured the subscribers that their gifts had produced tangible results. So too the voluntary hospitals embodied a distinctive set of social arrangements: a line of inequality was drawn between the donors and the recipients of charity; above that line, that is, among the subscribers, there were further social gradations, both by size of donation and by traditional rank; and yet, as we shall see, there was theoretical equality with respect to the management of the given hospital itself.

In the long term the voluntary hospitals acquired massive importance, in both their medical and charitable aspects. On the charitable front their contribution, though outweighed in the nineteenth century both by the burgeoning dispensaries and by the new Poor Law hospitals, was nevertheless considerable, not least because large-scale industrial firms came to be enrolled as subscribers. In medical terms, the voluntary hospitals became pre-eminent both as centres of medical innovation and as sites of medical education,[18] and they maintained their elite position until they were finally nationalised in 1948, as part of the creation of the NHS.

In their original, eighteenth-century setting, these hospitals belonged firmly within the 'bourgeois public sphere' as Habermas depicts it; we have seen this on general grounds, and the point is strengthened by several of their specific features. First, one of their defining characteristics was *public accountability*, associated with extensive use of the print medium. Further, when the subscribers met each year to receive the accounts and to elect a new committee, the humble tradesman who subscribed merely half a guinea had an equal voice with a lord, a bishop, a merchant or a captain of industry whose annual subscription could be several times that sum; this *formal equality* among the subscribers corresponds well with the picture that Habermas paints of the notional equality that prevailed within the bourgeois public sphere.[19] Again, the hospitals' ideology was in line with the Habermasian conception: for they studiously invoked the *public interest* as what they furthered.[20] In short, just as the 'English urban renaissance' in general corresponds well to Habermas's account of the eighteenth-century 'bourgeois public sphere', so this is particularly true of the voluntary hospitals.

Thus to recapitulate, the character of the 'bourgeois public sphere' should be illuminated by investigating the origins of any such hospital: in the present case, the Birmingham General Hospital, which stumbled into life between 1765 and 1779. I shall next outline the setting of the Hospital's foundation, which comprised not only Birmingham but also its county, Warwickshire, along with the singular institution that notionally linked the two, namely the Bean Club; I shall survey Birmingham, Warwickshire and the Bean Club from around 1750 to the late 1770s. The third section will examine the founding, abandoning and refounding of the Hospital itself, and the chapter will conclude by relating the findings to Habermas's concept of the *bürgerliche Öffentlichkeit*.

Birmingham, Warwickshire and the Bean Club, *c.*1750–80

In the late eighteenth century Birmingham, though not enfranchised in its own right, was to become effectively the political hub of Warwickshire, displacing the two enfranchised boroughs of Warwick and Coventry. There are several signs that this process was under way as early as the 1740s; of these I shall pick out just two, from the beginning and end of the decade.[21] First, in 1741 Thomas Aris founded the *Birmingham Gazette*, and although he had a rival in the form of *Jopson's Coventry Mercury*, which began publication in the same year, *Aris's* swiftly outstripped *Jopson's*, becoming not only the major newspaper of the Midlands but also the principal voice in Warwickshire affairs. Second, in May 1749 the Bean Club, a convivial association of 'high-flying' – that is, extreme – Tory gentlemen, led by a small but potent group of aristocrats, was refounded in Birmingham.[22] While the Club quickly acquired a national dimension, it was primarily oriented to Warwickshire, as is signalled by its close connection with the county's Parliamentary representation. Not only were both Knights of the Shire – Warwickshire's MPs – drawn from the Club's membership throughout the next several decades; in addition, the selection of those representatives was controlled by the same men who supplied the Club's leadership, that is to say, Barons Craven and Leigh and, from the mid-1750s, the Earl of Denbigh. Conversely the equally aristocratic family of Finch, holders of the Earldom of Aylsford, whose Toryism was of a far more moderate kind, were excluded throughout the 1750s and 1760s both from the Bean Club and from determining the representation of the county.[23] The Bean Club, then, was the key social forum for the clique of high Tories who effectively ran Warwickshire, and the fact that the Club initially based itself at Birmingham was a mark of the town's significance.

The reason for Birmingham's rising importance was of course the remarkable growth of its prosperity and population, which had been under way for several decades and was now gaining increasing momentum.[24] From its seventeenth-century base in iron-smelting, Birmingham capitalism was expanding in many directions: into gun-making, which had been under way since before 1700; to the working of metals in general, notably brass but eventually also silver and gold; into the production of metal buckles, buttons, trays and trinkets ('toys'), and thence into their decoration by such techniques as japanning; into the metal-dependent trade of printing, whence John Baskerville's famous typography; eventually, thanks to Matthew Boulton and James Watt, into the manufacture of steam-engines; and, meanwhile, as a result of the local demand for capital and for credit, into banking, notably through the firm of Taylor and Lloyd, the progenitor of Lloyds bank. Birmingham's numerous and thriving manufacturers large and small were a varied lot, comprising natives and immigrants, Anglicans and Dissenters, well-born men and self-made ones. This diversity can be illustrated schematically, at the upper reaches of prosperity, by the individual figures of Matthew Boulton and William Hutton. Boulton was a Birmingham-born Churchman who inherited his father's business in 1757 and expanded it mightily, building the vast 'manufactory' at Soho, near Handsworth, which became one of the wonders of the kingdom;[25] Hutton was an immigrant Presbyterian who began in 1750 as a book-pedlar with borrowed capital, yet by 1756 had opened his own paper warehouse, exploiting an opportunity arising from the town's expanding printing industry.[26]

The siting of the Bean Club in Birmingham reveals that Warwickshire Tories were showing an interest in the town at mid-century; the same was true of the Whig aristocracy, particularly the recently ennobled Archers of Umberslade;[27] and like any substantial English town at this period, Birmingham offered each party a natural constituency. On the one hand, the town had a high-Tory pedigree, perhaps indeed a Jacobite one,[28] whence its choice for the refounding of the Bean Club. On the other hand, although the great majority of the people of Birmingham as of other places belonged to the Church of England, and a few to its new Methodist offshoot,[29] there were several Dissenting churches:[30] a small congregation of Baptists,[31] a larger Quaker group and three Presbyterian meetings.[32] There was thus the potential for considerable conflict in Birmingham – as would become only too clear, and tragically so, in the anti-Priestley riots of 1791[33] – but at this stage in the town's history, that is to say, in the middle of the eighteenth century, four circumstances conspired to hold such tensions at bay. In the first place, Birmingham's burgeoning economy made for calm, by providing employment for the poor and niches for the enterprising of all persuasions. Second, its manorial government had evolved in such a way as to give both Dissenters and Anglicans a say in the running of the town,[34] and while the Birmingham Tories may not have been happy with this arrangement, they managed to tolerate it. Third, although Thomas Aris was a Tory and belonged to the Bean Club, his *Birmingham Gazette* cultivated a discreet rhetoric that avoided offending any section of his readership. Last but not least, Birmingham's potential electoral muscle had never been exercised, for it so happened that there had been no contest for Warwickshire's two Knights of the Shire since 1705. The Tory aristocrats and gentlemen of the county, who controlled its representation, had carefully avoided any by-electoral contest when sitting members died, and the handful of Whigs amongst the Warwickshire aristocracy had calculated that it would be fruitless to disturb what was called 'the peace of the county' by provoking such a contest at a general election. The absence of county electoral contests, combined with the fact that Birmingham was not enfranchised, meant that political differences never came into focus there in the way that they did, notoriously, in Coventry.

Although Birmingham prospered throughout the 1750s, the same cannot be said for relations between the town's Tories and the Bean Club, nor indeed for the Club itself.[35] Even in the early 1750s, the Club's link with Birmingham was weakening; by 1755 there were 387 members, yet only forty-two of these were from Birmingham; and, in that year, there emerged signs of tension between the Birmingham members and the country gentlemen. Just why this gap opened up between the Tories of Birmingham and of Warwickshire is not clear, but what can be said is that this presaged a wider decline in the Club's vitality. As early as 1753, the meetings were cut back from weekly to monthly; from 1756 onwards, fewer than half of these meetings were actually held, and the recruitment of new members plummeted; at the end of 1759 the monthly meetings were abandoned, leaving the annual anniversary meeting and dinner as the only occasions in the Club's calendar.

The decline of the Bean Club's momentum in the latter half of the 1750s reflected the fact that the Tory interest throughout the kingdom was disintegrating, under the impact of national political events: the breaking-up of the 'Old Corps' of Whigs; the emergence of Pitt; the impact of the fall of Minorca in 1756; and last but not least, the reform of the militia, which offered the Tory gentry opportunities for local office that had no precedent since the accession of George I in 1714.[36] Ironically, the collapse of proscription threw the Tories into disarray, by depriving them of their oppositional *raison d'être*. Thereupon, individual Tories went in a remarkable variety of different political directions,[37] and this process continued, and acquired new twists, after the accession of George III in 1760. It is thus intelligible that the Bean Club continued to be troubled into the 1760s. Its link with Birmingham remained feeble: symptomatic of this was the fact that after Thomas Aris died in July 1761, leaving the *Birmingham Gazette* to his son Samuel, no attempt was made to elect Samuel Aris as a member, even though he had inherited not only the newspaper but also his father's Anglicanism, his Toryism and his masterly editorial discretion. The Bean Club's failure to recruit so important a Birmingham Tory as the new editor of *Aris's Birmingham Gazette* suggests that its leaders had lost their political touch. And so they had, for throughout the 1760s the Club stumbled through a series of little catastrophes, repeatedly seeking to revive itself and yet falling back again, sometimes within a matter of months.

In sharp contrast with the Bean Club, Birmingham in the 1760s not only continued to expand rapidly but also embarked on a new self-assertiveness. The first sign of this was the publication in 1763 of James Sketchley's *Birmingham Directory*, one of the first provincial directories of the kingdom;[38] this was followed in 1765 by the project for the Birmingham General Hospital, to be considered in the next section; and as this was under way there came the successful launching of the Birmingham Canal Navigation, which was opened in 1768 to much rejoicing, and understandably so, for it almost halved the price of coal in the town.[39] But the climax of these developments came in March 1769, when Birmingham at long last came to play a role in Warwickshire politics. For a by-election held in that month returned Thomas Skipwith, a disaffected member of the Bean Club, as one of the two Knights of the Shire, and Skipwith owed his selection to the freeholders, to whom he had appealed directly by advertising his candidacy in the newspapers, in particular *Aris's Birmingham Gazette*.[40] This tactic, which was wholly novel in Warwickshire, had at a stroke unleashed the hitherto-dormant power of the Birmingham freeholders; Skipwith's selection as Member of Parliament, which was ritually completed at a county meeting held at Warwick on 29 March, was a triumph as much for the freeholders as it was for Skipwith himself.

Even though Skipwith himself was a gentleman and a Bean Club member, the effect of his campaign was to wrest the representation of Warwickshire from aristocratic and gentry control for the first time in living memory. This posed an unprecedented political threat to the high-Tory interest in the county, which had hitherto controlled the selection of the Knights of the Shire. And in response to that threat the Bean Club shook off its torpor and reinvented itself, beginning at the first available opportunity, that is, at the anniversary meeting of August 1769. The Club now adopted a new organizational form, by appointing two annual 'stewards', and, significantly, one of the two stewards chosen was none other than Thomas Skipwith, suggesting that a concerted effort was being made to heal wounds and close ranks in the wake of the by-election.[41] Initially this was no easy matter, because the next few months saw much pressure from Birmingham for a county petition in support of John Wilkes, and equally determined resistance from the county aristocracy, a passage of events which widened the rift between town and county.[42] But in the following year, when the Wilkes issue was dying down in the region, the attempt to re-establish the Club began to bear fruit, for ten new members were elected – and significantly, six of them hailed from Birmingham, including Samuel Aris himself, editor of the *Gazette*.[43] This was the beginning of a sustained and successful recruitment effort, which was targeted in particular to Birmingham. Between 1770 and 1773 the Club acquired fifty-one new members, that is to say, more than had been elected in the whole of the 1760s; over two-thirds of these (thirty-six of them) came from Birmingham, and these new Birmingham members included four merchants, two brass-makers, two mercers, two buckle-makers, two button-makers and a 'toyman', showing that there was now a policy of bringing Birmingham manufacturers into the Club.

These moves succeeded, for the quarterly meetings were revived in 1771, and subsequently, as John Money has shown, the Bean Club played a major role in the affairs of Birmingham and managed to create a more or less stable link between the town and the local landed interest,[44] principally of Warwickshire. Yet the Bean Club's links with both town and county were highly selective, for the Club continued to be deeply partisan in both politics and religion. Even though some of its individual members (such as Thomas Skipwith) had now forged new, Whig allegiances,[45] the Club as a whole remained specifically Tory: for strikingly, the Warwickshire Whig aristocratic families of Greville, Conway and Archer did not contribute a single member. Correspondingly, the Club continued to be exclusively Anglican; not a single Dissenter was ever elected to its ranks. And what is equally significant, the Club's Birmingham recruitment was still narrower than this, for there were some remarkable absentees even among Birmingham Churchmen: namely Matthew Boulton and the gun-maker Samuel Garbett, the town's two most eminent entrepreneurs. On the face of it, both Boulton and Garbett were supremely qualified for membership of the Bean Club, not just as leading capitalists but also in political terms: for Boulton was thoroughly conservative in outlook,[46] and his business partner John Fothergill had joined the Club in 1761, while Garbett had a longstanding link with Lord Denbigh. Yet neither Boulton nor Garbett was ever admitted – an omission that seriously weakened the Club's pretensions to leadership in Birmingham. The reason for their exclusion can readily be surmised: despite their Anglicanism and their conservative views, Boulton and Garbett were unfit, for each of them was also closely associated with Dissenters.[47]

It can be seen that Birmingham during the 1760s and 1770s brought into play a complex array of political interests, involving differences of locality, class, party, religion and family. Such were the circumstances of the founding of the Birmingham General Hospital, which took place in two stages: from 1765 to 1768, and from 1776 to 1779.[48]

The making of the Birmingham General Hospital

When a Birmingham hospital was proposed in the autumn of 1765, the circumstances were apparently favourable in three ways. First, the town was going from strength to strength as we have seen. Second, charitable help to the poor was particularly needed at this time, since local grain prices had been rising almost continuously for over a year and a half.[49] Third, in the summer of this year the Bean Club had experienced one of its little revivals of the 1760s;[50] and this was propitious for the intended Hospital because Dr John Ash, the leading spirit behind the Hospital proposal, was also a longstanding and well-respected member of the Club, which gave the Hospital's activists good reasons to hope for landed support. Sure enough, the Hospital was initially backed by a broad coalition of local interests, with the effect that funds came in quickly. In short, the Hospital had every prospect of success. Yet as we are about to see, the initiative failed disastrously, so much so that it took ten years to revive it.

It seems to have been the launch of a county infirmary in Staffordshire in 1765 that stirred some of Birmingham's leaders to initiate the hospital proposal. On 30 September 1765, through a letter published in *Aris's*, the town's Overseers of the Poor mooted the idea of a Birmingham hospital, in emulation of their Staffordshire neighbours.[51] No doubt part of their motive was to find a way of catering for the medical needs of Birmingham's numerous immigrant poor, many of whom would have been entitled to relief only in their home parishes, not in Birmingham itself.[52] Hence the specific proposal that was put forward in *Aris's* five weeks later, on 4 November 1765:

> A General Hospital for the relief of the sick and lame, situated near the town of Birmingham, is presumed would be greatly beneficial to the populous country about it, as well as [to] that place.[53]

The proposed Hospital was called 'General' to demonstrate that its benefits would be available to all, not just to natives of Birmingham or for that matter of Warwickshire, and the reference to 'the populous country about it' alluded to the fact that Birmingham's hinterland extended to Staffordshire, Worcestershire and to some extent Shropshire. The advertisement went on to call a public meeting on 21 November 'of the nobility and gentry of the neighbouring country, and of the principal inhabitants of this town', in order to 'consider of proper steps to render effectual so useful an undertaking'.

To all appearances this initial meeting was auspicious. It was attended – as the next issue of *Aris's* reported – by 'a considerable number of gentlemen both of the country and the town';[54] a subscription to fund the proposed Hospital was opened on the spot; donations totalling over £1,100 were 'sent in' on the day from some sixty-eight wealthy benefactors;[55] and in addition, over £200 per annum was pledged in subscriptions. Equally encouraging, though of course not mentioned in *Aris's*, was the fact that this support came not just from both 'country' and 'town' but also from a broad politico-religious spectrum within the Birmingham elite. Donations from the town were headed by the firm of Boulton and Fothergill (50 guineas), and came also, typically in sums of 10 or 20 guineas, from longstanding members of the Bean Club;[56] from moderate Churchmen such as Samuel Garbett and the attorney Joseph Carles; from the Quakers Samuel Galton and Sampson Lloyd; and from such Presbyterians or Unitarians as John Taylor (Lloyd's partner in the then-incipient bank) and William Russell. As for the 'country', this was represented by the Earls of Aylesford and Dartmouth, along with both of their wives; by baronets such as Sir Roger Newdigate (30 guineas);[57] by gentlemen such as Richard Geast;[58] and last but not least, by the two Knights of the Shire for Warwickshire – William Bromley and Sir Charles Mordaunt – who each gave 30 guineas, this however after most of the other benefactions (sixty-four of the sixty-eight) had been received.

The participation of both Warwickshire MPs draws attention to a curious and significant feature of the Hospital's landed support: despite the care of its activists to represent it as a regional initiative, not a county-specific one, almost all of its 'country' benefactors hailed from Warwickshire. Indeed the only significant landed contribution from outside the county came from the Earl and Countess of Dartmouth (50 guineas between them),[59] who were seated in Staffordshire, and there were several contingent reasons for Dartmouth's particular involvement.[60] Why was it that, apart from Dartmouth and one or two gentlemen, the Hospital failed to draw in landed backing from outside Warwickshire? Part of the reason was that Worcestershire and Shropshire already had county infirmaries, both established in the late 1740s, and Staffordshire was now following suit as we have seen, so that the available support in these counties was already committed elsewhere. Yet a deeper consideration was probably at work: namely that gentlemen and aristocrats throughout the region were oriented primarily towards their own counties. This localism may have involved an element of etiquette, in which case Dartmouth was breaching that etiquette. But it also made political sense: for although Birmingham had a considerable immigrant population, very few of these immigrants would have had freeholds in Worcestershire, Staffordshire or Shropshire, with the effect that there were not many votes to be gained in Birmingham for elections in any of those counties. Conversely, county loyalties lay behind the fact that the two Warwickshire MPs added their contributions once the Hospital had already amassed substantial support: for it was part of the recognized duty of Knights of the Shire to lend their backing impartially to any initiative arising within their respective counties, provided that the given project was not actively opposed there by some contending interest.

Thus the Birmingham General Hospital was immediately propelled towards becoming – contrary to its name and to the original intention – the *de facto* county infirmary of Warwickshire. In order for this to succeed, it would be necessary to maintain the double coalition that was manifested in the initial group of benefactors: between the Birmingham elite and the Warwickshire gentry, and between Churchmen and Dissenters within the town.

In the next few weeks and months the project seemingly continued to thrive. By 9 December the benefactions had reached over £1,900, and the promised subscriptions had come to £600 a year.[61] Further, by 16 December about a hundred small tradesmen from Birmingham had been enrolled as subscribers, mostly pledging an annual guinea or two apiece,[62] and this expansion of the Hospital's base of support was no doubt helped by the fact that its proceedings were being reported in *Aris's*. Thus encouraged, the subscribers met on Christmas Eve, agreed to build a hospital, and appointed a thirty-one-member committee to superintend this. And the composition of this committee reflected the broad base of the Hospital's support: its members came equally from the landed classes and from Birmingham (sixteen and fifteen men respectively), while those from Birmingham comprised nine Churchmen and six Dissenters.[63] Less than three months later (March 1766) the committee purchased a seven-acre site just north of the town, a plan was promptly commissioned, and work started on the building in the summer of 1766.[64]

Yet it swiftly turned out that the funds were insufficient, partly because the builders over-ran their original estimate. As a result the building had to be boarded up in November 1766, just when the structure had almost been completed.[65] Thereafter the project limped ahead for another year and a half,[66] beset by a squeeze between rising costs and insufficient income, which was met by a series of temporary expedients:[67] notably the bankers, Taylor and Lloyd – who were also amongst the Hospital's trustees, as we have seen – supplied a loan against future subscriptions. Eventually, in May 1768, the hospital was said to be ready 'for the immediate reception of patients';[68] but in fact this was whistling in the wind, for no such 'reception of patients' took place. The enterprise had now run into serious difficulties, for over £2,000 was owing to the bank, and the promised subscriptions were not coming in. Some help came in September from a three-day music festival, which raised almost £800, but this still left the Hospital massively indebted. And what was equally significant, the meeting of trustees scheduled for the first day of the festival (7 September) went unrecorded in the minute-book.[69] Perhaps the meeting was simply inquorate; more probably, the trustees were now unable to agree among themselves as to how to proceed; but whatever the reason, this signalled a collapse in morale, for at this point, that is, in September 1768, the operation was effectively suspended,[70] and the building was closed again, this time with no prospect of completing it. An initiative that had begun so brightly had become an ignominious failure: the hospital now existed solely as a debt that lay on the books, accumulating interest, and a boarded-up building that stood as a mute reproach to all concerned.

What had gone wrong? The hospital's governors probably made a tactical mistake in building a full-scale infirmary at the outset, rather than starting in small premises and then gradually expanding,[71] and the upward drift of the costs suggests that they were unlucky, or perhaps unwise, in their choice of builders. Above all, however, what let them down was that the hoped-for backing from the Warwickshire landed interest did not materialize, for the initial lead of a dozen or so gentlemen did not produce any wider financial support from the landed interest. Furthermore, the sixteen landed gentlemen on the building committee seem to have played no active part in its proceedings: from an early stage the Birmingham members were left to manage the Hospital on their own, and, indeed, as we shall shortly see, the gentlemen may even have withdrawn from the project altogether within as little as three months.

The first sign of the problem was implicit in the list of initial supporters, specifically at aristocratic level. For that list included only two lords, the Earls of Aylesford and Dartmouth – both probably recruited by Matthew Boulton[72] – and since Lord Dartmouth was seated in Staffordshire, Aylesford was the sole Warwickshire noble who backed the Hospital. Furthermore, Aylesford was in Warwickshire terms a political eccentric, for his moderate Toryism set him apart from the high-Tory peers who had long controlled the representation of the county (Craven, Leigh and Denbigh), yet cannot have endeared him to the local Whig lords (the Earls of Warwick and Hertford, and their junior partner Baron Archer). This, then, was not only a very narrow aristocratic base but was also an unpromising nucleus for drawing in further support – either from the aristocracy itself, both Whig and Tory, or from the gentry, who of course were overwhelmingly Tory. And the absence of support from Craven, Leigh and Denbigh reveals that Dr John Ash had been unable to make effective use of his Bean Club connections to draw in the landed interest.

Sure enough, the weakness of landed backing became apparent as early as March 1766 – that is, when the site for the Hospital was acquired – and this in two ways. For one thing, the set of twelve trustees who were now appointed to hold the land on the Hospital's behalf consisted wholly of Birmingham men: not a single gentleman lent his name, even in a token capacity. Hence the suspicion that by this time the sixteen gentlemen on the committee had withdrawn. For another, when announcing the purchase of the site the committee entered a plea that *'the nobility and gentry who are inclined to promote this universal charity, and have not yet signified their intentions, are earnestly requested to send their benefactions'*.[73] The wording of this appeal makes it clear that the landed interest was failing to support the Hospital – this within three months of constituting the committee, and well before the problem with the building costs emerged. The same pattern recurred after that problem had been announced: for in the following year, 1767, an appeal for a second tranche of benefactions brought in £180 or so from some sixteen Birmingham men, but not a single contribution from the aristocracy or the gentry.[74] And further proof of the Hospital's inability to recruit landed support came in May 1768 – that is, when the Hospital was allegedly ready 'for the immediate reception of patients', though in fact it was in desperate straits. At this time the committee sent two separate and carefully worded personal appeals to seven aristocrats and two gentlemen.[75] The fact that the governors could only come up with the names of two gentlemen to approach shows that Ash could not deliver so much as the hope of support from members of the Bean Club, while the list of seven peers was highly deficient, omitting as it did the most eminent Warwickshire lords of both political sides (the Tory Baron Craven, the Whig Earl of Hertford). And equally telling was the response, or rather the lack of it: for both letters fell on deaf ears.[76]

Now the Hospital's failure was not solely due to the collapse of landed support, for by this time its Birmingham backing had also subsided alarmingly. This is particularly revealed by the contrasting fortunes of the Birmingham Canal Navigation – a 'cut' from Birmingham to Wolverhampton, aimed principally at bringing in cheap coal from the Staffordshire collieries. The Navigation was set up in January 1767, that is, just after the Hospital was first boarded up (November 1766); within the ensuing seven months (January to August 1767), it drew in capital of £50,000,[77] most of it from inhabitants of Birmingham, including the very men who were promoting and running the Hospital project. At this time the Hospital could have cleared its debts with a modest £2,000 or so; yet as has been mentioned already, an appeal made in June brought in a mere sixteen benefactions, which between them amounted to a paltry £180. And since twelve of these donors belonged to the Hospital committee, while another had been among those who contributed in 1765,[78] it can be seen that this appeal brought only three more Birmingham men[79] to support the Hospital – whereas the Canal had over a hundred shareholders. In part, the dramatic divergence between the fates of the two initiatives reflected the very different attractions of profit on the one hand and charity on the other, but it is unlikely that this was the sole reason at work, since the Canal's success was by no means guaranteed in advance. In all probability, the decline in support for the Hospital in Birmingham was itself a result of the failure to secure any significant backing from the landed interest. For the project had from the outset sought to draw in the aristocracy and gentry; the failure to achieve this, which by this time (1767) was only too apparent, must have eaten into the morale of the Birmingham activists themselves, whence the fact that only about half of them contributed to their own appeal in June; the thinness of landed patronage implicitly stigmatized the project in the eyes of Birmingham at large, which was why hardly anyone else contributed at this time.

The final attempt to garner support for the Hospital in the 1760s, namely the music festival of 7–9 September 1768, though seemingly a success, actually set the seal on the Hospital's failure to draw in landed backing. An advertisement in *Aris's* reported that the festival attracted a 'concourse of nobility and gentry from this and the neighbouring counties', which 'gave the whole a most splendid appearance, and at the same time showed their desire to concur with the inhabitants of this place in support of a charity so beneficial and extensive'.[80] Yet there is every reason to suspect that this account greatly exaggerated the degree of 'support' from the 'nobility and gentry'. For one thing, the seven committee members who had organized the festival were all Birmingham men: that is, not a single gentleman had been involved, just as none of them had been named as land trustees two years before. For another, as we have already seen, the festival raised less than £800, which fell far short of the Hospital's debt. Further, the occasion cannot have induced any of the local 'nobility and gentry' to drum up any further support from their friends, since the Hospital's proceedings thereupon closed. And strikingly, the only 'nobility' who were actually *named* as being present were the same two Countesses who had backed the Hospital in the first place, namely Dartmouth and Aylesford.[81] The fact that the Hospital's aristocratic patronage was still limited to the families of Dartmouth and Aylesford – both of them, in different ways, outsiders in Warwickshire affairs – confirmed how narrow was its 'support' from the 'nobility', and doubtless from the gentry as well.

To sum up, the reason that the Birmingham General Hospital failed in 1765–8 was that its hoped-for coalition between town and country interests was weak from the outset and soon collapsed. As for its other, complementary dimension of coalition – that is to say, *within* the town, between Birmingham Churchmen and Dissenters – this seems to have held together throughout these troubled three years, albeit with one qualification: the Dissenters on the committee were more active, or perhaps more persistent, in their support for the Hospital than were the Churchmen.[82] It seems, therefore, that the Churchmen among the Hospital's Birmingham activists were especially discouraged by the withdrawal of the landed gentry – which is intelligible, since the gentry were of course their co-religionists.[83] By the time the festival took place, it will be recalled, the Hospital's land trustees were unable to decide how to proceed; and it is possible (though this is speculation) that they were divided on confessional lines.[84]

Now the Hospital's failure to recruit landed support mirrored a difficulty that had long been experienced by the Bean Club. As we saw earlier, the Club's links with Birmingham had faded within a few years of its refoundation in 1749 and remained feeble throughout the 1760s; conversely, the Birmingham initiative for the Hospital now proved unable to forge links with the landed gentlemen who belonged to the Club. But if these were two sides of the same problem, that problem acquired an additional twist in the case of the Hospital, thanks to the prominence of Dissenters among its leaders; and against this background, it is instructive to recall the subsequent development of the Bean Club and to compare this with what happened to the Hospital project. We have seen that in the wake of the 1769 by-election, the Bean Club was revived on a new basis, involving the election of annual stewards; the intended recouping of Thomas Skipwith, the new Knight of the Shire; the successful revival of quarterly meetings in 1771; and the recruitment of Birmingham members on an unprecedented scale.[85] Here at last was an institutional link between Birmingham and the landed interest of Warwickshire, which in theory could have made it possible to revive the Hospital project. But no such revival took place at this time, and the reason is not far to seek: the Bean Club had always been specifically Anglican and Tory, and it remained within these limits, whereas the Hospital rested on an alliance between Churchmen and Dissenters.[86]

It is thus perhaps significant that the first sign of renewed interest in the Hospital was the work of a Dissenter. In 1774 – that is, some six years after the Hospital's closure in 1768 – a young and pious Birmingham Baptist named Mark Wilkes (apparently no relation of his famous namesake) attempted to bring the project back to public attention by publishing an imaginary *Dialogue between the Hospital and the New Play House*.[87] It has been claimed that this piece sold 'an immense number of copies', and that it effectively shamed 'the public' into reviving the Hospital;[88] yet this is doubtful, for it was another two years before any attempt was made to reactivate the Hospital. Nevertheless, such an attempt was indeed made – whether prompted by Wilkes's dialogue or by some other stimulus is unclear – in September 1776, and this was the beginning of a process of revival that eventually attained success. A reconstituted committee solicited funds, organized another music festival, negotiated over the Hospital's debts and completed and furnished the building. Yet even now this was a protracted struggle, which took three years to reach completion, for it was not until September 1779 that the Hospital was finally opened for the admission of patients. [89]

There is not space here to trace these developments, but what we must notice is the social composition of the reconstituted Hospital committee. This time, the initial leadership came solely from Birmingham, for *every one of the sixteen landed or titled men who had served on the ill-fated committee of 1765 had now dropped out*, and no others were found to replace them. In contrast, over half of the Birmingham men who had been involved in 1765 (eleven out of twenty-one) were still active in 1776–9,[90] and twenty-three new activists had now been recruited, *all of them from Birmingham*. Thus, although the size of the core group was much as it had been before – thirty-four men, as compared with thirty-one in 1765 – its composition was radically different. Further, the strong contribution of Dissenters was maintained and indeed increased: four Dissenters from the 1765 committee were still involved,[91] while of the new activists, at least nine and probably ten were Dissenters.[92] Thus in all, Dissenters now comprised some thirteen or fourteen of the Hospital's thirty-four activists. In confessional terms, this was precisely in keeping with the retreat of the landed gentry, all of whom of course belonged to the Established Church. It is no surprise to find, therefore, that the Hospital once again had only limited success in attracting landed backing: its successful revival rested almost exclusively on benefactions and subscriptions from Birmingham itself. In effect Birmingham's leaders had learnt the lesson of self-reliance.

Nevertheless the Hospital did now manage at long last to acquire a Warwickshire aristocratic patron. And the man they found to back them was one whose politics were precisely in line with the strong presence of Dissenters on the new committee: namely the sixth Baron Craven, who was now of Whig allegiance. Curiously enough, Craven had begun his political life as a Tory, [93] as was to be expected in view of his family's tradition; but after succeeding to the barony in 1769, he had gradually migrated in a Whig direction,[94] a move that achieved its consummation in 1780, when he became the co-patron (along with Lord Archer) of the Dissenting corporation of Coventry.[95] Thus when Craven became the first President of the Birmingham General Hospital in 1779, this was precisely in line with the position that he had reached by the late 1770s; the fit between Craven's politics and the Hospital's confessional basis illustrates the fact that party and religion remained intertwined.[96]

Conclusion

What lessons concerning Habermas's concept of *bürgerliche Öffentlichkeit* – the 'bourgeois public sphere' or 'bourgeois publicness' – might emerge from this case-study? I want to draw out three points.

First, the question arises as to the *limits* of 'bourgeois publicness' in any given historical setting. What raises this issue is the fact that the Birmingham General Hospital's institutional closure in 1768 was accompanied by another kind of closure: the Hospital immediately *disappeared from the public arena*, and it remained so to speak out of sight for several years – and this despite the physical presence of the boarded-up building. This conspiracy of silence was remarkably widespread, taking in at least three distinct sets of interests: the country gentlemen who stopped subscribing; the Hospital's creditors; and, last but not least, Samuel Aris, the editor of the *Gazette*, who seems to have dropped all mention of the Hospital as soon as the problems began to emerge. While Habermas's stress on 'publicness' helps to bring this issue into prominence, this episode of silence conversely reveals that 'publicness' was not automatic but contingent in any given setting.

Second, the case of Birmingham in the 1760s and 1770s suggests that the public sphere was an arena not just of 'rational-critical debate' – the aspect that Habermas stressed – but also of difference and of contest. Habermas tended to minimize this agonistic character of the public sphere, because he sought to portray that 'sphere' as a single shared interest, over against the state; but while this may indeed have been the case over the long term and in an emergent manner, it is probably at odds with what happened in any specific setting. Rather, the 'bourgeois public sphere' – certainly in eighteenth-century Britain, and arguably in the French and German settings as well – was differentiated, and this in complex ways: not just by gender and class (as Habermas recognized, up to a point),[97] but also as between town and country, and by confessional differences. As John Money has shown, both the Bean Club and the General Hospital came to play prominent roles in Birmingham's public life,[98] yet these rested on very different constituencies: the one was constituted by an alliance between urban and landed elites, united by the bond of religion; the other rested on an alliance between Churchmen and Dissenters, united by their shared interest in furthering the emerging civic interest of Birmingham itself; and although a few men (notably Ash and, after 1779, Craven) belonged to both groups, the two remained largely distinct. Furthermore it may be suspected that the 'bourgeois public sphere' in general was actually *constituted* by the clash of different interests, in which case an adequate understanding of that 'sphere' will require us to recapture the dynamics of struggle within it.[99]

Third, the persistent importance of confessional divisions in Birmingham during the 1760s and 1770s raises the question as to the role of religion in Habermas's story, and here we encounter a curious paradox. On the one hand, religion was depicted as part and parcel of *repräsentative Öffentlichkeit*[100] – the earlier form of 'publicness' that, according to Habermas's analysis, preceded the development of *bürgerliche Öffentlichkeit* – and indeed as emblematic of it;[101] and what was more, the Reformation was assigned the leading role in the transition from *repräsentative Öffentlichkeit* to *bürgerliche Öffentlichkeit*.[102] On the other hand, when Habermas came to describe the subsequent development of the *bürgerliche Öffentlichkeit* itself, religious themes were systematically written out of his account: for instance when considering Britain, Habermas referred to the Exclusion Crisis of 1679 only in order to dismiss from consideration the very issue that had prompted that crisis, namely the Catholicism of James, Duke of York.[103] I shall not attempt to explain the contradiction between these two utterly different roles that Habermas assigned to religion – first as the prime mover in the genesis of *bürgerliche Öffentlichkeit* (though a highly abstract and stylized prime mover),[104] then as a complete irrelevance in the development of that form of *Öffentlichkeit*. Nor is this the place to suggest how Habermas's concept of the *bürgerliche Öffentlichkeit* might be modulated so as to accommodate religion, though I suspect that this could be done. What is clear is that some such modulation of the concept is required, both because the coherence of Habermas's entire conception is at stake and because religion was a vital aspect of eighteenth-century Britain, the very polity that Habermas took as his 'model case'.

The burden of my argument has been that Habermas's conception of the *bürgerliche Öffentlichkeit* stands in need of enlargement and enrichment: not only to embrace the founding of new institutions (this, it will be recalled, was my initial premise), but also to take account of differences and contests within the *bürgerliche Öffentlichkeit*, and especially to deal with religious issues. The theme of religion in particular will surely require considerable modification of Habermas's picture. But the converse may also apply: that is, a *rapprochement* between religion and the concept of the *bürgerliche Öffentlichkeit* may perhaps shed new light upon early-modern religion itself. And, in that case, historians of the early-modern period may still have much to learn from Habermas's *Strukturwandel der Öffentlichkeit*, forty years after that work was published.

Acknowledgements

For help with this chapter I wish to thank Jon Hodge, Sarah Kattau, Josephine Lloyd, John Money, Mike Woodhouse, David Wykes and the staffs of the Birmingham Central Reference Library (BCRL), the Warwickshire County Record Office (WCRO) and the Brotherton Library, University of Leeds. Special thanks go to Steve Sturdy both for his helpful comments and for his editorial patience.

Notes

1 Cf. A. Wilson, 'The politics of medical improvement in early Hanoverian London', in A. Cunningham and R.K. French (eds), *The Medical Enlightenment of the Eighteenth Century*, Cambridge: Cambridge University Press, 1990, pp. 4–39, at p. 7.

2 J. Habermas, *The Structural Transformation of the Public Sphere: An Inquiry into a Category of Bourgeois Society* (German original 1962), trans. T. Burger with the assistance of F. Lawrence, Cambridge: Polity Press, 1989, p. 57.

3 See for instance M.D. George, *London Life in the Eighteenth Century* (orig. pub. 1925), Harmondsworth: Penguin, 1966, and D. Andrew, *Philanthropy and Police: London Charity in the Eighteenth Century*, Princeton: Princeton University Press, 1989.

4 P. Borsay, *The English Urban Renaissance: Culture and Society in the Provincial Town 1660–1800*, Oxford: Clarendon Press, 1989.

5 Cf. Habermas, *Structural Transformation*, pp. 20–22, 27, 31–2, 38–9, 58–62.

6 Voluntary hospitals began in 1719 in London, and in 1737 in the provinces; dispensaries began in the 1770s.

7 In the provinces only some nine or ten dispensaries were founded before 1800, as against twenty-eight hospitals. On dispensaries see I. Loudon, 'The origins and growth of the dispensary movement in England', *Bulletin of the History of Medicine*, 1981, vol. 55, pp. 322–42, and R. Kilpatrick, '"Living in the light": dispensaries, philanthropy and medical reform in late eighteenth-century London', in Cunningham and French (eds), *Medical Enlightenment*, pp. 254–80.

8 These are listed in J. Woodward, *To Do the Sick no Harm: A Study of the British Voluntary Hospital System to 1875*, London, Routledge, 1974.

9 For overviews see Andrew, *Philanthropy and Police*, and S. Lawrence, *Charitable Knowledge: Hospital Pupils and Practitioners in Eighteenth-Century London*, Cambridge: Cambridge University Press, 1996.

10 The usual approach is to construct a composite picture by using selected examples from different localities; see R. Porter, 'The gift relation: philanthropy and provincial hospitals in eighteenth-century England', in L. Granshaw and R. Porter (eds), *The Hospital in History*, London: Routledge, 1989, pp. 149–78; K. Wilson, 'Urban culture and political activism in Hanoverian England: the example of voluntary hospitals', in E. Hellmuth (ed.), *The Transformation of Political Culture: England and Germany in the Late Eighteenth Century*, Oxford: Oxford University Press, 1990, pp. 165–84; P. Langford, *Public Life and the Propertied Englishman 1689–1798*, Oxford: Clarendon Press, 1991, pp. 493–500. For an attempt at a comprehensive survey, which yielded only crude and broad-brush results, see A. Wilson, 'Conflict, consensus and charity: politics and the provincial voluntary hospitals in the eighteenth century', *The English Historical Review*, 1996, vol. 111, pp. 599–619.

11 An example of such a study is W. Brockbank, *Portrait of a Hospital 1752–1948*, London: Heinemann, 1952.

12 H. Marland, *Medicine and Society in Wakefield and Huddersfield 1780–1870*, Cambridge: Cambridge University Press, 1987; M.E. Fissell, *Patients, Power and the Poor in Eighteenth-Century Bristol*, Cambridge: Cambridge University Press, 1991; J. Lane, *Worcester Infirmary in the Eighteenth Century*, Worcester Historical Society Occasional Publications No. 6, Worcester, 1992; A. Borsay, *Medicine and Charity in Georgian Bath: A Social History of the General Infirmary, c.1739–1830*, Aldershot: Ashgate, 1999.

13 J. Money, *Experience and Identity: Birmingham and the West Midlands, 1760–1800*, Manchester: Manchester University Press, 1977.

14 The Bath General Hospital got going in 1742 but only after four previous initiatives that went back to 1711; the county hospitals of Lincolnshire, Norfolk and Berkshire all failed in the early 1740s and were not revived until a generation or more later (Borsay, 'Cash and conscience', p. 208; Wilson, 'Conflict, consensus and charity', pp. 601–2).

15 This is attested at Winchester, Exeter and Leicester. See respectively A. Clarke, *A Sermon Preached in the Cathedral Church of Winchester, before the Governors of the County-Hospital...at the Opening of the Said Hospital*, London, 1737, pp. 20–2, and the attached 'A Collection of Papers', pp. 8–11; J. Caldwell, 'Notes on the history of Dean Clarke's Hospital 1741–1948', *Reports and Transactions of the Devonshire Association for the Advancement of Science, Literature and Art*, 1972, vol. 104, pp. 175–92, at pp. 176–7; and Porter, 'The gift relation', p. 154, quoted in Wilson, 'Conflict, consensus and charity', p. 604.

16 For more detailed accounts see Porter, 'The gift relation'; Borsay, 'Cash and conscience'; and Wilson, 'Conflict, consensus and charity'.

17 See the diagram in Wilson, 'The politics of medical improvement', p. 12.

18 Though in London, the three endowed hospitals of St Bartholomew's, St Thomas's and Guy's were even more important: see Lawrence, *Charitable Knowledge*.

19 Habermas, *Structural Transformation*, p. 36.

20 So too Habermas's account fits with the geographical and cultural associations of the voluntary hospitals: not only were they always located in towns, but more particularly they were commonly associated with forms of polite culture that were moving away from court patronage and towards a market orientation. Emblematic of this was the benefit performance of Handel's Messiah in 1749 for the London Foundling Hospital: see R.K. McClure, *Coram's Children: The London Foundling Hospital in the Eighteenth Century*, New Haven: Yale University Press, 1981.

21 For another such sign see note 27 below.

22 The original records of the Bean Club have not been found; I have used the transcripts in W.K.R. Bedford, *Notes from the Minute Book of the Bean Club, 1754–1836*, 1889, BCRL 131399, and J.B. Stone, 'Annals of the Bean Club, Birmingham', MS of *c.*1900, BCRL 345313.

23 Here my account differs from the standard view, which is that the Warwickshire representation in the 1750s and 1760s was managed by Baron Craven and the Earls of Warwick, Aylesford and Hertford: L. Namier and J. Brooke, *The House of Commons 1754–1790*, 2 vols, London: HMSO, 1964, vol. 1, p. 399, and Money, *Experience and Identity*, p. 171. The issue is discussed in A. Wilson, 'The peace of the county: Warwickshire, Birmingham and the Bean Club, 1746–1774' (forthcoming).

24 W. Hutton, *An History of Birmingham*, Birmingham, 1780 and 1783; reprinted with an introduction by C.R. Elrington, Wakefield: EP Publishing, 1976; C. Gill, *History of Birmingham*, vol. 1: *Manor and Borough to 1865*, London: Oxford University Press, 1952; Money, *Experience and Identity*.

25 See for instance S. Smiles, *Lives of Boulton and Watt*, 2nd edn, London: John Murray, 1866; H.W. Dickinson, *Matthew Boulton*, Cambridge: Cambridge University Press, 1937; R.E. Schofield, *The Lunar Society of Birmingham: A Social History of Provincial Science and Industry in Eighteenth Century England*, Oxford: Clarendon Press, 1963.

26 See Elrington's introduction to Hutton, *History of Birmingham*.

27 In 1746 – that is, the year before his ennoblement as first Baron Archer – Thomas Archer purchased the lordship of the manor of Birmingham at a cost of £1,700 (Hutton, *History of Birmingham*, p. 181); in 1752 his younger brother Henry Archer helped to set up a Birmingham Court of Conscience for the recovery of small debts.

28 E. Cruickshanks, *Political Untouchables: The Tories and the '45*, London: Duckworth, 1979, p. 107.

29 Hutton, *History of Birmingham*, pp. 124–5.

30 Ibid., pp. 116–21.

31 BCRL, BC/1 and BC/2.

32 The Old Meeting dated from the 1690s, the New Meeting from 1730, and the Carr's Lane Meeting split off from the Old Meeting in 1748: Hutton, *History of Birmingham*, pp. 116–18.

33 Money, *Experience and Identity*, pp. 222–4.

34 See J.T. Bunce, *History of the Corporation of Birmingham, with a Sketch of the Earlier Government of the Town*, vol. 1, Birmingham: Cornish Brothers, 1878, and Hutton, *History of Birmingham*, pp. 196–202.

35 What follows is discussed more fully, with supporting references, in Wilson, 'The peace of the county'.

36 J.R. Western, *The English Militia in the Eighteenth Century: The Story of a Political Issue 1600–1802*, London: Routledge, 1965, *passim*; L. Colley, *In Defiance of Oligarchy: The Tory Party 1714–60*, Cambridge: Cambridge University Press, 1982, p. 285.

37 M. Peters, 'The *Monitor* on the constitution, 1755–1765: new light on the origins of English radicalism', *The English Historical Review*, 1971, vol. 86; Colley, *In Defiance of Oligarchy*, pp. 288, 360 n. 67.

38 This directory is not extant; for its existence see J. Hill, *The Bookmakers and Booksellers of Old Birmingham*, Birmingham: privately printed, 1907, p. 65.

39 Hutton, *History of Birmingham*, p. 266.

40 For accounts of this by-election see Money, *Experience and Identity*, pp. 171–2, and Wilson, 'The peace of the county'.

41 Equally significant, the other steward was William Craven, the new Lord Craven (the sixth Baron), who immediately before his accession to the peerage had been in contention with Skipwith at the by-election. (Craven had been forced to withdraw because by a remarkable twist of fate, his uncle and namesake, the 5th Baron Craven, died on 17 March, whereupon the barony passed to him, making him ineligible to serve in the Commons. On the sixth Baron Craven see further below, at note 95.)

42 Money, *Experience and Identity*, pp. 172–3; and cf. pp. 106–7, 169.

43 All these members were elected on 11 September 1770.

44 Money, *Experience and Identity*, pp. 100–1 and *passim*.

45 For Skipwith see ibid., pp. 208–10 and F. O'Gorman, *The Rise of Party in England: The Rockingham Whigs 1760–82*, London: Allen & Unwin, 1975, pp. 320, 430–1, 596 n.19. Skipwith's so-to-speak leftwards political move was echoed in the early 1770s by Sir Charles Holte; and later in the decade Lord Craven, the sixth Baron Craven, went even further in the same direction (see below, at note 95).

46 Money, *Experience and Identity*, *passim*.

47 Garbett's partner Dr John Roebuck was in the late 1740s a trustee of the Presbyterian New Meeting, and in the 1760s Garbett was on very friendly terms with the Unitarian John Taylor and the Quaker Sampson Lloyd, partners in the firm of Taylor and Lloyd: Hill, *Bookmakers and Booksellers of Old Birmingham*, p. 89, and R.S. Sayers, *Lloyds Bank in the History of English Banking*, Oxford: Clarendon Press, 1957, pp. 6–7. For Boulton see Schofield, *The Lunar Society*, and Dickinson, *Matthew Boulton*.

48 For accounts of the Hospital's origin and development see J. A. Langford, *A Century of Birmingham Life*, vol. 1, Birmingham, 1968, pp. 153–74; Gill, *History of Birmingham*, vol. 1, pp. 130–1; and Money, *Experience and Identity*, pp. 9–11.

49 Money, *Experience and Identity*, p. 166.

50 Between May and August 1765 three meetings were held (as many as in the previous three years) and ten new members were elected (as many as in the previous four years).

51 *Aris's*, 30 September 1765.

52 For titles to settlement and relief see R. Burn, *The History of the Poor Laws, with Observations*, London, 1764, pp. 106–7; G.W. Oxley, *Poor Relief in England and Wales 1601–1834*, London: David & Charles, 1974, pp. 19–21; and K.D.M. Snell, *Annals of the Labouring Poor: Social Change and Agrarian England 1660–1900*, Cambridge: Cambridge University Press, 1985, *passim*, particularly pp. 71, 77.

53 Langford, *Birmingham Life*, p. 154, punctuation modified.

54 *Aris's*, 25 November 1765.

55 Birmingham General Hospital Quarterly Board of Governors Minute Book 1765–1842, entry for 21 November 1765, BCRL, MS. 1423/1. Some of these

benefactors had probably been present at the meeting, while others sent their gifts through the hands of friends.

56 Samuel Birch (elected 1751) and Richard Hicks (elected 1753).

57 On Newdigate see Money, *Experience and Identity*, p. 2.

58 One of the refounding members of the Bean Club in 1749; of Blythe Hall, a few miles north-east of Birmingham. Another Richard Geast, presumably his son, was to join the Club in 1775; his address was given as Birmingham.

59 This was the third Earl, William Legge (1731–1801), grandson of the second Earl, with whom he has sometimes been confused. The third Earl succeeded on 15 December 1750, but did not take his seat in the House of Lords until 31 May 1754; see A. Collins, *The Peerage of England*, 3rd edn, 5 vols in 6, London, 1756, vol. 3, p. 344.

60 Dartmouth's seat of Sandwell-Hall was only four miles from Birmingham; he was both a neighbour and a confidant of Matthew Boulton (see Money, *Experience and Identity*, p. 58), whose firm was, we have seen, one of the strongest supporters of the Hospital; Dartmouth may have been cultivating a Birmingham connection at this time, for when the Birmingham Canal Navigation was launched two years later, he was to be a major shareholder.

61 *Aris's*, 9 December 1765.

62 Ibid., 16 December 1765.

63 The Dissenters were Samuel Galton, John Kettle, Sampson Lloyd, Dr William Small, John Taylor and John Taylor Junior.

64 Langford, *Birmingham Life*, pp. 155–7.

65 Birmingham General Hospital Quarterly Board of Governors Minute Book 1765–1842, p. 19 (Friday 7 November 1766), BCRL, MS. 1423/1.

66 Birmingham General Hospital Committee of Trustees Minute Book 1766–84, entries for 1766–8, *passim*, BCRL, MS. 1423/2.

67 For instance, the secretary agreed to have his salary held back for a year, and as will emerge below, further benefactions were solicited.

68 BCRL, MS. 1423/2, 3 May 1768.

69 BCRL, MSS 1423/1 and 1423/2.

70 Save only that three further meetings were held: on 13 September, mainly to take out insurance on the building; on 22 November, which meeting was adjourned, supposedly for three months; and on 2 May 1769, when the secretary was requested to bring in exact accounts of the moneys owing: BCRL, MS. 1423/1.

71 As for instance at Manchester (see Brockbank, *Portrait of a Hospital*).

72 See Money, *Experience and Identity*, pp. 58 (Dartmouth; cf. note 60 above), 175 (correspondence with Aylesford's Countess).

73 Langford, *Birmingham Life*, pp. 156–7.

74 The appeal was made on 1 June 1767; its outcome was reported in *Aris's*, listing the individual donations (this probably in an attempt to shame others into contributing), on 25 January 1768. See Langford, *Birmingham Life*, pp. 157–8.

75 BCRL, MS. 1423/1, entry for 3 May 1768.

76 No reply to either letter was recorded in the minutes, and none of the recipients thereafter became a benefactor. A fitting emblem of the indifference of the county aristocracy is supplied by Lord Denbigh. Denbigh was a prime candidate to approach, for in his youth he had made a point of cultivating a Birmingham interest, and he was associated with two of the Hospital's leading activists (Samuel Garbett and Henry Carver); yet so little did he care about the Hospital's plight that he did not even trouble to record its communication in his letter-book: WCRO, CR 2017/C243.

77 C. Hadfield, *The Canals of the West Midlands*, Newton Abbot: David & Charles, 1969, pp. 63–4.

78 Mr Francis Goodall (5 guineas).

79 William Bentley (10 guineas), Edward Hector and James Farmer (5 guineas each).

80 *Aris's*, 12 September 1768, quoted in Langford, *Birmingham Life*, p. 159.
81 Cf. above, at note 72. After the Thursday morning performance of music from Handel and Boyce, held in St Phillip's Church, these Countesses (it was reported) 'very obligingly stood to receive at the church door for the benefit of the charity'.
82 Thus the appeal made in 1767 drew in contributions from five of the six Dissenters, but from only about half of the others (including contributions from relatives, such as Francis Garbett Esq., whom I take to have been related to Samuel Garbett); the Dissenters were disproportionately prominent on the little sub-committee that organized the music festival of 1768, contributing as they did three of its seven members (Dr William Small, John Taylor Esq., and Mr John Taylor Junior; others on the sub-committee were Dr John Ash, Henry Carver Junior, Mr Brooke Smith and Isaac Spooner Esq.).
83 Nevertheless, at least two of the three new donors in 1767 (note 79 above) were Churchmen: Edward Hector, a Bean Club member since 1751, and William Bentley, who was to be elected to the Club in 1774.
84 Above, at note 69. The Churchmen could well have been suspicious of the double role played by John Taylor and Sampson Lloyd, that is, as members of the committee and as the Hospital's bankers. Conversely the Dissenters may have resented the fact that members of the Established Church had delivered far less support to the Hospital than they themselves had produced.
85 Above, at note 43.
86 An emblem of the contrasting approaches underlying the Hospital and the Club is the case of Matthew Boulton. As a manufacturer, Boulton was in fierce rivalry with John Taylor, and there was no love lost between them in commercial matters (Taylor to Boulton, 16 July 1772, BCRL, Matthew Boulton papers, 256/42); yet Boulton served alongside Taylor on the Hospital committee, and he was to remain staunch in his support for the Hospital. But precisely because he associated freely with Dissenters like Taylor, he was excluded from the Bean Club, as we have seen (above, at note 47).
87 The full title was *Poetical Dream, Being a Dialogue between the Hospital and the New Play House*. See Langford, *Birmingham Life*, pp. 160–1.
88 J.W. Showell in *Aris's*, 1856, quoted in Langford, *Birmingham Life*, p. 162.
89 See the extracts in Langford, *Birmingham Life*, pp. 162–7.
90 Dr John Ash, William John Banner, Matthew Boulton, Henry Carver, Samuel Galton, John Kettle, Sampson Lloyd, Francis Parrott, Joseph Smith, John Taylor and John Turner.
91 Samuel Galton, John Kettle, Sampson Lloyd and John Taylor.
92 Known Dissenters were Samuel Galton Junior, Samuel Harvey, William Hunt, Michael Lakin, Charles Lloyd, Sampson Lloyd Junior, John Richards, John Rickards and William Russell, while a possible case was Samuel Freeth. What is particularly striking is that several of these new men – five or six of them – came from the Presbyterian Old Meeting, which had not contributed a single member to the original committee: Harvey, Hunt, Lakin, Richards, Rickards and possibly Freeth (perhaps the husband of Martha Freeth of the Old Meeting). Members of the Old Meeting have been identified from the MS. Register of their resolutions, 1771–91, in BCRL.
93 In the 1769 by-election he had initially offered himself against Skipwith, and his candidacy had been backed by Lord Denbigh: see note 41 above.
94 Perhaps under the influence of his wife: Money, *Experience and Identity*, p. 78 n.76.
95 Craven had attained a more liberal stance by 1774 (signalled by his backing Lord Guernsey as prospective candidate for the Warwickshire election), and he opposed the American war in 1775. See Money, *Experience and Identity*, pp. 69, 78 n. 67, 78 n. 76, 175–6, 216 n. 58.
96 At the same time, the question needs to be asked as to why Craven, only very lately a Whig, was chosen in this role, rather than the Earl of Hertford, the Earl of

Warwick or Baron Archer, all of whose Whig allegiances were of much longer standing. This is connected with a larger puzzle that I have not yet resolved: why was it that no effective links had developed between these Whig aristocrats and the Dissenters among the Birmingham elite? This is all the more of a conundrum in view of the Archers' earlier interest in Birmingham (note 27 above). There was at least one such link, between John Taylor and Lord Warwick, which is attested in 1769 and had no doubt developed earlier, but this merely intensifies the question as to why the Hospital made so little of connections like this. For the Taylor–Lord Warwick connection, see S.H.A. Hervey (ed.), *Journals of the Hon. William Hervey, in North America and Europe, from 1755 to 1814; with Order Books at Montreal, 1760–1763. With Memoir and Notes*, Suffolk Green Books, No. 14, Bury St Edmunds: Paul and Mathew, 1906, p. 217.

97 See for instance Habermas, *Structural Transformation*, pp. 33, 55–6.

98 Money, *Experience and Identity*, pp. 9–11, 100–1 and *passim*.

99 It is important to register that what we might call the 'internal' relations of the public sphere were themselves contingent upon 'external' relations with the state, at least in the setting that has been considered here. What defined an aristocrat was his family's membership of the House of Lords; what made a man a gentleman, in the full sense of the word, was his appointment to the county Commission of the Peace, an appointment that was made by the Crown; and what gave force to religious divisions was that the Church of England and this alone was *Established*, that is, formally united with the state. Thus the conflicts within the 'public sphere' lead us not away from the state but back towards it: cf. my 'A critical portrait of social history', in A. Wilson (ed.) *Rethinking Social History: English Society 1570–1920 and its Interpretation*, Manchester: Manchester University Press, 1993, pp. 9–58, at pp. 13–20.

100 In the English translation, *repräsentative Öffentlichkeit* has been variously rendered as 'representative publicness' (Habermas, *Structural Transformation*, pp. 10, 11), as 'the publicity of representation' (p. 9), and as 'the publicity that characterized representation' (p. 8); in view of the difficulties of translation, it seems safest to stick to Habermas's German words. Speaking approximately, *repräsentative Öffentlichkeit* was a ceremonial display of the status of those who held power (pp. 7, 8). More precisely, *repräsentative Öffentlichkeit* was a display of the *virtues* held to be associated with that power: qualities such as 'excellence, highness, majesty, fame, dignity, and honour' (p. 7, apparently quoting Carl Schmitt; cf. the next note). This was quite different in kind from 'representation' as we tend to think of it, that is, 'representation in the sense in which the members of a national assembly represent a nation, or a lawyer represents his clients' (p. 7). Rather, what was represented was the ensemble of noble virtues; the way that this ensemble of virtues was represented was through the being of the ruler. Habermas suggested that *repräsentative Öffentlichkeit* took a succession of different forms – first courtly-knightly, then Renaissance-humanist and finally monarchic-aristocratic (pp. 9–11).

101 Habermas, *Structural Transformation*, pp. 8–9. This phase of Habermas's argument leaned heavily on the writings of Carl Schmitt, published in the 1920s and 1930s.

102 Ibid., pp. 11–12.

103 Ibid., p. 63. Again, when Habermas turned to France its Catholicism was not even noticed; the 1685 revocation of the Edict of Nantes was registered merely in a footnote and even there only obliquely (p. 263, n.23 to p. 67); the religious concerns of the early *philosophes* were mentioned only to dismiss these as non-political (p. 68). And with respect to Germany Habermas excluded all mention of religion, not only from his initial discussion of its political development (pp. 71–3), but also from his subsequent account of the thought of both Hegel and Marx (pp. 117–29).

104 Habermas described the Reformation as bringing about, or as equivalent to (it was not clear which), 'the so-called freedom of religion' (ibid., p. 11).

5 Between separate spheres

Medical women, moral hygiene and the Edinburgh Hospital for Women and Children

Elaine Thomson

Habermas's exploration of the development and meaning of the public sphere was one of his earliest projects. Locating the origins of the public sphere in the critical political debates of the coffee house and salon culture of eighteenth-century Europe, Habermas charted its development and transformation into the twentieth century. Within this extended historical process, he suggests, from the middle of the nineteenth century (perhaps as a result of the 1848 revolutions) the bourgeois state began to monitor and restrict areas of private life in order to maintain the stability of society. By the early twentieth century, this trend had resulted in the emergence of the welfare state. The critical and informed public debate that had originally found its expression in public opinion had been replaced by the views of an uncritical mass public, whose opinions were neutralized by the consumption of mass media and manipulated by commercial and party political interests.

Despite the persuasiveness of Habermas's general arguments, a more detailed and specific inquiry into the historical development of the public sphere is required if any full understanding of its construction is to be arrived at. This is especially so with regard to issues of gender. Habermas has not adequately addressed the questions posed by the exclusion of women from the public sphere, nor explored the gender dimensions of the public/private split. The entry of women into bourgeois public life, via philanthropy and the professions, should form an integral part of any full analysis of the public sphere. Habermas implies that the political power inherent in public opinion was denatured over time and, from the mid-Victorian period, was rendered impotent by the gradual emergence of a coercive welfare state. However, an exploration of women's entry into the public sphere raises the question of how power within that sphere is constructed, and by whom. From the later nineteenth century middle-class women, so long without a voice or a role in the public sphere, were able to take part in the construction of middle-class institutions – such as medicine and public health – which can be interpreted as being coercive and repressive. Indeed, medicine has frequently been pinpointed as being an institution that has been, and still is, especially repressive to women.[1] To understand the contradictions and complexities inherent in the emergence of new institutions of power and surveillance in the late nineteenth and early twentieth centuries, the role of women – traditionally the inhabitants of the private world – in that process must be engaged with. In turn, the impact that women's entry to the public world had on their own self-definition, particularly within the professions, must also be considered.

Medicine as a profession sits in an ambiguous position with regard to the public and private worlds. Medical authority is based on knowledge of private bodily functions, while knowledge of the body and medical advice about personal health and illness necessarily involve an opportunity for those who create that knowledge to monitor and regulate private behaviour. In addition to this, as Habermas implies, the emergence of state-sponsored public health schemes in the early twentieth century made the surveillance and regulation of private lives by the medical profession and the state far more persuasive and coherent. Because of this link between the public and the private worlds, medicine was one of the first professions to which women won access. Thus, women's entry to the medical profession in the late Victorian period, and their subsequent practice of medicine, provides an instructive case study in helping our understanding of the structure and continuing development of the public – and private – spheres.

The first section of this chapter will examine how women's role in the medical profession was shaped by their response to the notion of separate spheres. Following on from this, medical women's involvement with public health measures to combat venereal diseases in Edinburgh will be explored. This includes their involvement with the propaganda campaigns of the National Council for Combating Venereal Diseases (NCCVD) and their role in the treatment of in- and outpatient cases at the Edinburgh Hospital for Women and Children (EHWC). This analysis will illustrate how the medical women entered the public sphere, and served it, while still holding on to many of the perceptions about women's traditional private role that they carried with them when they entered the medical profession in the 1870s. The final section will consider how, by the 1920s, women doctors in Edinburgh were adopting a more pragmatic attitude towards their involvement with medicine and public health, which was more in tune with the political impulses of the public sphere than with the traditional female virtues of the private sphere.

Women's mission to women in nineteenth-century Edinburgh

The notion that men and women occupied distinct 'separate spheres' formed a powerful ideology throughout the Victorian period. It assumed that women would remain in the home and would devote themselves to all things domestic, while men were concerned with the public world of business, commerce and the professions.[2] Public discourse in Edinburgh during the late nineteenth century was uncompromising on the subject. 'It is only when each sex works faithfully in its own department, that the wheels of existence run smoothly', wrote *Chambers's Journal* in 1887. 'The domestic sphere – all that concerns the care of the house and the household and the management of the children – pre-eminently is the woman's kingdom.'[3] Indeed, it was conceded that women possessed only one characteristic in which they were superior to men: their innate moral sense.[4]

Many women accepted the restrictions posed by the notion of separate spheres. Those who did not, however, were nonetheless forced to confront them whenever they sought to enter the male-dominated arena of public life. Women activists (both feminists and philanthropists) chose either to reinterpret or to ignore these boundaries in their efforts to open up for themselves areas of activity within the public sphere.[5] Male institutions (such as the universities) and professions (such as medicine) inevitably had to be engaged with on their own terms if women were to succeed in their objective of breaking down, or at least eroding, the distinctions between public and private.

One such engagement was the campaign for the medical education of women. Under the leadership of the charismatic and vocal Sophia Jex-Blake, a campaign of direct action was carried out in Edinburgh from 1869 to 1873, as women sought to enter Edinburgh University Medical School for the purposes of qualifying and practising as doctors. The medical women addressed the notion of 'separate spheres' by stressing women's fitness to compete on equal terms as men.[6] At the same time, they emphasized women's special moral qualities as further evidence of women's fitness to practise this most intimate of professions. The medical women used these subtly opposing discourses to the same end: to carve out a distinctive position for themselves within the public sphere.[7]

By following these arguments, however, the medical women implicitly denied themselves a place alongside men in the public sphere of voluntary hospitals and clinical laboratories. Instead, women doctors emerged as the champions of preventive medicine and domestic hygiene. Thus, where they did succeed was in finding a place for themselves in medicine as the intermediaries between the public and private worlds.[8]

Throughout their campaign for medical education, hygiene and preventive medicine had been emphasized by the medical women as being areas of knowledge that they, as women, were most suited to dispense among their 'sisters' at large. Their personal understanding of women's bodies and their innate sensitivity to the needs of wives, mothers and children meant that women physicians alone could ask the right questions and thus provide the best care for this particular constituency.[9] Women (specifically working-class women) were ill-informed about the rules of hygiene, and 'poor health' among the working class was the result of 'ignorance of sanitary laws'.[10]

From the early 1870s, many medical women were actively involved in the dissemination of knowledge of 'practical physiology' among women at large. Jex-Blake gave public lectures on physiology and hygiene in Edinburgh in that city's series of 'Health Lectures for the People', which ran from 1882 to 1886. She also lectured on the importance of hygiene for women at the London School of Medicine for Women from 1878 to 1889, and published a pamphlet on *The Care of Infants*, which stressed the importance of a knowledge of hygiene and physiology for mothers and nurses. Other medical women, such as Louise

Atkins, Eliza Walker Dunbar, Edith Pechey, Frances Hoggan and Alice Ker, wrote and lectured on subjects such as 'Womanhood and Advanced Womanhood', 'The Hygienic Requirements of Sick Children', and 'Swimming and its Relation to the Health of Women'.[11]

Implicit in any emphasis on the need for hygienic instruction is the notion that individuals failed to maintain their health by adopting incorrect personal habits or through ignorance. The medical profession, however, could claim to offer the best advice with regard to how to correct one's erroneous or misguided life-style. Indeed, it was implicit in the medical women's rhetoric that only if working-class women followed the advice of the trained medical expert would health be restored and maintained, homes made happy, children robust, husbands content and 'half the vice and crime known to our police officers' dispelled.[12] The practice of medicine by women doctors at the Edinburgh Hospital for Women and Children reflected this preoccupation with hygienic instruction. Through fostering individual responsibility for personal health, the medical women carried the benefits of hygiene instruction into the wards of their Hospital, ensuring that their message of moral hygiene was brought to bear directly on their patients.

Sophia Jex-Blake founded the EHWC in 1878. Initially a dispensary, it expanded to become a six-bed cottage hospital in 1884. The Hospital was staffed by women doctors only, and remained so until its closure in 1984. In this early period, the EHWC was crucial for the training of medical women.[13] A further claim to distinction lay in the fact that, while the Hospital relied to an extent on charitable donations to remain afloat, patients were as far as possible treated and accommodated on a provident basis.[14] This meant that, rather than receiving their hospital care for free, patients were expected to pay at least a proportion of the cost of their treatment, either as a one-off payment or by paying regular contributions into a provident fund.[15] Those who made use of the services of the Edinburgh Hospital were thus considered to be independent, paying patients, rather than the grateful objects of a beneficent charity. Running their hospital in accordance with the principles of self-help, rather than as a paternalistic charity, was an extension of the medical women's emphasis on support (both by and for women) and the responsibility of the individual for her own health.

The practice of medicine at the Hospital echoed this outlook. From 1885 the medical women successfully put into operation a caring and supportive clinical regime that emphasized the tenets of hygiene and physiology as a means to achieving and maintaining good health. Working in a poor part of town among working-class women, the physicians at the Edinburgh Hospital recognized that exhaustion and poor diet were the main causes of illness among this particular constituency. In the Hospital, medication was kept to a minimum, and the regularity of the bowels and of the metabolism in general emphasized as the surest way of achieving a lasting recovery from illness. The hygienic regime central to the health care offered there involved such prescriptions as the avoidance of stimulants (including tea), healthy eating, exercise and fresh air, lots of rest, and respite from back-breaking domestic chores, demanding children and violent or abusive husbands.[16]

By establishing themselves as moral and hygienic instructors to their working-class patients, the medical women in Edinburgh tapped into a distinct public discourse concerning the moral reform of working-class domesticity, laying claim to a public role as the guardians of private morality and hygiene.[17] Despite the paternalism of this stance, however, the medical women interpreted their role as being non-judgemental, and even non-moralistic, in the sense that they emphasized the more supportive, caring and compassionate side to their self-prescribed role. The medical women listened to working women's problems, offered rest, good food and a quiet environment as a means of recovering from illness, fatigue and anxiety caused by their everyday lives. In this way, although emerging as the agents of moral reform, the role of the medical women at the EHWC was based upon a regime of sympathy and support to their 'suffering sisters' in the (respectable) working class.[18] As a special health service, this moral regime was unique in hospital care in the city at this time, and served to justify women's practice of medicine in the city.[19]

In terms of securing a public identity and role within the medical institutions of Edinburgh, however, the development of the Edinburgh Hospital as a place for working-class women to find rest, care and hygienic advice opened up few opportunities for women doctors. Ultimately, it proved to be a professional dead end. On their own admission, opportunities for female doctors were hard to come by in Edinburgh. Even by the early twentieth century, although as well qualified as their male counterparts in the profession, resistance to women doctors, especially in the voluntary hospitals, remained well entrenched.[20] In addition to these prejudices, a surfeit of well-qualified doctors in Edinburgh, combined with the limitations of the medical women's practice at the EHWC, meant that female physicians continued to find it difficult to thrive in the city.[21] By 1900, after over twenty years in the medical profession, women doctors at the Edinburgh Hospital were still struggling to find a place for themselves in medical practice.[22]

After a rather ambitious move to larger premises in 1900, the EHWC began a steady decline into what became little more than a nursing home for women with chronic or debilitating illnesses. As a public institution it had failed to secure public support to allow it to thrive and prosper into the twentieth century. Unable to maintain a sufficient number of paying patients, and struggling to attract voluntary contributions from the public at large, by 1918 the EHWC had sunk into serious debt. Rescue for the medical women – both financial and professional – came in the aftermath of the First World War with the growth of government-sponsored measures to reduce the incidence of venereal diseases (VD).

Medical women, venereal diseases and NCCVD propaganda

The emergence of VD as a public health issue was a consequence of the mobilization of troops during the First World War. Government concern over the problem led to the adoption of measures proposed by the Royal Commission for the Treatment of Venereal Diseases in 1916. The Commission suggested that two measures should be implemented conjointly to reduce the incidence of VD. A propaganda campaign was to be conducted under the auspices of the NCCVD, with the support of the medical profession and the public health authorities. This was to be carried out in tandem with the setting up and running of VD treatment centres up and down the country.[23]

Rather than encouraging the use of prophylactics to control the spread of VD, the NCCVD encouraged individuals to lead chaste sexual lives and to regulate themselves and their own sexual behaviour. Personal behaviour – drinking, 'immoral conduct' and 'flirting' for instance – increasingly became open to censure, and could be blamed for the spread of venereal disease and thus linked to the decline of the British race, nation and empire.[24] 'Venereal disease...can be conquered in one of two ways, by cure and by prevention', declared a typical NCCVD pamphlet, 'and the latter is the best way. It is the doctor's business to cure it, it is the business of every man and every woman – it is *your* business – to prevent it.'[25] Prevention was to be achieved through the dissemination of advice on health and hygiene via public lectures and films, and the distribution of pamphlets, posters and leaflets. Influential groups, such as nurses, teachers and social workers, were also to be targeted with specific lectures, so as to broaden the scope of the propaganda to include those professionals who might come into contact with the public, either through health care or as educators.

In the previous century the notion that an ignorance of hygiene and the 'laws of life' could lead to illness and disease had generally referred to such things as overtiredness, tight corsets, lack of stewed fruit in the diet and poorly ventilated bedrooms. With its emphasis on prevention, the NCCVD emphasized that the medical understanding of hygiene also encompassed social and sexual practices. Private behaviour was increasingly seen to have public consequences.[26] It was within this extended remit of hygienic advice that the medical women in Edinburgh were able to find a role for themselves in the propaganda campaigns of the NCCVD and in the treatment centres set up by the local authorities.

On behalf of the NCCVD, members of the medical profession were enlisted to lecture to the public on the evils of VD and to point out the incorrect habits that could result in the spread of this most personal and private of problems. In Edinburgh, women doctors, most of them associated with the EHWC, eagerly volunteered themselves to lecture to the public and to various groups of health professionals and teachers, on such subjects as 'Responsibility of Citizenship', 'Marriage and Parenthood' and 'Renewal of Life'.[27] Short films, slides and music often accompanied these lectures. The lecture 'Love, Marriage, Parenthood' used films of 'pollen germinating' and 'orchard blossoms' to the accompaniment of 'a little quiet music' as a preliminary to the revelations of the horrors of life with VD. One of the central messages of the lecture was the responsibility of women in the maintenance of the physical and moral health of the species. To the accompaniment of a slide of Venus, motherhood was described as 'the best work we can do for our country'. Alcohol and sexual misconduct were clearly connected, and a slide depicting a scene 'outside a public house' was accompanied by the question 'what beauty of motherhood can be found there?' Slides of syphilitic babies ('doomed!'), victims of general paralysis of the insane ('the "Happy" victim') and 'congenital imbeciles' ('the worst effects...imbecility, idiocy!') were displayed, before the lecture turned 'to the story of hope!', which detailed the 'splendid efforts' of the medical profession in diagnosis and cure. Having also discussed the importance of a 'noble sex life' for men, the evils of 'lazing and loitering about the streets' for the young and the bracing benefits of cycling and other wholesome outdoor pursuits in general, the lecture closed 'with a few words on the power of womanhood to save the next generation' and a slide picturing the Madonna.[28] Leaflets were distributed at these and other similar lectures, with such instructive titles as *Ignorance, The Great Enemy*; *What Mother Must Tell*; and *Sex in Life: Young Women*. Other, less circumspect, titles included *How Girls Can Help in the Fight Against Venereal Disease; VD and its Effects* and *Dangers of VD*.[29]

Clearly, the burden of responsibility for checking the spread of VD was seen to rest mainly with women. 'Every workshop, every factory, every club, is what the girls and women there make it', urged Dr Mary Douie, author of *How Girls Can Help*. 'And you can help the men', she continued, 'they are largely what women make them.'[30] As in the previous century, women were responsible for their own health, for the health of their children, of their husbands, and also of their male and female friends, acquaintances and colleagues. Again, drawing on arguments that stressed their moral superiority to men, women doctors pressed their claim to be the best suited to take the question of the public need for sexual hygiene into the private sphere of the home.

In the public arena of NCCVD propaganda campaigns, the medical women strongly endorsed and colonized the paternalistic medico-moral discourse of discipline and surveillance advocated by the NCCVD and the city's Department of Public Health. Indeed, the medical women took over the bulk of lectures for the NCCVD in Edinburgh, the majority of which were aimed at women (and thus, they suggested, should rightly be delivered by women doctors). For instance, Dr Mary MacNicol, the physician in charge of the VD ward at the Edinburgh Hospital, lectured for the NCCVD from 1918. In this year alone she spoke to the College of Nursing, the Queen Mary's Army Auxiliary Corps (QMAAC), the Voluntary Health Visitors, the Women Citizens Association, and to two groups of teachers and social workers.[31] Mrs Chalmers Watson was on the consulting staff of the Edinburgh Hospital, and had been a physician there from 1905 to 1906 and again from 1916 to 1920.[32] From 1918 she was at the forefront of NCCVD activity as a lecturer and administrator in Edinburgh, and had been active in promoting the role of the medical women in the struggle against VD from the very outset of the campaign.[33] She was Honorary Secretary of the Scottish Branch of the NCCVD, and their main spokesperson in negotiations with the Public Health Department with regard to the lectures, films, pamphlets and books that were distributed throughout the city from 1918.

The determination of the medical women to engage fully with Edinburgh health officials' medico-moral discourse of surveillance and discipline can be illustrated by their attitude to the problem of those who defaulted on their treatment. One of the main hindrances to the eradication of VD, as perceived by the NCCVD, the medical profession and the Department of Public Health, was the defaulter.[34] The Annual Reports of the Medical Officer of Health (MOH) in Edinburgh repeatedly stressed the need for controls to prevent the infected from defaulting on their treatment, which took up to two years of painful injections to fully effect a cure. Those defaulters who were singled out as especially problematic were men (whose careless behaviour infected their wives and children) and 'the problem single girl'. The Scottish Branch of the NCCVD supported the MOH in his preoccupation with these two groups. Yet this moral stance was by no means universally accepted. A number of national feminist groups, such as the Medical Women's Federation, the Women's Freedom League and the Association for Moral and Social Hygiene, opposed the imposition of compulsory VD controls, arguing that forcible treatment could lead to concealment and would simply intensify the problem by driving it underground. Despite the opinion of these feminist groups, the Edinburgh medical women gave their full support to the prevailing medical opinion in the city that compulsory controls were a necessity if innocent women and children were to be protected. In particular, medical women in local groups, such as the Edinburgh Women's Citizens Association, voiced their support for VD controls, despite the firm opposition of the Medical Women's Federation.[35]

The rhetoric of the MOH and the NCCVD was strongly paternalistic, and intensely critical of those who failed to allow themselves to be effectively treated and cured. Women, or rather 'single girls', were pinpointed as needing special surveillance and discipline if they were to cease being the vectors of venereal diseases. Indeed, such was the outrage and alarm of the MOH on the matter that he saw fit to mention the 'infected single girl' as a monstrous source of disease and immorality in every Annual Report from 1919 to 1930. 'Problem girls', he explained, were unmarried women who had 'fallen into disgrace at home', had attended hospital for treatment, but 'on leaving…have no place to go…drift back to their old habits…[and end up] returning to the gutter'.[36] Most such 'infected single girls' were regarded as 'morally deficient' and 'many' were condemned as 'mentally deficient'. Although they were such imbeciles that they did not understand that they had to attend the VD clinic regularly, they were not 'sufficiently so' to be locked up in an asylum out of harm's way.[37]

The medical women of the NCCVD in Edinburgh echoed this moral stance, emphasizing the 'mental and moral deficiency' of those who defaulted on their treatment, or who engaged in sexual practices that resulted in infection. Here too, 'single girls' were pinpointed as vectors of 'the social evil'. Mrs Chalmers Watson, for example, on lecturing to a group of social workers in 1919, cautioned that 'high grade mental defectives suffering from Venereal Diseases…a large proportion of whom join the ranks of prostitutes, are really moral imbeciles and should be under control'.[38]

The treatment of venereal diseases at the EHWC

If the Edinburgh medical women adopted the moralistic paternalism of other public health reformers in their propaganda for the NCCVD, they would significantly modify that stance in their own dealings with women VD patients. In addition to the importance of propaganda, the Royal Commission on Venereal Diseases had also proposed that special VD treatment centres should be set up at the voluntary hospitals, without cost to the patient (being funded 75 per cent by central government and 25 per cent by local rates).[39] Furthermore, treatment for those infected had to take account of the fact that some, at least, were innocent of any charges of wanton sexual indulgence and unchecked licentiousness. These 'innocent victims' (and even the MOH made a cursory note that such women did exist) had a right to be treated with the maximum of discretion and respect. It was as the 'innocent victims' of this wave of male-borne venereal diseases that married women and children were seen to be especially in need of forms of medical care that operated with discretion and minimized the risk of stigma. Furthermore, it was argued, the intimate nature of the disease meant that distress and embarrassment to the patient would be minimized if women doctors carried out medical examination and treatment.

In 1919, therefore, the Edinburgh Hospital, with its all-female staff, was singled out by the Town Council Public Health Department as the ideal institution for the treatment of VD among married women and children in the city.[40] Despite some initial reluctance at the prospect of their Hospital becoming an annex in the government's public health schemes,[41] the Executive Committee decided that the Hospital's grave financial situation meant that such a generous incentive could not be rejected.[42] A VD ward, with three cots and twelve beds, was duly established in early 1919.[43] Outpatient clinics were also set up (on Tuesday afternoons) at the EHWC itself, and at the Hospital's Dispensary at 25 Grove Street. Dr Mary MacNicol, who as we have seen was already offering lectures for the NCCVD, was appointed to take care of this branch of the Hospital's in- and outpatient work, her salary being paid by the Town Council.[44]

From the establishment of its VD ward, the Edinburgh Hospital found that the demand for its services in this department was greater than had initially been expected.[45] The Annual Reports noted that the VD ward 'with its special adaptation to the needs of married women and children' met a demand 'hitherto unrealised or neglected'.[46] Furthermore, although established with the needs of married women primarily in mind, the Hospital VD ward did not treat this constituency exclusively. Although most unmarried mothers or 'single girls' received their treatment at the Royal Infirmary or the Simpson Memorial Maternity Hospital, some were treated at the Edinburgh Hospital. In contrast to the attitude of the MOH and the rhetoric of the NCCVD towards 'single girls' or unmarried mothers, however, whether the patients at the Edinburgh Hospital were married or not, the Annual Reports always describe those being treated for venereal diseases in its wards as 'innocent', rather than mentally or morally deficient.[47]

A similar degree of sensitivity is evidenced in the attitude of the Edinburgh Hospital towards the defaulter. The MOH and the NCCVD regarded the 'problem' of defaulters as one of the most frustrating aspects of VD treatment. The Annual Reports of the EHWC were pleased to point out that the ever-decreasing number of such women was one of their VD ward's more important achievements.[48] The sympathy and discretion offered by the medical women was emphasized as being especially important to infected married women, and vital in minimizing the risk of defaulters. Determination to play down the VD work at the EHWC is made apparent by the decision not even to mention venereal diseases (other than euphemistically) from 1923.[49] However, the female defaulter and the female who was rapidly re-infected were perceived to be a problem by the medical women at the Edinburgh Hospital, although they were not singled out for recrimination in the Annual Reports. For example, Drs MacNicol and Chalmers Watson emphasized the need for a refuge home for these women.[50] Furthermore, Drs MacNicol and Liston (who was the clinical assistant special-izing in VD of women at the Royal Infirmary) attempted to liaise with the Edinburgh Magdalene Asylum on the matter, although they were unsuccessful in their petition.[51]

The ambivalence of the medical women's attitude between support and surveillance with regard to the treatment of VD and the question of tackling the notorious defaulters is highlighted by the employment of a 'Lady Almoner' at the Edinburgh Hospital from 1924. The main purpose of the Lady Almoner was to track down those women who had defaulted on their treatment, make 'inquiries into the reasons for any failures to attend', and keep them under surveillance in order to minimize the risk of them defaulting again. She was then able to monitor patients in their home environment, 'report...on home condi-tion' and garner 'knowledge of their circumstances'. On the basis of this 'knowledge', she was then qualified to offer them 'advice and help of practical value' with regard to personal and sexual hygiene.[52]

The main emphasis of the work of the Almoner's Department at the Edinburgh Hospital was on dispensing hygienic advice to single women and to married women and mothers. The Almoner's mission to police and monitor those who defaulted on the VD treatment, however, remained discreet. Specific references to venereal diseases are absent from the accounts of the Almoner's Department in the Hospital's Annual Reports. Furthermore, throughout the 1920s and 1930s, the VD work of the Almoner was further obscured by being blended in with the advice-giving work of the mother and baby clinics that the Hospital offered to the working and working-class women of Edinburgh throughout this period.[53] Moreover, although the Almoner was represented as offering an important service for married women, she was pinpointed as being of particular value to 'the unmarried mother', who had 'special difficulties as to her own future and that of her child'.[54]

Unlike the Annual Reports of the MOH, however, no judgements were made about the moral character or 'imbecility' of such unmarried women. Rather, all women were to be taught physiology, hygiene and the 'laws of health' – the very subjects that the medical women had advocated in the 1870s and 1880s as being vital knowledge for women at large. 'All mothers will be welcome, and will be able to obtain medical treatment, and learn the value of fresh air and sunshine and proper food and clothing in the prevention of disease', the Annual Report for 1923 announced optimistically. 'Thus one more step will be taken to make their households healthy and happy, and to banish rickets and preventable diseases from their homes.'[55] 'Preventable diseases' by the 1920s, however, also included venereal diseases.[56] 'This beneficent work in the Prevention of Disease is a real economy', declared the Annual Report in 1926 with reference to instruction on measures that would prevent the onset of 'specific diseases' (i.e. venereal diseases). '[F]or to tend the victims of disease in hospital is a costly task and the bill a heavy one.'[57]

From the outset, the medical women operated their services for VD-infected women with sympathy and discretion, avoiding the condemnation of infected single mothers, referring to their patients as 'innocent victims' with 'special difficulties' and combining advice on sexual hygiene with information more generally on the 'laws of health'. And yet, tensions soon arose between the more intimate aspects of the medical women's practice at the Hospital and the practicalities of acting as the moral agents of public health. The appointment of the Lady Almoner suggests that the medical women's public discourse of moral hygiene, and the bureaucracy that supported this discourse, increasingly encroached upon the space in which the medical women attempted to maintain a less judgemental and disciplinary moral practice. The work of the dispensary and its Almoner's Department indicates that keeping working-class patients under surveillance in their own homes had become an essential aspect of the medical women's regime of preventive and curative medicine.[58] Although the VD work of the medical women at the EHWC was to be carried out with the maximum of sensitivity, therefore, VD cases increasingly became construed as objects of public surveillance and control. This was at odds with the medical women's language of sympathy and support, and with the image of the Edinburgh Hospital as a home-from-home convalescent hospital for respectable working-class women. Thus, increasingly, the medical women's public presentation of their work at the Hospital was concealed behind such euphemisms as 'specific diseases' and subterfuges such as omitting to mention the treatment of unmarried girls or single mothers. In the treatment of VD cases, the Hospital itself had, in a sense, become a private world, its activities withdrawn from the public gaze and dissociated from public discourse.

Conclusions

The construction of power within the public sphere is a complex process, with public institutions such as VD provision in the 1920s emerging as sites of political mediation between different interest groups. The establishment of the VD schemes in Edinburgh heralded the emergence of new institutional and political structures in the arena of public health to which women doctors could success-fully address themselves. It is significant also that these were institutions with supervisory and coercive powers – unlike the Edinburgh Hospital, which, run on the provident system, relied upon the support of women philanthropists and patients for its success.

From 1919, therefore, a different moral economy began to impinge on the work and attitudes of the medical women: a moral economy of public health surveillance and medical management. This new morality provided the medical women with an invaluable source of income for their hospital, as well as opening up new opportunities for professional development (in public health, for instance) in the years after the First World War. Women doctors radically reinterpreted the traditional gendered definition of the limits of the public sphere for their own political ends. As the moral guardians of society, and as the main occupants of the domestic world of the private sphere – roles which they had inherited from their Victorian forebears – the medical women of the early twentieth century portrayed themselves as the ideal moral agents to take the concerns of the Public Health Department into the private sphere of the home. They adopted a strong moral tone in their participation in public health debates, such as in their support of the campaign for compulsory controls and their lectures for the NCCVD, and portrayed themselves as the ideal agents of moral surveillance. They set up dispensaries and employed a Lady Almoner to monitor and report on working-class sexual health. As a result, medical women in Edinburgh made themselves indispensable to the Town Council's schemes for the eradication and prevention of VD. Indeed, these state-funded schemes enabled the medical women to maintain their hospital and extend their medical mission to women, both of which had been faltering due to lack of voluntary support.

Ironically, however, it was this very extension of the medical women's public influence that ultimately compromised their peculiarly feminine role of domestic support and sympathy. The notion of women's mission to women, which had characterized the medical women's rhetoric in the nineteenth century, was increasingly eroded by more pragmatic, career-oriented concerns. At the Edinburgh Hospital, in contrast to the strong moral tone of their NCCVD propaganda, the medical women adopted a much softer rhetorical approach, one that was in keeping with the sensibilities of the respectable working-class women who sought treatment there. However, their dependence on public funds inevitably led to a growing involvement with disciplinary forms of practice. The surveillance and criticism of working-class women's behaviour, in turn, inevitably brought with it the imposition of a middle-class moral code onto working-class practices of personal hygiene, social and sexual behaviour. In effect, the medical women's participation in schemes for the control and treatment of VD can be interpreted as an alliance with a coercive state that began to supplement, if not totally displace, the politics of feminine solidarity as a route to professional status for medical women in Edinburgh.

Notes

1 Many historians have discussed the role Victorian science and medicine played in authorizing and perpetuating notions of women's inferiority. Examples include L. Duffin, 'The conspicuous consumptive: woman as invalid', in S. Delamont and L. Duffin (eds), *The Nineteenth-Century Woman, Her Cultural and Physical World*, London and New York: Croom Helm, 1978, pp. 26–56; Carroll Smith-Rosenberg, 'Puberty to menopause: the cycle of femininity in nineteenth-century America', in M.S. Hartman and L. Banner (eds), *Clio's Consciousness Raised: Perspectives on the History of Women*, New York and London: Harper & Row, 1974, pp. 23–37; L. Jordanova, *Sexual Visions: Images of Gender in Science and Medicine between the Eighteenth and Twentieth Centuries*, New York and London: Harvester Wheatsheaf, 1989; O. Moscucci, *The Science of Woman*, Cambridge: Cambridge University Press, 1990; C. Gallagher and T. Laqueur (eds), *The Making of the Modern Body*, Berkeley and London: University of California Press, 1987; C.E. Russett, *Sexual Science: The Victorian Construction of Womanhood*, Cambridge, MA and London: Harvard University Press, 1991; Carroll Smith-Rosenberg, 'The hysterical woman', *Social Research*, 1972, vol. 39, pp. 652–78.
2 For a succinct overview of these discussions, see J. Lewis, *Women in England 1870–1950: Sexual Divisions and Social Change*, Brighton: Harvester Wheatsheaf, 1984.
3 Anon., 'The higher education of women. II. The question of its advantages', *Chambers's Journal*, 1887, vol. 4, pp. 134–7, p. 134. See also Anon., 'What woman is fitted for', *Westminster Review*, 1887, vol. 7, pp. 64–75.
4 '[W]omen's excellence over man is…in the sphere of wisdom, and love, and moral power', wrote Dr Thomas Laycock in 1869. T. Laycock, *Mind and Brain*, vol. 2, 2nd edn, London: Simpkin, Marshall & Co., 1969, p. 483. Women's wondrous moral influence on society was still being stressed in the early twentieth century. See Anon., 'The progress of woman', *Quarterly Review*, 1902, vol. 195, pp. 201–20.
5 F.K. Prochaska, *Women and Philanthropy in Nineteenth-Century England*, Oxford: Clarendon Press, 1980; O. Checkland, *Philanthropy in Victorian Scotland*, Edinburgh: John Donald, 1980; C. Blake, *The Charge of the Parasols: Women's Entry to the Medical Profession*, London: Women's Press, 1990.
6 Margaret Todd, *The Life of Sophia Jex-Blake*, London: Macmillan: 1918, p. 262.
7 G. Rose, 'The struggle for political democracy: emancipation, gender and geography', *Environment and Planning*, 1990, vol. 8, pp. 395–408. As Mary Ann Elston has suggested, the medical women 'argued not for equal rights to compete with men in the public sphere, but for access to it in order to better pursue their feminine interests and talents'. See M.A. Elston, 'Women doctors and the British health services: a sociological survey of their careers and opportunities', University of Leeds, unpublished PhD thesis, 1986, pp. 130–2. See also E. Thomson, 'Women in medicine in late nineteenth and early twentieth-century Edinburgh: a case study', University of Edinburgh, unpublished PhD thesis, 1998, pp. 29–45. Prochaska has explored the same themes in his *Women and Philanthropy*.
8 Cf. Pamela Gilbert's discussion of Octavia Hill's housing reform work, in the present volume.
9 Sophia Jex-Blake, *Medical Women a Thesis and a History*, 2nd edn, Edinburgh: Oliphant, Anderson & Ferrier, 1886, p. 48.
10 Ibid., pp. 50–1.
11 Thomson, 'Women in medicine', pp. 107–12.
12 John Hughes Bennett, 'Physiology for women', *Nature*, 1871, no.5, pp. 72–3; Jex-Blake, *Medical Women*, p. 44.
13 Thomson, 'Women in medicine', pp. 62, 211–12. Leith Hospital appointed a female House Physician in 1891 and the Royal Hospital for Sick Children appointed women as Registrar and Resident Physician in 1897, but this was by no means the beginning of a widespread trend. It was not until the early twentieth century that other hospitals in Edinburgh provided the necessary training for female doctors. Leith Hospital Annual

Report 1891, Lothian Health Services Archive (LHSA), Division of Special Collections, Edinburgh University Library, LHB6/1/1–32, p. 16; and Royal Hospital for Sick Children Annual Report 1897, LHSA LHB5/2/11–42; p. 6.

14 Edinburgh was home to a vast number of medical hospitals and charities: four 'Royal' hospitals, seven special hospitals, three municipal hospitals, eighteen dispensaries, four convalescent homes and sundry other 'medical charities' were also at work in the city. Edinburgh Charities Registration Union, *First Annual Report and Handbook of Edinburgh Charities and Benevolent Institutions*, Edinburgh, 1888, pp. v–vii.

15 Members paid 2s 6d every quarter, plus the cost of medicines, in order to gain free medical treatment as and when they needed it. Non-provident patients were expected to pay a proportion of the cost of their treatment at the Dispensary or Hospital. Those who could not afford to pay had their fees met by the 'free bed fund'. Edinburgh Charities Registration Union, *First Annual Report*, pp. 17–18.

16 Thomson, 'Women in medicine', pp. 123–65.

17 The patient records from the Hospital frequently note pieces of health-giving advice for discharged patients, such as 'great caution as to food', 'warn[ed] against constipation and unsuitable diet' and – an impractical piece of advice to a dressmaker – 'only to go out in sunshine...[and] to give up dressmaking'. See ibid., p. 152.

18 Ibid., p. 196.

19 E. Thomson, 'Sick and tired of being sick and tired: working class women and the Edinburgh Hospital, 1885–1900', *Review of Scottish Culture*, 2000–1, vol. 13, pp. 66–73.

20 See above note 13.

21 Thomson, 'Women in medicine', pp. 207–11.

22 Edinburgh Hospital for Women and Children (EHWC), Executive Committee Minutes, vol. 3, 4 Nov. 1903, LHSA LHB 8/1/3, pp. 146–8. By 1900 there were nineteen women doctors practising in Edinburgh. Fourteen of that number had links with the Edinburgh Hospital. Thomson, 'Women in medicine', pp. 61–2.

23 L. Bland, '"Cleansing the portals of life": the venereal disease campaign in the early twentieth century', in M. Langan and B. Schwarz (eds), *Crises in the British State, 1880–1930*, London: Hutchison, 1985, pp. 192–208, at p. 193.

24 M. Douie, *How Girls Can Help in the Fight against Venereal Disease*, London: NCCVD, 1918, p. 5. The links between the NCCVD and the Eugenics Education Society were strong. See, for example, Leonard Darwin, 'The Eugenics Education Society and VD', *Eugenics Review*, 1916–17, vol. 8, pp. 213–17.

25 M. Douie, *Sex in Life: Young Women*, London: NCCVD, 1918, p. 33.

26 For a full discussion of the emergence of the 'medico-moral coalition' and the surveillance of sexuality, see Frank Mort, *Dangerous Sexualities: Medico-Moral Politics in England Since 1830*, London and New York: Routledge & Kegan Paul, 1987.

27 NCCVD Report, Edinburgh City Archives, Public Health Committee Files, March 1919–October 1919, DRT 14 box 34.

28 Syllabus of a lecture entitled 'Love, Marriage, Parenthood', NCCVD to Town Clerk 23 October 1919, Edinburgh City Archives, Edinburgh Town Clerk's Department, Public Health Committee, Venereal Disease, General File, January 1918–31 December 1919, box 34, 36e.

29 NCCVD to Town Clerk, 22 January 1919, re: leaflets to be distributed. Edinburgh City Archives, Edinburgh Corporation Town Clerk's Department Public Health Committee, Treatment of Venereal Diseases, 31 October 1916–28 February 1919, PH 15.

30 Douie, *How Girls Can Help*, p. 11. Mary Douie was one of the first women to graduate from Edinburgh University in 1897. She studied medicine at the London School of Medicine for Women from 1897 and worked for the Professor of Physiology at Toronto University from 1907. By 1918 she was writing and lecturing for the NCCVD. *Proceedings of the Imperial Social Hygiene Congress*, May 12–14, 1924, p. ii.

31 Report of the NCCVD to the Town Clerk, 9 April 1919, Edinburgh City Archives, Edinburgh Corporation Town Clerk's Department Public Health Committee,

Venereal Diseases, General File, January 1918–31 December 1919, box 34, 36e: Report and Mrs Chalmers Watson's Report of the Conference of Members of the Propaganda Committee of the National Council held on 18 June 1918, p. 4, Edinburgh City Archives, Public Health Committee Files, January 1918–December 1919, DRT 14 box 34. Dr MacNicol continued to lecture on the subject of VD throughout the 1920s. See, for example, Edinburgh Women Citizens Association Syllabus, 1922–3; Edinburgh Women Citizens Association Syllabus, 1926–7; Edinburgh Women Citizens Association 10th Annual Report 1927–8, pp. 15–16: Edinburgh Public Library (EPL), Edinburgh Room.

32 Mrs Chalmers Watson was one of Edinburgh's most prominent medical women. She had been educated at the Medical College for Women in Edinburgh in the 1890s, and had been one of the first two women to graduate in medicine from Edinburgh University. I. Venters, 'Mrs. Chalmers Watson: a pioneer in medicine', *Scotsman*, 8 August 1936. EHWC Annual Reports 1905–6 and 1920–3.

33 NCCVD Social Workers Course, Syllabus of Lectures, 22 February 1919, Edinburgh Corporation Town Clerk's Department Public Health Committee, Edinburgh City Archive, Treatment of Venereal Diseases, 31 October 1916–28 February 1919, PH 15. Note from the MOH to the Town Clerk re. the work of the NCCVD, 25 October 1918, Edinburgh Town Clerk's Department, Public Health Committee, Venereal Diseases, General File, January 1918–31 December 1919, box 34, 36e.

34 Roger Davidson has discussed the attempts of the medical profession in Scotland to eliminate defaulters. See R. Davidson, 'Venereal disease, sexual morality and public health in interwar Scotland', *Journal of the History of Sexuality*, 1994, vol. 5, pp. 267–94, especially pp. 280–4. See also *idem*, '"A scourge to be firmly gripped": the campaign for VD controls in interwar Scotland', *Social History of Medicine*, 1993, vol. 6, pp. 213–36.

35 For a discussion of the position of women doctors with regard to VD controls see Bland, '"Cleansing the portals of life"', pp. 199–200.

36 Medical Officer of Health for Edinburgh (MOH) Annual Report 1920, EPL, Edinburgh Room, p. 54.

37 MOH Annual Report 1928, p. 77.

38 Mrs Chalmers Watson's Report of the Conference of Members of the Propaganda Committee of the National Council, held on 18 June 1918, p. 4. Edinburgh City Archives, Public Health Committee Files, January 1918–December 1919, DRT 14, box 34.

39 Report of the Royal Commission on Venereal Diseases, *Edinburgh Medical Journal*, 1916, ns. vol. 16, pp. 323–4. EHWC Executive Committee Minutes, vol. 4, 11 June 1918, pp. 247–9.

40 EHWC Annual Report 1919, LHSA LHB8/7/22–52, p. 4. See also MOH Annual Report 1919, p. 55. History of the VD Department at the Bruntsfield Hospital and Elsie Inglis Memorial Maternity Hospital, n.d., Miscellaneous Papers, LHSA LHB8/11/2/5.

41 EHWC Medical Committee Minutes, 1912–19, 4 October 1918, LHSA LHB8/5/1–3.

42 EHWC Executive Committee Minutes vol. 4, 11 June 1918, pp. 247–9.

43 EHWC Medical Committee Minutes, 1919–27, 25 March 1919. Increased VD work at the dispensary in connection with the Town Council's scheme meant that it needed to be properly equipped for the work. It was suggested that the basement should be fitted out to deal with VD patients in isolation from those patients who were not suffering from venereal diseases. The Town Council authorized and paid for such a refit by November of 1919. EHWC Executive Committee Minutes, vol. 4, 15 July 1919, p. 279. See also Edinburgh Town Council Public Health Sub-Committee, Edinburgh City Archives, 1917–19, SL 26/2/1, 4 March 1919, p. 205.

44 EHWC Medical Committee Minutes, 28 October 1919. Dr MacNicol was paid 'one guinea a week' for her treatment of VD cases.

45 By the mid-1920s the Hospital was treating 146 patients a year for VD as inpatients, in addition to 336 at special VD outpatient clinics that were run at the Hospital and at the Dispensary. EHWC Annual Report 1925, p. 8.
46 EHWC Annual Report 1919, pp. 5–6.
47 EHWC Annual Report 1924, p. 3.
48 EHWC Annual Report 1924, p. 8.
49 From 1923 those women being treated for VD in the Hospital are described in the Annual Reports as suffering from 'specific diseases'. See MOH Annual Report 1924, p. 59, and EHWC Annual Report 1924, p. 5.
50 NCCVD conference notes, Edinburgh Corporation Town Clerk's Department, Public Health Committee, Venereal Diseases, General File, January 1918–31 December 1919, box 34, 36e.
51 Edinburgh Magdalene Asylum Sub-Committee Minute Book, 1901–22, 12 May 1920, and 14 July 1920 (no pagination), EPL Edinburgh Room.
52 EHWC Annual Report 1924, p. 7.
53 Thomson, 'Women in medicine', pp. 205–42.
54 EHWC Annual Report 1930, pp. 6–7.
55 EHWC Annual Report 1923, p. 3.
56 EHWC Annual Report 1925, p. 10.
57 EHWC Annual Report 1926, p. 4. MOH Annual Report 1919, p. 24.
58 As David Armstrong has observed, the dispensary was no longer simply a place where people came for treatment. Under the auspices of the state and, in this context, in the hands of the medical women, it now 'radiated out into the community. Illness was sought, identified and monitored by various techniques and agents in the community; the dispensary building was merely the co-ordinating centre'. D. Armstrong, *Political Anatomy of the Body: Medical Knowledge in Britain in the Twentieth Century*, Cambridge: Cambridge University Press, 1983, p. 8.

6   British voluntary hospitals and the public sphere

Contribution and participation before the National Health Service

Martin Gorsky, Martin Powell and John Mohan [*]

> We hope to induce all who are concerned for the Miseries of the poor laborious Part of Mankind...to join in promoting and further extending an Undertaking...calculated for their Relief, and thereby for the good of the Community in general.
>
> (*An Account of the Bristol Infirmary*, 1739)[1]

> It is pleasing to note that in some instances the industrious working classes have evinced their gratitude for benefits received, or in the prospect of relief, when overtaken by sickness and disease, have manifested a desire to support it by accumulative contributions in small sums.
>
> (*The State of the Bristol Infirmary*, 1846)[2]

> The community no longer regards hospital care as charity and the Almoner, in her capacity as assessor of patients' payments no longer dispenses but collects.
>
> (*Annual Report of the Bristol Royal Infirmary*, 1947)[3]

These three extracts chart the changing relationship between a large provincial hospital and the public who supported it over the course of two centuries. The first is from one of its earliest reports and epitomizes the approach to funding and treatment adopted at the inception of the British voluntary hospital movement.[4] Within the 'community' that the infirmary served, the 'worthy contributors' were clearly differentiated from the recipients: 'our poor brethren', 'the sick and needy'.[5] Only the labouring poor were assumed to require institutional care, while the benefit for the donor lay in the externalities the hospital provided. The second, from the mid-nineteenth century, provides an early glimpse of the impending transition in the nature of the voluntary hospitals' finance and utilization. Alongside the philanthropy of urban elites they began to rely also on the funds of the workers who expected to use the institutions themselves.[6] By the 1920s such payment by patients had been systematically organized, either through mass contributory schemes or by means testing carried out by almoners, so that the stamp of paternalism associated with admission regimes based on subscriber recommendation had all but disappeared.[7] The third extract is from the Infirmary's final report, produced in the interval between the passage of the National Health Service Act and the 'appointed day' on which the voluntary hospitals were to be nationalized. The Almoner's Department was to be renamed the Welfare Department, prompting the observation that public opinion now rejected the notion of hospital care as charitable dispensation. Currently a right founded upon contribution, it was shortly to become a right founded upon citizenship alone.

At first glance, this narrative of broadening entitlement might be fitted comfortably within an analysis of welfare development that emphasizes the leading role of democratization and the expansion of citizenship.[8] However, a central feature of the present 'crisis' of the welfare state has been the conviction that it has engendered a passive citizenship rather than the active engagement anticipated by its founders.[9] Conservatives have highlighted the tendency of state welfare to encourage dependency, as an 'excess of democracy' fosters ever-growing claims by special interest groups for costly benefits.[10] Left and right alike have drawn attention to the way in which individuals have been thwarted by the bureaucratic rigidity and professional self-interest that drive up costs and prevent them from obtaining the welfare goods they need.[11] Within the NHS part of the rationale for organizational reform since 1991 has been the concern with 'provider capture' (by doctors and administrators) of the service, at the expense of the citizen.[12] More broadly, the influence of communitarian ideas has been instrumental in undermining the concept of citizenship that emphasizes rights over duties.[13] Within the history of social policy a particularly influential notion is that of the 'citizenship of contribution'. This was advanced by Finlayson in a reworking of the idea of citizenship that aimed to restate the significance of voluntary action. Drawing on the rhetoric of voluntary-sector leaders Finlayson suggested that the active, contributing citizen embodied characteristics of individual initiative, self-reliance, freedom of choice in social action and a genuine engagement in public affairs – all virtues absent from the welfare state's 'citizenship of entitlement'.[14] This perspective accords closely with arguments in favour of the revival of civil society as a panacea for the problems faced by the welfare state. Thus stakeholding is held to promote greater personal involvement in such areas as thrift and education, while voluntary and mutual associations are admired for those features that statutory arrangements are thought to lack. For example, they enrich democracy through encouraging civic participation and forging bonds of trust; they empower users, offering them a greater range of choices over their welfare requirements; and they provide an outlet for the fundamental human ethical impulse of reciprocal altruism.[15]

The concerns voiced in the late twentieth century about the role of the citizen in the welfare state therefore invite a reconsideration of earlier arrangements. The aim of this chapter is to analyse the changing 'citizenship of contribution and entitlement' in British hospitals prior to the establishment of the NHS. Its concern is the scope for participation offered by the pre-1948 health services, with their mixed economy of voluntary and local government providers. In particular it will discuss the extent and implications of the reorganization of hospital finance and utilization suggested by the opening quotations. Did the broadening of contribution to hospitals genuinely provide new channels by which the 'community' formulated views and policy in the way hinted at above?

A helpful framework for addressing these issues is provided by Jürgen Habermas in his *The Structural Transformation of the Public Sphere*.[16] Habermas's account of the emergence and decline of the bourgeois public sphere is rather different from accounts that concentrated on incremental gains in political and social rights. Instead, the capacity of the active private citizen to engage in critical debate was undermined in the nineteenth century as political discourse was captured by organized interest groups. Where Marshall argued that the 'instruments of modern democracy (newspapers, political meetings etc.) were fashioned by the upper classes then handed down...to the lower', Habermas sees instead the debasement of the media through 'the publicist self-presentations of privileged private interests'.[17] Though popular assent was intermittently obtained in the electoral process for the actions of the state apparatus, this did not amount to 'substantive democracy' entailing 'genuine participation of citizens in the process of political will-formation'.[18] Quiescence resulted from passivity – 'civic privatism' – as people set aside political engagement to enjoy the fruits of advanced capitalism, in the form of money, leisure time and security.[19] Habermas analyses the 'social-welfare state' from a Marxian perspective as the agent of class compromise. Thus the state, acting in the interest of 'private goals of profit maximisation' bears responsibility for the collective commodities of social consumption, to alleviate the worst, and politically most dangerous, effects of the mode of production. Though the direction of social reform was originally set by the activity of the labour movement it also served to produce surplus value through developing the infrastructure, and to buttress civic privatism through alleviating social risk.[20]

The role of the voluntary sector is only intermittently developed in this schema. In the classic age of the bourgeois public sphere it was the voluntary arena of clubs and cultural institutions that, alongside the press and new public spaces, provided the forum for private citizens to engage in debate and decision-making. Habermas does not deal specifically with the subsequent trajectory of charitable voluntary associations in his account of the disintegration of the public sphere. His emphasis is placed rather on the capture of media and cultural outlets by the leisure industry, the undermining of the autonomy of the family, the penetration of the private sphere of social welfare by the state and the increasing grip on public debate by 'private bureaucracies, special interest groups, parties and public administration'.[21] However, his later work suggests that he sees an enduring role for voluntarism in the twentieth century as a locus of popular participation. Following Claus Offe, he identifies citizens' initiatives and neighbourhood associations as destabilizing forces that threaten civic privatism by politicizing the public realm.[22]

It is therefore of considerable interest to place the history of the British hospital within Habermas's account. His juxtaposition of the ideal of a critically reasoning public with the reality of civic disempowerment invites a pessimistic reading of the changing contours of the right to hospital treatment. However, empirical findings that apparently point to broadening participation in the 1920s and 1930s raise difficulties for the chronology of 'disintegration' that he advances. Habermas has suggested that under the 'social-welfare state' the public sphere might only be reactivated 'on an altered basis...under the mutual control of rival organisations committed to the public sphere in their internal structure as well as in their relations with the state and each other'.[23] Did the arrangements for the shaping of hospital policy before 1948, both in local government and the voluntary sector, evince these features?

Changing patterns of hospital funding

As Eley has noted, Habermas's depiction of the emergent public sphere in the eighteenth and early nineteenth centuries has been both amplified and authenticated by urban, political and social historians writing since the publication of *Structural Transformation* in 1962.[24] A wealth of findings have appeared on the efflorescence of voluntary institutions of the middling classes in the provincial city, some emphasizing their role in ameliorating the stresses of rapid urban growth and others their centrality to the formation of middle-class identity.[25] The voluntary hospitals were among the most heavily capitalized and widely supported of these ventures and they shared various characteristics that Habermas claimed for the new literary and political institutions. These included the leading role of urban middle-class elites, from whom the majority of subscribers and donors were drawn, and who staffed the management boards. Transparent financing was ensured by the publication of audited accounts in the hospitals' annual report, conforming to what Habermas called 'the mandate of publicity'.[26] Participatory democracy was enshrined in quarterly or annual meetings at which qualifying 'governors' (typically the annual subscribers) were entitled to vote on policy. These features distinguished voluntary hospitals from traditional charitable endowments administered by closed corporate bodies with their taint of venality.[27] And, as Kathleen Wilson argues, in their commitment to accountability they represented a model of a more open politics, standing in radical contrast to the Hanoverian state.[28] Of course, not all subscribers were actively involved; some were motivated less by civic engagement than by the desire to assert status in the social pecking order or to wear the badge of political partisanship.[29] However, the essence of the Habermasian public sphere – 'private people gathered together as a public...articulating the needs of society' – was clearly discernible: in trustee meetings to develop hospital rules, in governors' elections of doctors to honorary posts, in sermons that expounded the rationale of provision, and in the individual decisions of subscribers when approached by those who sought their patronage and an admission note.[30] The voluntary hospital can also be said to have mediated between state and society in respect of poverty. By delineating a section of society – the industrious poor – which the public considered worthy of philanthropic aid it effectively consigned other groups, like the elderly, the mobile and those with chronic and infectious diseases, to the statutory authorities.[31]

It is also possible to see in voluntary hospital history the disintegration of the bourgeois public sphere that Habermas placed in the later nineteenth century. Central to this process was the diminishing role of the private citizen, the lay subscriber, and the growing dominance of interest groups in the making of policy.

The 'medicalization' of the hospital, in the sense of an orientation towards treatment founded upon medical science rather than philanthropic succour, was already under way in the Georgian era, with the formalization of teaching arrangements and of systematic clinical observation.[32] Henceforth hospital doctors exercised ever greater control over admissions and medical policy, owing to the enhanced authority of the profession, and the growth of the hospitals' capital assets, which allowed the expansion of patient capacity beyond the limits placed by the annual subscriptions.[33] Tensions between consultants and trustee bodies persisted, with many hospitals preferring to assign their medical staffs to a sub-committee that acted in an advisory capacity to the lay governing boards.[34] Nonetheless, their unhesitating willingness to fund the cost of 'scientific research and discoveries of swifter and better ways of healing' suggests that lay trustees still worked within a dominant paradigm established by the medical profession.[35] At the same time hospital infrastructure became larger and more complex, mirroring developments in factories and office buildings. Electrification, the mechanization of laundries, lifts and communications, the increasing specialization demanded of medical nursing and ancillary staff, all demanded a greater level of managerial oversight than the charitable visitor could provide. Governors became more absorbed in the intricacies of management, employing salaried staff to deal with issues like fund-raising, record-keeping and accounting, so that hospital administration emerged as a profession, with its standardized procedures, its own journal and its own particular concerns.[36] The broad involvement of donors in hospital management therefore gave way, leaving governorship 'in the hands of a small, wealthy clique'; some were highly committed, others more like 'the big business man who dashes in for five minutes and is out in four'.[37]

The consolidation of control by interest groups at the expense of the active citizen occurred within the context of a changing pattern of contribution to the voluntary hospital. The long-run shift in the composition of different income sources, with charity in decline and patient payment and provident schemes on the rise, was first demonstrated by Pinker, with reference to four sample years.[38] Figure 6.1 presents a fuller sequence, showing the components of income between the late nineteenth century and the Second World War. Its source is a series of yearbooks produced by voluntary sector advocates, beginning in 1889, which provide a systematic collation of annual income statistics.[39] The first striking feature of the graph is the relative decline of the 'charity' component, which here includes sums raised through donations, legacies, entertainments and collections. By contrast income from patients, in the form of mass contributory schemes or direct payment for services, expanded from a minor element to the point in 1938 where it was the source of about half of all income. 'Other' income embraces interest earned on assets and subventions from the state or local authorities; its share remained fairly stable at first, and then rose in the 1920s when additional funds were granted by the Exchequer for the treatment of tuberculosis, venereal disease and maternity and child welfare. The 'subscriptions' category refers to sums pledged annually, and at the start of the sequence it accounted for about a quarter of total income. If it were possible to extend the series back

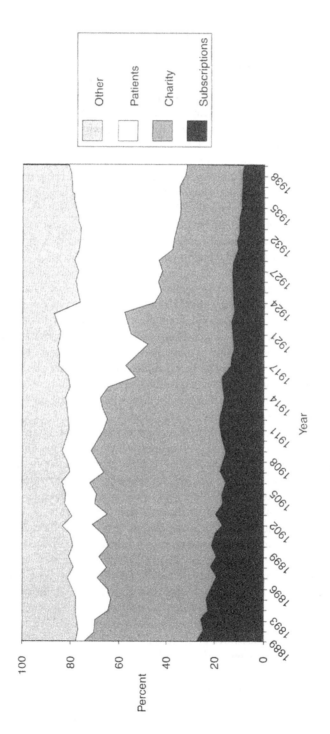

Figure 6.1 Composition of income of voluntary hospitals in England, Wales and Scotland, 1889–1938

further the role of subscription would have been even larger, as it was not unusual for hospitals in their early years to draw as much as half their income from this source.[40] Thus part of the decline in significance of charity as an element of hospital income was the demise of the actively involved philanthropist, who as subscriber and governor had been the one-time lynch-pin of the public sphere.

In fact, the diminishing role of the private charitable citizen was rather more advanced than the national pattern of income suggests. Consideration of subscription details in the annual reports of individual hospitals reveals that it was no longer only the lay philanthropist who made this type of gift, but institutions also. Table 6.1 examines the 'subscriptions' category in six general hospitals situated in Newcastle, Aberdeen, Bristol and London, separating the sums given by private individuals from those given by institutions, mostly firms, but also friendly societies, schools, corporations, parishes and clubs.[41] In all cases other than London's Royal Northern the proportion subscribed by firms was on the increase, and for two of the hospitals the trend may be viewed from 1831 to emphasize the scale of growth. Over the long run hospital subscription was less and less the preserve of the lay voluntarist and increasingly dominated by firms, for whom it was both an act of charity (for which, from 1921, tax relief could be claimed) and a means of ensuring hospital provision for their employees.[42] There was distinct variation between the metropolis and the provinces, with subscriptions in the northern cities almost entirely paid by institutions, those in Bristol more evenly distributed and those in London still predominantly from individuals. This may reflect the greater availability of pay beds in the capital, and the resilience of philanthropy on the part of its aristocratic and business elite.[43]

In terms of absolute numbers then, private charitable subscribers represented only a tiny proportion of the population by the 1930s. For example, in Newcastle around 400 persons subscribed to the Royal Victoria Infirmary (RVI), whose departments and medical school served a catchment of around 1 million people,

Table 6.1 Institutional subscriptions as percent of all subscriptions

| | Hospital | | | | | |
	RVI	*ARI*	*BRI*	*BGH*	*RR*	*RN*
1831	40		24			
1851	60		25			
1891	60	69	34	42	14	37
1901	67	73	35	47	14	22
1911	72	90	33	43	21	32
1921	87	88	48	47	29	23
1931	86	89	45	50	38	15

Key: RVI: Royal Victoria Infirmary, Newcastle-upon-Tyne; ARI: Aberdeen Royal Infirmary; BRI: Bristol Royal Infirmary; BGH: Bristol General Hospital; RR: Royal Richmond Hospital; RN: Royal Northern Hospital.

while in Bristol about 6,000 persons subscribed to the Royal and the General, which between them served a city of nearly 400,000 as well as its adjoining counties. This contrasts with the situation in eighteenth-century cities, where the numbers recorded in subscription lists suggest the majority of middle-class families were local infirmary benefactors.[44] As the significance of the individual subscriber fell, so hospitals began to abandon the use of the subscriber's prerogative to admit non-emergency patients by a signed note.[45] Some did so before 1900, and well before contributory insurance was significant; an early example was Newcastle's RVI which in 1888 became a 'free' institution, in which admission depended only on the doctor's assessment of medical need and the constraints of the waiting list.[46] More generally, hospitals retained the formal existence of the subscriber's note, on the grounds that the abolition of the privilege could deter potential donors.[47] Of the 111 London hospitals listed in *Burdett's* yearbook in 1928, 52 per cent preserved the subscriber's note system, though only eight institutions used it exclusively; the rest combined notes with free admission and/or patient payments.[48] Thus despite formal retention the practice fell into disuse: in Gloucestershire Royal Hospital, which recorded mode of admission in its annual report, 53 per cent of inpatients were admitted by subscribers' notes in 1875, falling to 11 per cent in 1900, and to 0.3 per cent (11 patients) by 1935.[49]

What all this suggests is that the input of the lay subscriber – the private citizen in the public sphere – was being superseded, both by institutional givers and by the various forms of patient payments. This shift to a reliance on funds received from patients or potential patients was by no means an even process, and Figure 6.2 maps the geographical variations, based on the income statistics of the largest voluntary hospitals recorded in the hospital yearbooks.[50] At the turn of the century the patient contribution was relatively undeveloped, initially flourishing in the North-East and the Midlands. By the 1930s a similar regional distribution was apparent, although now hospitals in the South and East Anglia had joined those areas where income from patients was more significant. Common to all these places was the insufficiency of traditional funding sources for financing the expansion deemed necessary to meet perceived demands. However, the means adopted to elicit payment from the broad mass of hospital users varied considerably. Most fundamentally, hospitals might choose either to concentrate on organized low-cost contributory schemes, some with a pre-payment element, or on extracting fees from patients at the point of service. This is an important distinction, because only the former method carried rights of participation. The aggregate figures furnished in the yearbooks do not separate the two methods, so Figure 6.3 draws on the annual reports of twelve large hospitals to illustrate the different approaches.[51] In London the contributory schemes' impact was dispersed due to the large concentration of hospitals, and there a policy of charging, either according to means or at full cost in private wards, was pursued.[52] Aberdeen drew on both workplace arrangements and a system of 'patients' donations', while in Oxford the Radcliffe Infirmary opted for an insurance scheme, begun in 1920, based on a subscription of 2d weekly.[53] In

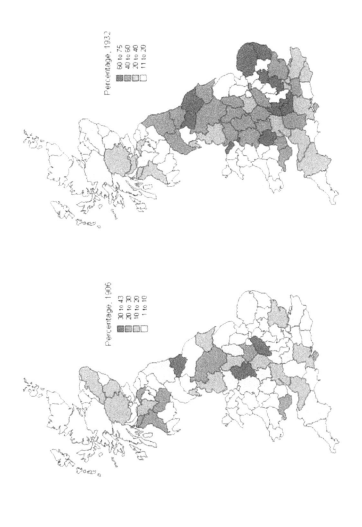

Figure 6.2 Proportion of voluntary hospital income derived from contributory schemes or patient payments, 1906 and 1932

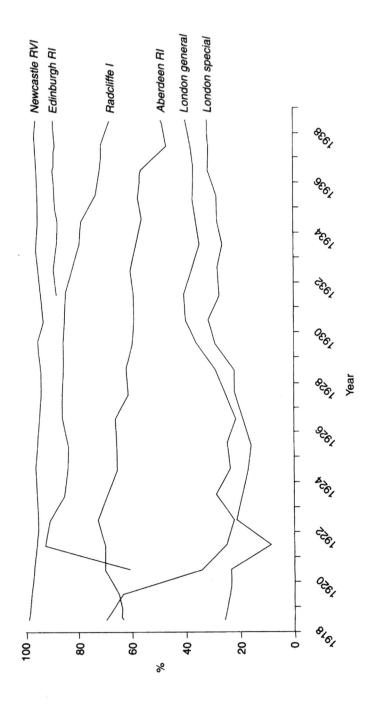

Figure 6.3 Contributory schemes as a proportion of income from patients in selected British voluntary hospitals, 1918–38

Edinburgh the Infirmary only countenanced direct payment by maternity patients, and relied instead on its 'League of Subscribers', established in 1917 by the managers and the local Trades Council.[54] Newcastle's RVI had built up its workplace schemes after abandoning subscriber admission. Their base had initially been in the city's engineering and munitions firms, but early in the century schemes were promoted in the coalfields of Durham and Northumberland, and by 1938 they provided 58 per cent of all income.[55]

As indicated in Figure 6.1, it was not until the late 1910s that a distinct shift from philanthropy to mass payment occurred nationally. Workmen's contributions had begun in about the 1850s, when rising real wages permitted a greater degree of saving and insurance. Later some had been formalized in the Hospital Saturday funds, whereby a single day was designated for an annual works collection.[56] The late nineteenth century also saw private patients accepted in voluntary hospitals for the first time, and by 1910 there were 502 pay beds in London's hospitals.[57] Meanwhile, factories, mines, shipyards and workshops proceeded to develop contributory arrangements whereby regular sums were given direct from wages. Figure 6.2 hints that these appeared first in areas whose industries had a tradition of collective workplace organization, though individual cases show that it was proselytizing by the hospitals that was the spur: for example Newcastle's success in pioneering contributory funds was attributed to the hospital's programme of 'education, education, and still more education' to inform local trades unionists about the RVI's functions.[58] However, these early developments were relatively insignificant. The real watershed was the financial hardship suffered at the end of the First World War, when the hospitals confronted a backlog of delayed spending on infrastructure, coinciding with spiralling prices, the influenza pandemic and the collapse of charitable gifts due to heavy taxation. This was the point at which many institutions first employed almoners, either to vet prospective patients and elicit part payment according to income, as in Bristol Royal Infirmary, or to persuade free patients to join a contributory scheme, as in the RVI. The 1921 report of the Cave Committee, which the government had appointed to enquire into hospital finance, also prompted those institutions still without contributory schemes to implement them. Rapid growth followed: in Edinburgh for example the League of Subscribers began by contributing about £4,000 in 1919, rising to over £20,000 ten years later, by which time it had more than 100,000 members from 1,418 separate businesses each paying 1d a week.[59] Private payment of all kinds grew too, with London's pay bed complement rising to 2,260 by 1938.[60]

Contribution and participation

This lengthy empirical detour shows that the history of hospital support conforms to Habermas's account of the withdrawal of the private citizen from the public sphere. However, the nature of this transition in the British voluntary hospitals raises a problem for another aspect of his thesis. For Habermas, the 'refeudalization' of the public sphere led directly to the twentieth-century social-welfare state, whose policies were not determined by consensus arising from rational-critical debate, but by the wishes of powerful interest groups.[61] Perhaps with Bismarckian social security legislation in mind, he characterized state welfare as an arrangement imposed from above without due public discussion. Its over-riding purpose was the 'pacification of class conflict', by which the burdens created by late capitalist conditions of work were made 'subjectively bearable'. While acknowledging its superiority to earlier poor-law arrangements, he insisted on the loss of individual autonomy in the process of 'juridification' which entitle-ment to welfare benefits entailed, a process involving 'the bureaucratization and monetarization' of social relations.[62] This may be an appropriate analysis of the situation in German hospitals, where, by the 1920s, public hospital bed capacity exceeded that of the voluntaries by a factor of seven, where the prestigious university hospitals had long been state-run, and where patient costs were met principally from insurance funds, municipal payments and private fees.[63] The British hospital, by contrast, did not respond to the demise of bourgeois philan-thropy by surrendering to state control as in Germany, or by turning predominantly to private fees as in the United States.[64] Instead it reinvented and reinvigorated its sources of voluntary support through the development of the workers' contributory schemes.

The inception and expansion of contributory schemes prompts us to ask how far Habermas's account of the refeudalization of the public sphere is applicable to the case of British hospitals. Were the contributory schemes anything more than a voluntary version of the state-dominated and bureaucratic system of hospital funding that developed in Germany? Or do they signify instead the revival of the public sphere that stood between the state and the individual, offering a rational public a democratically accountable forum for critical debate, to which hospital governors were genuinely responsive? Put another way, did the new citizenship of contribution bring with it genuine participation of the type suggested by Finlayson?[65] Earlier verdicts are mixed. Trainor notes that workmen hospital governors in the late-Victorian Black Country largely acqui-esced with the wishes of hospital trustees, playing 'no more than a supporting role' in key decisions.[66] Cherry argues that where contributory schemes were associated with individual hospitals conflict over policy could arise and the influ-ence of their representatives could be felt.[67] A contemporary perspective, delivered in the influential 1937 report of Political and Economic Planning, noted that as a scheme grew larger and more bureaucratic, so its 'sense of responsibility to its constituents is likely to diminish'.[68] A bleaker judgement was famously passed by Aneurin Bevan in the second reading of the NHS Bill. Drawing on his experience in South Wales, the Labour health minister angrily contrasted the massive scale of the workers' financial contribution with their invisibility on hospital management boards: 'We had an annual meeting and a cordial vote of thanks was passed to the manager of the colliery company for his generosity...but nobody passed a vote of thanks to the miners.'[69]

The first issue to be resolved is whether the schemes can be regarded as genuinely voluntary organizations that sought to represent their members' views rather than simply elicit financial support. Certainly a number of schemes, such as those in Oxford, Gloucester and Winchester, did not pretend to be anything other than insurance or pre-payment arrangements, and, as noted above, there were considerable differences in the extent to which different hospitals relied on mass schemes at all, as opposed to direct payment.[70] But, in many cases, the hospital leadership made every effort to portray the contributory scheme as bringing the principle of voluntary subscription within the means of the low-paid. Terms such as 'free-will offerings' were used to describe the sums raised, so that they should not be confused with a form of insurance or pre-payment; instead they were held to denote 'civic spirit', and the affection in which ordinary citizens held 'their' hospital.[71] The cover of the League of Subscribers' report from Edinburgh Royal Infirmary (Figure 6.4) nicely captures the ethos of mutualism surrounding the schemes. In their more candid moments hospital managers acknowledged the subscribers' expectation of a 'quid pro quo' – free treatment when required – but it was still important to maintain publicly that these were entirely voluntary donations.[72] If specific entitlements *had* been given then the basis for other philanthropic gifts would be undermined and the spectre raised of doctors claiming payments for their services. However, the implication of this stance was that the characteristic voluntary sector procedures of subscriber democracy had to be built into the schemes. One approach was to admit workmen governors who would attend the Annual General Meeting and exercise voting rights in elections to the board of management. In Newcastle's RVI, one workman governor could be sent for each £10 contributed by an individual workplace, resulting in healthy representation from the ship-builders Swan Hunter, the munitions firm Armstrong Whitworth and from the miners of Durham and Northumberland. The Edinburgh League of Subscribers had its own executive and an AGM at which two League members were elected managers on the hospital board. All subscribers had rights to vote and nominate candidates for the management board and the executive, which was empowered to consult 'upon any matter concerning the business and work of the League'.[73] The AGMs were advertised in the local press: in 1930 270 members turned out to cast their votes and discuss the dire state of the Infirmary's waiting list.[74] This was clearly not 'civic privatism'.

Contributory schemes could therefore provide a real conduit for popular opinion. To assess the extent to which they actually facilitated democratic outcomes, the next problem is to identify the issues that affected members. As the previous example hints, the availability of beds when required by patients/contributors was a prime concern. There was good reason for limited provision to loom large as a problem in this period. The enthusiasm of 'every man and woman, irrespective of class' for hospital attendance 'to the maximum extent' had risen in the late nineteenth century.[75] However, this burgeoning demand confronted the uneven geography of voluntary hospital distribution, the legacy of its unplanned and localist development. It can be shown that there were significant variations in bed provision, staffing and in-patient admissions at the county level.[76] Broadly London, the South-East, the South-West and the

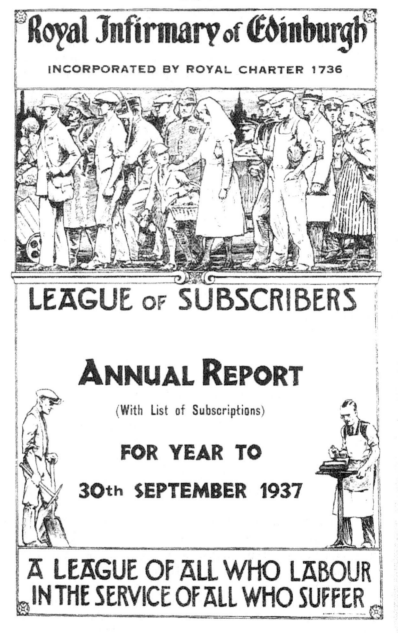

Figure 6.4 Cover of Edinburgh Royal Infirmary *League of Subscribers Annual Report*, 1937

Midlands were the best served parts of England, and in Scotland the central urban belt, as well as some of the thinly populated Highland counties. Individual cities such as Oxford, with bed provision of 5.7 per 1,000 persons in 1931, may be compared with Merthyr, with a bed level of 1.35.[77] The broadening of the funding base eased this situation to some extent, with the mean number of beds per 1,000 persons in the British counties rising from 0.8 in 1901 to 1.1 in 1921 and to 1.4 by 1938. However, the overall growth in provision was not accompanied by a significant narrowing of regional differences: the coefficients of variation (which indicate the extent of differences between counties) stood at 0.7 in both 1901 and 1921, falling to only 0.6 by 1931.[78]

The problem of insufficient accommodation raised two questions for contributory scheme members beyond that of their own financial input. First, what was their relationship to be with hospitals in the statutory sector? In the 1920s they generally would not countenance using a Poor Law infirmary, but with the emergence of the municipal general hospital after 1929 the prospect arose of using public institutions to ease pressure on waiting lists.[79] This raised a further difficulty: local authorities were empowered to charge patients who had not been referred to hospital through the relieving officer. If contributory scheme patients were charged, they would be paying twice for the service they had expected to receive in 'their' voluntary hospital; if not then the local authority was effectively subsidizing the voluntary sector. Different towns resolved the issue in their own way. In Liverpool the municipal hospitals gave free treatment to members of the local scheme, the Merseyside Hospitals Council, at a cost far in excess of sums received back from the scheme.[80] In Edinburgh however the repeated efforts of the League of Subscribers to persuade the Infirmary Board and the City Council to reach such an agreement came to nothing, and contributors sent to the municipal hospital to clear the ERI's waiting list became liable for the charges levied there. Despite clear and repeated articulation of the wishes of users, policy did not alter, in this case because the rivalry and ill-feeling between the leaders of the voluntary and public hospitals prevented compromise.[81] The League itself was reluctant to advocate a full pre-payment scheme at a level acceptable to both hospitals, as this would have meant increasing the subscriptions on a scale many could not afford.[82]

A second issue arising was the acceptability of introducing pay beds for private patients. Rather than viewing this as a sensible means of bringing in additional funds, contributory scheme members worried that it breached the principle of free treatment and extended provision in a way that did not benefit them.[83] For instance, in 1935 managers of the Sunderland Royal Infirmary proposed to augment income by designating some wards entirely for fee-paying patients. Workmen's representatives opposed this on the grounds that the full facilities of the hospital should be devoted to 'poor people who could not afford to pay fees'; however, they failed to block the change.[84] The Board of the Edinburgh Royal Infirmary also had a torrid time trying to sell the principle of pay beds to the League of Subscribers. At the 1936 AGM Lord Fleming asked rhetorically:

> If you say 'free treatment for all'…that would mean that a man with an income of £3,000 or £4,000 would be entitled to go into the Royal Infirmary and not pay a penny. I would ask you all to consider whether you are in favour of that sort of thing. (Cries of 'Yes' and 'We are'.)

A voice from the floor then informed the managers: 'If there is any intention of making charges to the poorer classes for treatment…the League of Subscribers are not going to have it.'[85] This stance deterred the Infirmary from implementing formal charges until the opening of the new Maternity Pavilion in 1939, although it continued to benefit from 'patients' donations'.

In addition to these core concerns the contributors' relationship to the hospital could give rise to various other issues. For instance, many schemes were initially attached to a single hospital, and this posed a difficulty for members who found themselves having to enter another institution, due perhaps to labour mobility or residence.[86] The solutions arrived at were either to extend the number of hospitals covered by the scheme or to make a series of mutual agreements with neighbouring schemes allowing for a transfer payment when the member of one entered the hospital of the other.[87] In this case it was in the interest of hospital governors as much as members to develop such arrangements as they increased income, and by 1939 a network of inter-scheme contracts was developing.[88] A more contentious issue was the attitude of contributors to the medical staff. In 1936 the Court of Governors of the Sunderland Royal faced a serious split, when the workmen governors moved to dismiss a doctor who had made himself unpopular with miners through his treatment of industrial injury claims. As in the pay bed case the previous year, they were unsuccessful.[89]

These are anecdotes drawn from only a handful of individual cases, but they do suggest a broad conclusion about the capacity of contributory schemes to operate as a 'sphere of ongoing participation in a rational-critical debate concerning public authority'.[90] Their representative structures did permit popular views to be aired and potentially to influence policy. However, the extent to which they were actually able to effect change remained circumscribed. This was because decisions were taken by hospital boards, which, despite permitting limited representation of the mass contributors, remained dominated by local elites and medical professionals.[91] For instance, in Edinburgh the twenty-eight-strong Board of Management included seven workmen governors, alongside four from the Royal Colleges of Surgeons and Physicians, two from the University Senate, five members of local professional associations and six from the ordinary subscribers.[92] A similar situation obtained in hospitals that had pioneered the contributory principle: in the RVI, of the forty-four members on the hospital committee in 1901 only twelve were nominated by the works governors, and this in-built minority persisted into the inter-war period. Where contributors sought to change the balance of power the status quo was easily defended. In Aberdeen an attempt at the 1920 AGM to achieve 'sectional representation' for workers on the Board of Directors was brushed aside, and henceforth the only record of dissent on the part of mass contributors was a dispute over whether granite should be used in the building of the new Infirmary.[93] In Sunderland, workmen aggrieved at the repeated rebuffs sought to alter their representation on the Board, where they were outnumbered two to one by the charitable subscribers and the honorary staff, to reflect more accurately their financial contribution. Again they failed, admonished by the Chairman that the Board's job was to 'do their best for the Infirmary and not simply to represent a sectional interest'.[94] The problem then did not lie in the suppression of rational debate or the absence of publicity, but rather in the inflexible power structure that perpetuated the hierarchical character of voluntarism and protected the interests of doctors.

Conclusions

Situating the history of British voluntary hospitals within Habermas's account of the rise and transformation of the public sphere yields a rather pessimistic insight into the role of the citizen in the formulation of policy. In many respects the disappearance of the private subscriber, the emergence of institutional contribution and the administrative development of the hospital did illustrate the disintegration of the public sphere, in the sense of private people conferring 'in an unrestricted fashion…about matters of general interest'.[95] However, these changes also presented the possibility of a revivified public sphere in the early twentieth century associated with the broadening of financial contribution and the appearance of workmen governors, coupled with the enduring tradition of open accounting and statistical reporting. In practice, though, this reconstituted public sphere was not fully successful in promoting debate and consensus. The local case studies point instead to the retention of power in hospital government by established trustee bodies and medical staff, allowing the express wishes of the mass contributors sometimes to be over-ruled.

Nonetheless, it would be hard to argue that the broadening of entitlement to hospital care in this period was not a benign development. The erosion of the idea of hospital medicine as charitable dispensation increased access for a public enthusiastic about institutional treatment. Nor are these changes incompatible with Habermas's speculative vision of the good society 'bringing about social relations in which mutuality predominates and satisfaction does not mean the triumph of one over the repressed needs of the other'.[96] They did not arise directly from a new 'citizenship of contribution' on the part of hospital subscribers; this was curtailed by the often sclerotic power structure of the voluntary hospitals. Instead their proximate causes were the financial necessities that underpinned the decline of hierarchical charity in the voluntaries. However, mass contribution did reshape popular expectations about services, cost and social stigma.[97] As the introduction suggested, both political rhetoric and private policy documents now laid claim to a distinct shift in public opinion regarding the right to hospital treatment. Moves towards an integrated hospital system which presaged the NHS were made in the name of 'an informed public' – a public that now put the quality of treatment before a commitment to voluntarism and which was 'beginning to feel that the hospitals belong to them, that they go there by right of citizenship'.[98]

To what extent did the NHS facilitate citizen participation in hospital management, and the representation of the interests of users of the service? Voluntary fund-raising in support of hospitals has consistently been encouraged, but NHS authorities have arguably lacked democratic accountability, as was feared by proponents of local government control in the wartime debates. Although local authorities were granted the right to nominate some members to health authorities from 1974, they are no longer able to do so, and management boards of health authorities now consist of a small number of executive directors balanced by appointed non-executives. Consumer representation was not institutionalized until the establishment of Community Health Councils in 1974. Although these were largely reactive bodies with few powers, they had a statutory right to be consulted on changes to the delivery of services and they could therefore put a case for those most affected. The recent NHS Plan[99] argues that the health service must be 'designed around the patient'. It claims that 'for the first time patients will have a real say in the NHS'. However, the document proposes the abolition of Community Health Councils, and there are concerns about the efficacy of the proposed complex and unwieldy alternative arrangements. Discussions about health care provision are therefore characterized by limited public debate. There are occasional high-profile campaigns about the closure of individual hospitals, spilling over into the electoral arena, as in the recent election of an MP on a single-issue platform concerning the closure of a hospital in Worcestershire, but apart from these there seems little public concern about the erosion of participation. In this sense, civic privatism, in Habermas's terms, may be said to be in the ascendant, and despite occasional proposals for the reinvigoration of participation in and control of hospitals[100] there seems little prospect of this situation being reversed.

Acknowledgements

The authors gratefully acknowledge the financial support of the Leverhulme Trust.

Notes

* The order in which the authors' names appear reflects their respective contributions to the paper.
1 *An Account of the Bristol Infirmary from the First Institution to this Time*, Bristol, 1739, p. 4.
2 Bristol Record Office (BRO) 35893/21/a, *The State of the Bristol Infirmary*, Bristol, 1846.
3 BRO 35893/21/r, Bristol Royal Infirmary, *Annual Report of the Bristol Royal Infirmary*, Bristol, 1947.
4 B. Abel-Smith, *The Hospitals 1800–1948: A Study in Social Administration in England and Wales*, London: Heinemann, 1964, pp. 5–6, 36; A. Berry, 'Community sponsorship and the hospital patient in late eighteenth century England', in R. Smith and P. Horden (eds), *The Locus of Care: Families, Communities, Institutions, and the Provision of Welfare since Antiquity*, London: Routledge, 1998, pp. 126–50.
5 Josiah Tucker, *A sermon preach'd in the parish church of St James in Bristol*, London, 1746, pp. 4, 26.

6 S. Yeo, *Religion and Voluntary Organizations in Crisis*, London: Croom Helm, 1976, pp. 211–18.
7 S. Cherry, 'Before the National Health Service: financing the voluntary hospitals, 1900–1939', *Economic History Review*, 1997, vol. 50, pp. 305–26.
8 As formulated by T.H. Marshall in his classic essay on citizenship and social class, the winning of social rights in the twentieth century followed on the extension of civil rights in the eighteenth and the gradual widening of the franchise in the nineteenth. T.H. Marshall, *Citizenship and Social Class: And Other Essays*, Cambridge: Cambridge University Press, 1950. However, Marshall's thesis is generally examined in the context of statutory rather than voluntary provision. Moreover, fifty years on from Marshall the relationship between democracy and social rights has come to seem more problematic.
9 I. Culpitt, *Welfare and Citizenship: Beyond the Crisis of the Welfare State?*, London: Sage, 1992.
10 Summarized in H. Heclo, 'Toward a new welfare state', in P. Flora and A. Heidenheimer (eds), *The Development of Welfare States in Europe and America*, New Brunswick: Transaction Books, 1984, pp. 383–406, at pp. 398–401.
11 P. Hirst, *Associative Democracy: New Forms of Economic and Social Governance*, Cambridge: Polity, 1994; D.G. Green, *Re-inventing Civil Society: The Rediscovery of Welfare without Politics*, London: IEA Health and Welfare Unit, 1993.
12 C. Ham, *Public, Private or Community: What Next for the NHS?*, London: Demos, 1996.
13 D. Selbourne, *The Principle of Duty: An Essay on the Foundations of the Civic Order*, London: Sinclair-Stevenson, 1994; M. Ignatieff, 'Citizenship and moral narcissism', *Political Quarterly*, 1989, vol. 60.
14 G. Finlayson, *Citizen, State and Social Welfare in Britain, 1830–1990*, Oxford: Clarendon Press, 1994, pp. 8–9.
15 R.D. Putnam, *Making Democracy Work: Civic Traditions in Modern Italy*, Princeton: Princeton University Press, 1993; P. Hoggett and S. Thompson, 'The delivery of welfare: the associationist vision', in J. Carter (ed.), *Postmodernity and the Fragmentation of Welfare*, London: Routledge, 1998, pp. 237–51; G. Mulgan and C. Landry, *The Other Invisible Hand: Remaking Charity for the 21st Century*, London: Demos, 1995, pp. 14–21.
16 J. Habermas, *The Structural Transformation of the Public Sphere*, trans. T. Burger, Cambridge: Polity Press, 1989.
17 Marshall, *Citizenship*, p. 25; Habermas, *Structural Transformation*, p. 195.
18 J. Habermas, *Legitimation Crisis*, trans. T. McCarthy, London: Heinemann Educational, 1976, p. 36.
19 Ibid., pp. 37, 58, 74.
20 Ibid., pp. 54–5; J. Habermas, 'Marx and the theory of internal colonization', in W. Outhwaite (ed.), *The Habermas Reader*, Oxford: Polity, 1996, pp. 283–304, at pp. 287, 290–1.
21 Habermas, *Structural Transformation*, pp. 141–75, quotation at p. 176.
22 Habermas, *Legitimation Crisis*, p. 72; P.U. Hohendahl, 'Critical theory, public sphere and culture. Jurgen Habermas and his critics', *New German Critique*, 1979, vol. 16, pp. 89–118, at pp. 116–7.
23 J. Habermas, 'The public sphere: an encyclopedia article (1964)', *New German Critique*, 1974, vol. 3, pp. 49–55, at p. 55.
24 G. Eley, 'Nations, publics and public cultures: placing Habermas in the nineteenth century', in N. Dirks, G. Eley and S. Ortner (eds), *Culture/Power/History: A Reader in Contemporary Social Theory*, Princeton: Princeton University Press, 1994, pp. 297–335, at pp. 301–2.
25 R.J. Morris, *Class, Sect and Party: The Making of the British Middle Class, Leeds 1820–1850*, Manchester: Manchester University Press, 1990; N. McKendrick, J. Brewer and J.H. Plumb, *The Birth of a Consumer Society: The Commercialization of Eighteenth Century England*, London: Europa, 1982; P. Clark, *British Clubs and Societies, 1580–1800: The Origins of an*

Associational World, Oxford: Clarendon Press, 2000; J. Barry, 'Bourgeois collectivism? Urban association and the middling sort', in J. Barry and C. Brooks (eds), *The Middling Sort of People: Culture, Society and Politics in England, 1550–1800*, Basingstoke: Macmillan, 1994, pp. 84–112; M. Gorsky, *Patterns of Philanthropy: Charity and Society in Nineteenth Century Bristol*, Woodbridge: Royal Historical Society, 1999.

26 Habermas, *Structural Transformation*, p. 232.

27 A. Borsay, '"Persons of honour and reputation": the voluntary hospital in an age of corruption', *Medical History*, 1991, vol. 35, pp. 281–94; K. Wilson, 'Urban culture and political activism in Hanoverian England: the example of voluntary hospitals', in E. Hellmuth (ed.), *The Transformation of Political Culture: England and Germany in the Late Eighteenth Century*, Oxford: Oxford University Press, 1990, pp. 165–84, at pp. 167, 180–2; Gorsky, *Patterns of Philanthropy*, p. 60.

28 Wilson, 'Urban culture', pp. 167, 180–2.

29 Gorsky, *Patterns of Philanthropy*, pp. 122–7, 195–200; J. Seed, 'From "middling sort" to middle class in late eighteenth- and early nineteenth-century England', in M.L. Bush (ed.), *Social Orders and Social Classes in Europe since 1500: Studies in Social Stratification*, London: Longman, 1992, pp. 114–35. See also Adrian Wilson's chapter in the present volume.

30 Habermas, *Structural Transformation*, p. 176.

31 Wilson, 'Urban culture', pp. 178–9; M.E. Fissell, 'The "sick and drooping poor" in eighteenth century Bristol and its region', *Social History of Medicine*, 1989, vol. 2, pp. 35–58.

32 G.B. Risse, *Hospital Life in Enlightenment Scotland: Care and Teaching at the Royal Infirmary of Edinburgh*, Cambridge: Cambridge University Press, 1986.

33 M.E. Fissell, *Patients, Power, and the Poor in Eighteenth Century Bristol*, Cambridge: Cambridge University Press, 1991; Gorsky, *Patterns of Philanthropy*, pp. 189–90; K. Waddington, *Charity and the London Hospitals, 1850–1898*, Woodbridge: Royal Historical Society, 2000.

34 K. Waddington, 'The nursing dispute at Guy's Hospital, 1879–1880', *Social History of Medicine*, 1995, vol. 8, pp. 211–30; *Burdett's Hospitals and Charities: The Year Book of Philanthropy and Hospital Annual*, London, 1901, pp. 69–74.

35 London Metropolitan Archives (hereafter LMA), H9/GY/A94/9, Guy's Hospital, *Annual Report*, 1928.

36 S. Sturdy and R. Cooter, 'Science, scientific management, and the transformation of medicine in Britain c.1870–1950', *History of Science*, 1998, vol. 36, pp. 421–66, at p. 425; B.L. Craig, 'The role of records and record-keeping in the development of the modern hospital in London, England, and Ontario, Canada, c.1890–c.1940', *Bulletin of the History of Medicine*, 1991, vol. 65, pp. 376–97; *The Hospital Gazette*, renamed *The Hospital* in the 1930s.

37 K. Waddington, '"Grasping gratitude": charity and hospital finance in late-Victorian London', in M. Daunton (ed.), *Charity, Self-interest and Welfare in the English Past*, London: UCL Press, 1996, pp. 181–202, at p. 197; British Library of Economic and Political Science, BHCSA 3/9, British Hospitals Association Proceedings, 1936–7, 1 April 1936.

38 R. Pinker, *English Hospital Statistics 1861–1938*, London: Heinemann, 1966, pp. 152–84. C. Braithwaite, *The Voluntary Citizen: An Enquiry into the Place of Philanthropy in the Community*, London: Methuen, 1938, observed the rise of income from these sources between 1924 and 1934; see also Political and Economic Planning (PEP), *Report on the British Health Services*, London: PEP, 1937.

39 *Burdett's Hospitals and Charities*; Order of St John (OSJ), *Third–Ninth Annual Report on the Voluntary Hospitals in Great Britain (excluding London)*, London, 1921–1928; Central Bureau of Hospital Information, *The Hospitals Yearbook*, issued under the auspices of the Joint Council of the Order of St John and the British Red Cross Society and the British Hospitals Association; c.100 hospitals submitted data 1889–1922, and c.750 after 1929.

40 For example: Bristol Infirmary, 1760, 53 per cent; Royal Hampshire County Hospital, 1818, 52 per cent; Royal Portsmouth Hospital, 1852, 55 per cent.

41 Annual Reports of: Royal Victoria Infirmary (RVI), Newcastle upon Tyne, Tyne and Wear Archives, HO/RVI/72/100–26; Aberdeen Royal Infirmary (ARI), Northern Health Service Archive, Grampian Regional Health Board, GRHB 1/7; Bristol Royal Infirmary (BRI), BRO 35893/21; Bristol General Hospital (BGH), BRO 40530/A/1/d; Royal Richmond (RR), Wellcome Library for the History and Understanding of Medicine; Royal Northern Hospital (RN), LMA H33/RN/A12.

42 Berry, 'Community sponsorship'; J.E. Stone, *Hospital Organization and Management (Including Planning and Construction)*, London: Faber & Gwyer, 1927, pp. 538–9.

43 M. Gorsky and J. Mohan, 'London's voluntary hospitals in the inter-war period: growth, transformation or crisis?', *Non-Profit and Voluntary Sector Quarterly*, 2001, vol. 30, pp. 247–75.

44 Gorsky, *Patterns of Philanthropy*, pp. 212–14.

45 *Hospital Gazette*, November 1928, p. 232.

46 G. Haliburton Hume, *The History of the Newcastle Infirmary*, Newcastle upon Tyne: Andrew Reid, 1906, pp. 84–7.

47 Public Record Office (PRO), Kew, MH/58/205, 'Minutes of Evidence to the Cave Committee', day 17.

48 *Burdett's Hospitals and Charities*, 1928.

49 Gloucestershire Record Office, HO 19/8, *Annual Report of the Gloucestershire Royal Hospital*, 1875, 1900, 1935.

50 *Burdett's Hospitals and Charities*, 1908; *Hospitals Yearbook*, 1934.

51 London general hospitals: Royal Northern, LMA H33/RN/A12/34; Prince of Wales General, LMA SC/PPS/093/47; West London, LMA SC/PPS/093/77; Queen Mary's Hospital for the East End, LMA SC/PPS/093/52. London special hospitals: Hospital for Sick Children, LMA SC/PPS/093/21; Queen Charlotte's Maternity, LMA SC/PPS/093/50; National Hospital for Consumption and Diseases of the Chest, LMA SC/PPS/093/13; National Hospital, Queen Square, LMA SC/PPS/093/43. Provincial general hospitals: Radcliffe Infirmary (RI), Oxford, Oxfordshire Health Archives; Edinburgh Royal Infirmary (ERI), Edinburgh Reference Library (ERL) YRA 987; see also note 41 for Newcastle RVI and Aberdeen RI.

52 Stone, *Hospital Organization and Management*, p. 218.

53 RI, *Annual Report*, 1920.

54 ERI, *Annual Report*, 1918; an almoner was appointed in 1939 with the opening of the new Maternity Pavilion.

55 RVI, *Annual Report*, 1938.

56 S. Cherry, 'Accountability, entitlement and control issues and voluntary hospital funding c.1860–1939', *Social History of Medicine*, 1996, vol. 9, pp. 215–233, at pp. 219–20.

57 Abel-Smith, *The Hospitals*, pp. 187–94, 338–9; King Edward's Hospital Fund (KF) for London, *Statistical Summary...for the Year 1910*, pp. 14–18.

58 'Cave Committee Minutes', day 15.

59 ERI, *Annual Report*, 1919, 1927, 1929.

60 KF, *Statistical Summary...1938* (1939), p. 86.

61 Habermas, *Structural Transformation*, pp. 195, 220–2.

62 Habermas, 'Internal colonization', p. 297, 299.

63 A. Newsholme, *International Studies on the Relation between the Private and Official Practice of Medicine*, vol. 1, London: Millbank Memorial Fund, 1931, pp. 139–40; in a cryptic comment in *Legitimation Crisis*, p. 71, Habermas admiringly contrasts the traditional 'classless hospital' with the planned health system.

64 R. Stevens, *In Sickness and in Wealth: American Hospitals in the Twentieth Century*, revised edn, Baltimore: Johns Hopkins University Press, 1999, pp. 30–9.

65 Finlayson noted the growth of the schemes but did not develop their implications for 'citizenship of contribution', in *Citizen, State and Social Welfare*, pp. 237, 273.

66 R.H. Trainor, *Black Country Elites: The Exercise of Authority in an Industrialised Area, 1830–1900*, Oxford: Clarendon Press, 1993, p. 329.

67 Cherry, 'Accountability, entitlement and control', pp. 225–8.

68 PEP, *Report*, pp. 236–7.
69 Hansard (*House of Commons Official Report, Parliamentary Debates*), 5th series, vol. 422, col. 47.
70 For example Royal Hants County Hospital (RHCH), *Annual Report*, 1921.
71 ERI, *Annual Report*, 1929; *Hospital Gazette*, July 1924, p. 137.
72 OSJ, *Fifth Annual Report*, p. 102; *Hospital Gazette*, January 1928, p. 6; *Hospital*, June 1932, p. 149.
73 ERI, *League of Subscribers Annual Report*, 1924.
74 Lothian Health Board Archive, Edinburgh University Library, Division of Special Collections, LHB1/18/2, 'League of Subscribers Minutes of Meetings 1930–1937', 25 November 1930.
75 *Burdett's Hospitals and Charities*, 1901, p. 69.
76 M. Gorsky, J. Mohan, and M. Powell, 'British voluntary hospitals, 1871–1938: the geography of provision and utilization', *Journal of Historical Geography*, 1999, vol. 25, pp. 463–482; J. Mohan and M. Gorsky, *Don't Look Back: Voluntary and Charitable Fundraising and Health Care in Britain, Past and Present*, London: Office of Health Economics, 2001.
77 Calculated from *Hospitals Yearbook*, 1933.
78 Gorsky *et al.*, 'British voluntary hospitals', pp. 468–74.
79 *Hospital Gazette*, November 1928, p. 223; April 1929, p. 62; *Hospital*, November 1936, p. 284.
80 PRO, MH 66/721, Dr Lethem, 'Liverpool Survey Report', p. 148 – cost: c.£75,000, receipts, £12,000.
81 ERI, *League of Subscribers, Annual Report, passim*, 1935–7, 1939–42, 1945.
82 'League of Subscribers Minutes of Meetings 1930–1937', 22 June 1937.
83 Cherry, 'Accountability, entitlement and control', p. 226.
84 Tyne and Wear Archives, 1381/111–2, Sunderland Royal Infirmary (SRI), *Annual Report*, 1935.
85 'League of Subscribers Minutes of Meetings 1930–1937', 25 November 1936.
86 *Hospital*, November 1934, pp. 290–2.
87 ERI, *League of Subscribers, Annual Report*, 1942–4; RHCH, *Annual Report*, 1923, 1931.
88 S. Cherry, 'Beyond National Health Insurance. The voluntary hospitals and hospital contributory schemes: a regional study', *Social History of Medicine*, 1992, vol. 5, pp. 455–82, at pp. 467–70.
89 SRI, *Annual Report*, 1936.
90 Habermas, *Structural Transformation*, p. 211.
91 *Hospital Gazette*, March 1929, pp. 1–2, 52; Cherry, 'Accountability, entitlement and control', p. 228.
92 ERI, *Annual Report*, 1938; the others were the chairman, the Lord Provost, a member of the Town Council and a representative of the Infirmary Managers.
93 GRHB 1/1/27, 'Royal Infirmary Minute Book', 1920, 1930.
94 SRI, *Annual Report*, 1937.
95 Habermas, 'Public sphere', p. 49.
96 J. Habermas, *Communication and the Evolution of Society*, trans. T. McCarthy, London: Heinemann Educational, 1979, p. 199.
97 Cherry, 'Accountability, entitlement and control', p. 232.
98 'The Future Development of the Voluntary System', office memo, 1938, PRO MH 80/24; Mo Hill, 'The Voluntary Hospitals of Great Britain, 1920–1940', 15 August 1940, PRO MH 80/24; 'The future of hospitals', *The Times*, 30 April 1937, p. 17, cols 2, 3; Somerville Hastings, *Hospital*, August 1934, p. 215.
99 Secretary of State for Health, *The NHS Plan*, London: The Stationery Office, 2000.
100 Hirst, *Associative Democracy*; Ham, *Public, Private or Community*.

7 Representing 'the public'

Medicine, charity and emotion in twentieth-century Britain

David Cantor

Disease campaigns were central to twentieth-century medicine. Crusades against cancer, tuberculosis, polio, venereal disease, AIDS, arthritis, asthma and other conditions raised huge sums for research, treatment and health education. They acted as a focus for professional struggles for power and authority. They lobbied government for better health resources. They enlisted millions of volunteers to raise money. They reached countless others through advertising and health education programmes. And they did much of this in the name of the public. They portrayed themselves as promoting the public's health, and as educating the public. They also claimed to be its protectors, saving it from disease and from itself, its ignorance and emotionality. It was to the public's generosity that they appealed for financial and political support. They competed with each other for the public's attention, and occasionally they also sought the public's advice on combating illness. Thus if disease campaigns were central to twentieth-century medicine, the public was central to such campaigns.

This chapter explores the representations of the public produced by one of Britain's major disease charities, the Empire Rheumatism Council (ERC), founded in 1936. The ERC was not a public institution in the Habermasian sense of an open site for all who wished to participate in opinion formation. It was in fact a relatively closed group dominated by clinicians and scientists interested in the rheumatic and arthritic diseases, and it was their portrayal of the public that dominated the organization. The public, these clinicians and scientists feared, tended to be resistant to science and medicine. This resistance, they suggested, was due to public ignorance, and this ignorance could only be countered, top-down, through educational programmes. Such a view of the public will be familiar to readers of the literature on what, in the 1980s and 1990s, came to be known as the 'public understanding of science'.[1] As their critics suggest, advocates of the 'public understanding of science' often portrayed the public as like an empty vessel of ignorance into which scientific and medical expertise could be poured through health education. However, the ERC's clinicians and scientists saw the public as not only ignorant, but also at the mercy of its emotions. In their view emotional vulnerability made the public prone to manipulation and delusion, which might hinder any attempt to get it to understand science or medicine. What follows is an exploration of the ways in which representations of especially the emotional general public functioned in medicine and charity between the 1930s and 1970s.

At first sight the ERC (renamed the Arthritis and Rheumatism Council for Research (ARC) in 1964)[2] might seem an unlikely candidate to shed light on such attitudes towards the public. It was a tiny organization when it started, working on what was often regarded as a dull and unexciting group of diseases. But the doctors who founded the organization were prominently involved in many other health and disease campaigns during the inter-war and post-war years, and the organization attracted support from leading figures in finance, industry, politics and the trades union movement.[3] For such reasons, the founders of the ERC did not see the public to which they appealed for support as defined solely by the rheumatic diseases, the collective label for arthritic and rheumatic conditions. They often compared the public's response to the rheumatic diseases to its response to other diseases, especially cancer. Despite being at the opposite end of the emotional spectrum (apathy in the case of arthritis; fear in the case of cancer), such responses suggested that the public was easy prey to exaggerated claims of cures by quacks promoted in the press, on radio and in advertisements. To the leaders of the ERC, such anxieties about the emotional manipulability of the public seemed eerily parallel to its emotional manipulation by agitators and fifth columnists during the industrial and political disputes of the 1930s, a worrying concern at the time when the vote had recently been extended to a broader populace, and war with Germany seemed a real possibility. Thus, the ERC's vision of the public was shaped by broader cultural concerns about mass culture, the media, democracy and commercialism as well as disease.

This chapter is not concerned with the 'real' general public, whatever that might be. To modify a comment by Raymond Williams, there is no 'general public', only ways of seeing it.[4] This chapter's focus is the *portrayal* of the general public, its construction as an entity and in the properties associated with this entity. It is also concerned with the ways in which the ERC/ARC used its portrayal of this entity to define its medical men, and 'its' disease, much as the historian D.L. LeMahieu explores the relationship between self-styled cultivated elites and mass-culture in inter-war Britain. LeMahieu shows how such elites used portrayals of the masses to define their own identity as elites.[5] For LeMahieu, where the masses were construed as a largely undifferentiated agglomeration, elites defined themselves in terms of individuality. Where the masses were defined as open to emotional manipulation, elites defined themselves as elevating the masses. Common images of the masses compared them to animals or children, images that self-styled elites never applied to themselves. So the portrayal of the masses cannot be treated in isolation. It is a relational concept: it is always defined in relation to something else. And much the same can be said of 'the public'. 'The public' was always constructed in relation to something else, and shared many of the same characteristics as 'the masses' and 'the crowd', though rarely the physical threat; related notions such as the 'public mind' or 'public opinion' referred to the nebulous world of perception or mentality more than the physical reality of the crowd.[6] In this chapter, the idea of 'the public' is explored in relation to the ERC/ARC's portrayal of itself as a collective entity, and to its portrayal of two powerful groups within the Council: doctors, and businessmen or industrialists.

If this chapter is about ways in which representations of the general public function to define doctors, diseases and patients, it is also about the meanings of 'emotion', by which I refer to concerns about a range of attitudes such as enthusiasm, optimism, pessimism, fear and hope. Throughout the period covered by the chapter, these attitudes were repeatedly evoked in discussions of the general public. Yet they were suspect qualities. They opened those subject to them to manipulation. They also made those subjects unpredictable. To the ERC/ARC's propagandists, the British population could be divided into two opposed pairs. The first pair separated those subject to emotions from those able to control their disruptive urges; the general public usually fell into the former category, while medicine, certain businessmen and the ERC/ARC itself fell into the latter. The British population could also be divided into a different pair: those who exploited the public's emotions and those who sought to manage them for a broader social good. The first category included quacks, the popular press, unscrupulous advertisers, political demagogues and those physicians and scientists misled by their own enthusiasms. The second category included the ERC/ARC and its component businessmen and medical practitioners.

In thus taking upon itself a responsibility for managing the public's emotions for the greater public good, the ERC/ARC was even prepared on occasion to resort to the kinds of sensationalist techniques of persuasion employed by advertisers and the popular press. Indeed, in 1937 it publicly endorsed a campaign by the *Daily Mirror* in which the paper attempted to raise public awareness with the screaming headline: 'Obey These Rules! Or – ANOTHER 25,000 WILL DIE NEXT YEAR!'[7] Sensationalism was thus a component part of the ERC/ARC's anti-rheumatism campaign, at the very time that the organization worried about the capacity of such forms of propaganda, if irresponsibly employed, to undermine its efforts to manage the public's emotions. To understand this apparent contradiction, it is necessary to realize that the ERC/ARC saw emotion as posing two quite different dangers, depending on the intensity of stimulation it provided the public.

On the one hand, emotion could be dangerous when it resulted from overstimulation, as when sensationalist advertisers or the popular press turned the heat too far up on the cauldron of public sentiment. In such circumstances the ERC/ARC saw its mission as being to dampen the emotional heat so as to better direct the public into what it saw as more productive channels. In its view, only a relatively emotionally contained public could be so directed. But, on the other hand, emotion – or the lack of it – could also be a danger for quite the opposite reason: it could result in depression, as for instance when the ERC/ARC argued that the general public exhibited apathy towards the rheumatic diseases that worked against their recognition as a public health problem. The ERC/ARC's attempts to manage the public's emotions were thus not only about suppressing overly heated urges. They were also about stimulating sufficient emotion to overcome depressive tendencies. It was all a question of balance. An emotional swing in either direction, the ERC/ARC believed, undermined any objective assessment of the dangers of rheumatic disease, making the public a danger to itself and to the ERC/ARC. This view of the dangers of emotion also suggested that there was something not entirely 'public' about this entity – the public. There were powerful emotional currents hidden deep within it that could surface when least expected and with unpredictable results. Only by vigilantly monitoring and managing these emotions could the public be motivated to act in its own best interest, and the knowledge and skills of the doctors who constituted ERC/ARC be deployed for what they argued was the greatest public benefit.

The public in the 1930s

How did the ERC in the 1930s portray emotion in relation to the public? In the first place, it seems to have been akin to a sort of mental illness. The ERC's fund-raisers often described the general public as a sort of disembodied mind subject to various pathological disorders. One fund-raiser wrote of 'a sort of curious apathy or coma [that] seems to possess the public mind, with the idea that nothing much can be done in the matter'.[8] She foresaw what she called a future 'awakening' when the public would recognize that the medical profession saw the disease as a serious medical problem and would demand adequate treatment facilities: 'The manifest duty of the rank and file of the public,' she concluded, 'and more especially of those who have benefited from treatment, is to join in promoting this propaganda.'[9] Others talked not so much of a 'public mind' as of a 'public interest', by which they meant a sort of mental attention, easily distracted by the momentous events of the late 1930s: the abdication of Edward VIII or the preparations for war against Germany, for example. Such mental distractions served to compound the problem of apathy.[10]

In all such discussions the public was portrayed as psychologically disturbed. It was – in their words – 'comatose', 'apathetic', 'easily distracted' or overly 'pessimistic'. To the ERC, such a disturbed population held inappropriate ideas about the rheumatic diseases. Its fund-raisers repeatedly contrasted the public's views of these conditions with the ERC's own medically sanctioned ideas. For example, from the ERC's perspective, there was a sort of perverse pride among those with the disease. As one ERC doctor put it: 'We have got to arouse public opinion to an intolerance of this complaint, to get rid of that mentality which is just a little proud of its "touch of rheumatism".'[11] To this fund-raiser, such displays of pride reduced people with rheumatism to the level of children. 'There are numbers of adult people,' he noted, 'who in such things have the outlook of the schoolboy who satisfies his self-importance by displaying yards of bandage over a very small scratch.'[12]

Thus, in the ERC's construction of the public, the rheumatic diseases were a sort of prized possession. At other times, these illnesses were just part of the family. One fund-raiser, for example, claimed that rheumatics displayed quite inappropriate parental feelings towards their disease. They turned it into a baby. She noted:

Many spoke of their rheumatism with the tenderness they would give to a new born child (laughter). They gave the impression they would not part with it if they could; it was the subject of every conversation, in fact they seemed to enjoy being miserable (laughter).[13]

Other fund-raisers saw themselves fighting not so much deviant parental emotions as corrupted sibling relations. As one noted, the ERC was waging a war 'against a deadly enemy to the nation, not against someone who ought to be a brother'.[14]

For the ERC, of course, rheumatic diseases were neither small schoolboy scratches nor members of the family. By characterizing the general public's view of this group of diseases as largely benign, the ERC was able to employ different images of them to cast itself in a leadership role. In its view, the rheumatic diseases were dangerous family interlopers, which killed or crippled, while the deluded public saw the disease as one of the family, fooled into a congenial and even loving relationship with the interloper. Only knowledgeable ERC practitioners could detect such interlopers. Indeed, for the ERC, images of acute rheumatism went beyond mere interlopers. The disease was an out-and-out killer, a 'masked killer' in fact: 'masked' because mortality from it went largely unrecognized by the public.[15] More broadly, all the rheumatic diseases were killers in a second sense: the disease was in the trenches, arraigned in warfare against the health of the patient whose body – containing 'dugout' for microbes,[16] as one newspaper put it – was also the frontline of defence against rheumatism's attack on the nation.

These images of death, war and killing defined appropriate roles for both the public and the doctors. Medical men were the heroes, their special expertise enabling them to track down the microbe lurking within the body and the dangerous killer who stalked unseen among the public. Pursuing a military theme, members of the ERC constituted what they called a 'General Staff',[17] and so members of the general public had a role as foot-soldiers in the 'war' against rheumatism, ordered to take back those dugouts where the microbes threatened. Of course, the bodies of individual members of the public were themselves the site of such battles. In neither role – as site of battle nor as foot-soldiers – were the public afforded much autonomy or agency.

Masked-killer and military imagery served also to underline the broader threat posed by the rheumatic diseases. They were a threat to the nation itself, especially its industrial, military and imperial strength. The dominant theme in the ERC's pre-war propaganda was that the rheumatic diseases undermined industrial and military efficiency, weakening the health of the workforce and of the armed forces as they prepared for war against Germany. In the ERC's view the future survival of the nation and Empire would depend on its ability to fight the rheumatic diseases that accounted for between one-sixth and one-seventh of sickness absence in the National Health Insurance scheme, costing £1,800,000 in sick benefit and 3,141,000 lost weeks of work among the insured population.[18] Such a fight would also help to encourage industrial and social harmony after the bitter industrial disputes of the 1920s, uniting employers and labour in a crusade against a common foe. Yet all this could be undone by the activities of hidden enemies, and the tolerance or apathy that protected them. This at the very time that concern emerged about the activities of other hidden enemies: political agitators and fifth columnists who sought to insinuate themselves into the British population just as rheumatism did. Indeed, one newspaper played with the idea of the disease as 'Fifth Column Rheumatism'.[19]

At the heart of ERC concerns about hidden enemies was a broader concern about the public's vulnerability to political or commercial manipulation. In the ERC's view, the public was apathetic because the disease lacked drama compared to killer diseases like cancer or tuberculosis. Hidden enemies were never keen on spectacle. They worked by blending into the population, secretly manipulating its emotions much as rheumatism did. Yet the ERC remained hesitant about dramatizing the disease. In its view, dramatic reporting was often the hallmark of the quack, the unscrupulous advertiser, the popular press and the demagogue. All relied on an appeal to the public's most basic emotions. They could plunge it into the depths of despair. They could raise hopes that could not be met. They could turn a crowd to anger and violence. In such ways, the rheumatism campaign highlighted ambivalences not only about popular participation in the rheumatism campaign, but also about the possibilities of democracy itself. As one fund-raiser noted, explaining the aims of the ERC's propaganda campaign: 'We should aim to secure recognition by every intelligent person – and in these democratic days we should act on the presumption that all are potentially intelligent.'[20] But only 'potentially' intelligent. Too often it seemed such higher faculties were undermined by the public's wayward emotional state: a danger to the nation and to its health so soon after extensions of the franchise in 1918 and 1928.

While emotion was a difficult category for the ERC, always threatening to lead the general public astray, in practical terms it needed to employ emotion to get its public health message across. If hidden enemies were to be exposed, dramatic reporting promised to sweep away the veil of delusion and apathy that sheltered them. Almost wistfully one fund-raiser noted that rheumatism did not – unlike the more prominent cancer – strike terror into the heart of the average man, as if such terror were to be welcomed.[21] But if it was to adopt the methods of commercial advertisers, the ERC's organizers believed that they had to avoid inducing the public delusions and mood swings that characterized much commercial advertising. One solution was to offer truth: 'Truth in Advertising'[22] as one fund-raiser put it, a slogan originally coined in America before the war, but recently revived in Britain as part of a broader attempt by some businessmen to counter what they saw as the worst extremes of commercial advertising.[23] But 'Truth' alone might not counter public delusions at least while less scrupulous advertisers, newspaper barons and quacks continued to manipulate the masses emotionally. So the ERC began to seek other ways of instilling means of self-control within the general public, often using itself or its component clinicians and businessmen as examples the public should follow.

The ERC's attempts to instil self-control often rested upon a binary opposition between the public and the organization. Its founders characterized the latter both by its opposition to all the public represented, and by its superiority to the public. In the ERC's view, if the general public was subject to emotion and delusion, the ERC embodied self-control, enlightenment and truth. If the public was apathetic and passive, the ERC was active and aggressive, engaged in what it called a ruthless, give-no-quarter war against the disease.[24] It was these very qualities of emotional self-control, enlightenment and channelled aggression that defined the nature of its superiority. And, at least to the ERC, such qualities marked it and its component businessmen and clinicians for leadership – leadership by example perhaps, but also a leadership with an authoritarian streak: recall the military images of disease that cast the ERC as the General Staff in charge of the conduct of battle. So, too, if the members of the public were marked by their homogeneity, passivity and failure, clinicians and businessmen were defined explicitly by their individuality, ambition and success.[25] 'Success' in this instance was defined at least in part in terms of their personal wealth or social connections to wealthy people. By contrast, the public was rarely associated with wealth. Indeed, to the ERC wealth had a sort of magnetism that marked its holders as leaders. 'In public appeals,' wrote the ERC's organizing secretary, 'the principle does not apply, "Take care of the pennies and the pounds will take care of themselves". The reverse is the case. It is the big money that draws in the small subscribers.'[26]

The fragmentation of the public

Thus the ERC employed the category of the general public in interlocking constructions of the roles of doctors, industrialists, disease and the organization itself. Of course such constructions were not isolated culturally. As LeMahieu and other historians of the 1930s have argued, writers, intellectuals and cultural critics of this period also defined their own identity in relation to associated notions such as the masses or the crowd.[27] In the case of the ERC, such self-definition was intimately related to the dominance within the organization of physicians engaged in elite private practice.[28] Such physicians tended to harbour deep suspicions of the influence of crowd psychology and the mass mind in twentieth-century society, preferring a return to the individual and a strengthening of the will to resist the siren call of the crowd.[29] By casting the public as a sort of mass mind subject to pathological disorder they tended to associate it with such a crowd mentality. In so doing they created a paradoxical 'public' role for themselves, as well as for those they termed the 'public men'[30] of influence to whom they turned for support. These 'public' figures were not part of the entity 'the public'. They had 'public' careers, 'public' reputations and engaged in 'public' service in the view of 'the public'. But they were not part of it. Their 'public' roles derived from their individuality, character, will and wealth, which would always separate them out from the mass general public. Such 'public' roles thus point to another tension in the ERC's attitude towards the public. The identity of these 'public' figures was defined in part by their differentiation from that entity 'the public'. As such, it was entirely unclear how public education (the education of 'the public') could succeed without dissolving the difference, since it would involve the public acquiring many of the characteristics of the 'public' figures they were supposed to emulate. The practicalities of public education appeared to be at odds with the symbolic role of 'the public' in defining elite identity. Or so it seemed, for all this was about to change. The creation of the National Health Service (NHS) in the 1940s began to undermine the centrality of elite private practice to medicine. It also began to undermine industrialists' support for medical charity, and with it the idea that the success of 'public appeals' depended on the 'big money' donor.

In these changed circumstances, the ERC redefined the nature of its supporters. If, in the 1930s, fund-raisers portrayed the businessman as enlightened, scientific and a direct manager of his workforce, by the middle of the 1950s the portrayal had changed. No longer was he portrayed as socially enlightened. No longer was he aware of the huge costs of the rheumatic disease to industry. And no longer was he treated as competent to provide advice on research, as he had been in the 1930s. The ERC portrayed businessmen as operating only on grounds of cold, rational self-interest. As one planning document put it in 1955: 'Industrialists are, by their very nature, hard hearted, and will only support a cause if they can see that it will ultimately benefit themselves.'[31] This is not to say that during the 1930s fund-raisers had portrayed all businessmen as enlightened or public-spirited.[32] Rather they had seen public spiritedness as the way business should go. Their opposition to and leadership of their more mean-spirited business brothers thus defined those who had already adopted such an enlightened attitude. But by the 1950s the socially enlightened businessman had more or less disappeared from the ARC's planning papers. Public-spiritedness had been replaced by hard hearts.

The roots of the changing image of the businessman went back to the creation of the post-war welfare state.[33] Fund-raisers repeatedly complained that the welfare state had undermined industry's support for charity. They also noted that increasingly business sponsorship depended less on the support of individual enlightened leaders of industries than on the advertising or marketing department of anonymous corporations. To add to these problems, the ERC's relative anonymity made it difficult to persuade either industrial leaders or their marketing managers to support the organization, while the emergence of three rival rheumatism charities in the 1940s and 1950s only seemed to confuse the issue further.[34] And even if industrialists were sympathetic to the ERC, fund-raisers saw Britain's slow economic recovery after the Second World War tightening the philanthropic purse-strings. The economic situation improved in the early 1950s. But by 1955 fund-raisers gloomily predicted another downturn in the national economy, and a consequent re-hardening of industrialists' hearts.[35]

Thus if in the 1930s the founders of the ERC had counterposed enlightened industrialists and scientists against an ignorant and emotional general public, by the 1950s the configuration had changed. Hard-hearted industrialists were now counterposed against a still emotional general public, while only scientists and doctors remained enlightened, socially or technically. The ERC also redefined the category 'the general public' after the war, still seeking ways in which this category could serve to define the organization itself. Recognizing the difficulties of attracting funds from rich industrialists and businessmen, it abandoned the earlier idea of the magnetic attraction of wealth. In common with many other large British research charities in the 1960s, it began to reassess the economics of fund-raising, turning from a strategy that used big money to attract small money, to develop more and more sophisticated means of attracting large numbers of small donations previously thought uneconomic. Many of these techniques involved little more than adopting, centralizing and co-ordinating methods that had been the mainstay of philanthropy for over a century – street collecting boxes, savings clubs, workplace collections, sponsored sports events and so on.[36] To do this, the ERC began to divide the public into more and more specialized groups starting tentatively in 1959 by targeting workers, and shifting soon after to housewives, who in the portrayal of affluence at the end of the 1950s drove Britain's consumer boom. By the middle of the 1960s, the now renamed Arthritis and Rheumatism Council for Research (ARC) seems to have broken down the general public into more and more specialized groups: sports lovers, fans of soap operas, theatre goers, cinema goers and, as one proposal put it, 'the cheque book-less reader of the Daily Mirror'.[37] None of these groups had been targeted systematically before, lost in the undifferentiated mass of the general public.

As it began to divide the public into smaller and smaller groups, it also began to adopt increasingly emotive, personalized advertising. For example, in 1959 the ERC's recently appointed advertising agency employed a very familiar linkage of emotion and the public. The agency urged them to abandon the old appeal to the rational self-interest of businessmen, and to start appealing on emotional grounds. To the agency, businessmen responded best to logical argument about the effects of rheumatism on industrial efficiency. Members of the general public by contrast responded best to emotional appeals.[38]

Gradually, the ERC/ARC began to adopt such ideas.[39] Thus during the 1960s a steady stream of radio and television personalities documented the impact of the rheumatic diseases in their lives, and the ERC/ARC devoted considerable efforts through movies and advertising campaigns to highlighting the tragic costs of rheumatism to children and the dire impact of disablement in the lives of ordinary people. Such emotive advertising was justified by the ERC/ARC's continued belief that the public was apathetic and comatose. Just as in the 1930s, emotional advertising offered the opportunity to shake the public out of such apathy, though the ERC of the 1930s had always feared that such publicity could stir the stockpot of public emotion in ways it found threatening. The ERC/ARC of the 1960s, however, seems to have been less concerned about the potential for loss of emotional control. Indeed, it began to recast the general public as self-restrained in ways that it had not done so before.

This new image of the emotionally restrained public seems to have emerged (albeit problematically) in many of the strategies that marked the ERC/ARC's discovery and sub-division of the general public. One strategy, for example, was an attempt to convert to charitable purposes what it regarded as traditional working-class activities, such as pub-going, savings clubs, bingo and the pools. In part this turn to working-class activities seems to have involved an attempt to reconceptualize at least certain working-class individuals as rational, level-headed chaps, concerned for their families and for their community. To these rational members of the general public the ERC/ARC suggested that charity was a form of investment or insurance, a protection for their families;[40] much as it suggested to rational industrialists that supporting research was a form of industrial insurance or investment, a protection for their business. What was new about this turn to the worker was that it occurred at a time of growing concern about the increasing militancy of the workforce, the late 1950s being the worst period of industrial confrontation for Britain since the 1920s. So the image of the rational level-headed worker protecting his family must be set against that other image of striking transport workers egged on by extremist union leaders.

Another strategy that marked the ERC/ARC's discovery and sub-division of the general public was to turn concerns about consumerism to its own advantage. It did this in two ways. First, in its efforts to get 'the public' to take the rheumatic diseases seriously it repackaged the old idea of them as a 'cost' to industry. This cost was now presented in terms of unwanted consumption of the national welfare, touching on broader anxieties about the costs of the welfare state. 'You see,' one ARC physician told the BBC's *World at One* programme in 1971, 'the great snag of the rheumatic diseases is that people cease to be producers and become consumers and go on being consumers of the national welfare for a very long time.'[41] The twist in the tale was that while it deplored such forms of consumption, it also encouraged them. Increasingly, the ARC saw patients as consumers of state-provided welfare who might be persuaded to lobby for more resources for this group of diseases[42] – the 'Cinderella' diseases without, as one paper put it, the fairy tale ending.[43] Thus in the late 1960s and early 1970s, the ARC began to highlight the uneven and often inadequate provision of rheumatological services throughout the country.[44] So it was that the organization both decried the costs of the rheumatic diseases and encouraged them.

Second, if the ERC/ARC played on anxieties about welfare consumption, it also played on anxieties about consumption in another sense. Increasingly, the ERC/ARC saw the general public as consumers of private-sector goods and services who might be persuaded to part with some of their newly acquired wealth as gifts to or purchases for charity. Yet in 1950s and 1960s Britain, consumerism often carried with it the danger of a loss of self-restraint. As consumers, individuals were always in danger of capitulating to desire or indulging in impulse, and the ERC/ARC encouraged such desires and impulses in its forays into bingo and the pools, even charity shops and Christmas cards.[45] For example, the traditional argument against gambling for charitable purposes was that it was the slippery slope to immiseration. It involved loss of self-control; it was 'corrupting' as one volunteer put it[46] – an image that also applied to the mania for bargain-hunting that allegedly swept Britain's growing number of charity shops. Yet the idea that activities like gambling and shopping were inevitably corrupting began to change in the 1950s and 1960s. As the historian Mark Clapson argues, social scientists pointed out that working-class gambling did not inevitably lead to ruination. It involved self-regulation and control, even a financial responsibility of sorts as when it was portrayed as an investment strategy.[47] The ERC/ARC and other charities encouraged such imagery when they portrayed playing bingo or the pools for a 'good cause' as a sort of investment for a healthy future.[48] Paradoxically, then, the desires and impulses encouraged by consumption also involved delaying and repressing immediate gratification. So, too, those desires and impulses associated with purchases at charity shops or jumble sales, or the promise of a win at a charity fête, could now be cast as investments for future health, especially given the ERC/ARC's increasing research focus. Investing in research was like investing for retirement – particularly because many of the rheumatic diseases were associated with middle or old age, and the results of research were not expected for some time.

The broadening of the ERC/ARC's appeal, however, raised some concern about the impact of emotive advertising on the general public, albeit not the ones that might have been predicted thirty years previously. In 1936 the concern was how far to push emotive advertising to shake the public out of its apathy about the rheumatic diseases; in 1966 it was how far the routine of fund-raising might undermine the emotive impact of any advertising. The ERC/ARC had created a new category of the general public, and its emotionality was potentially threatening. In its efforts to broaden its appeal, the ERC/ARC recruited a huge army of volunteer fund-raisers, organized on a regional and local basis throughout the country, and co-ordinated from central office in London. As Major Joe Hoddinott, the ARC's organizing secretary of the Western Counties Region, noted, research had 'been the field of the wealthy patron who sponsors the scientist, and now the place of the wealthy patron has been taken by organisations like my own'.[49] These thousands of volunteers were the ones who organized the countless charitable jumble sales, sponsored sports events, coffee mornings, charitable film shows and so on that characterized much fund-raising in the 1960s and 1970s. But it could be very hard work, and fund-raisers became concerned about what came to be known as compassion fatigue. As one volunteer, Mary Trevena, put it in 1966, describing the deadening effects of the sheer hard work and daily grind of volunteer fund-raising:

> Good causes can be as corrupting as gambling or gin; you can't see the wood (the actual object of your concern) for the trees (the mere mechanics of fund-raising).
>
> The urgent objective is achieved, the money comes in to help cope with desperate needs, but compassion seeps away.[50]

Thus the emotional lives of lay volunteers had to be monitored and managed. For Trevena, the urgent need was to maintain compassion in such volunteers, the sense of pity that poster children or other emotive subjects could evoke. And this could only be achieved through what she called 'direct personal involvement', which in the case of arthritis meant shaking people out of their continued apathy and ignorance of the rheumatic diseases: persuading them, in her words, that it 'can happen to them'. Such involvement in the lives of ordinary people not only countered the fact that the rheumatic diseases lacked 'a direct, urgent emotional appeal', as she put it, echoing sentiments from thirty years before. It could also help to restore a proper emotional balance in the volunteer helper. 'Direct involvement,' she concluded, 'can also move you to anger, a healthy emotion when it is aroused by unnecessary suffering or by sheer stupidity and insensitivity.'[51]

Continuity and change

The fragmentation of the public in the 1960s might be portrayed in terms of the emergence of a clearer, scientific understanding of the public by professional advertisers and marketing people who came to influence fund-raising at that time. Yet such a portrayal would misunderstand the ways in which such sub-categories of the public were themselves constructions of the time, serving particular interests and agendas. It would also misunderstand how the general category of the public persisted despite its simultaneous fragmentation. After more than thirty years, the public was still ignorant and still apathetic about this group of diseases, though the resonances of such claims had changed with the ARC's attempts to broaden its support.

First, the ERC/ARC continued to use the image of an ignorant public to assert the need for more research. Thus in 1967 it joined with one of its rival welfare organizations to launch an arthritis month, ostensibly because both organizations were, as the *Guardian* put it, 'so perturbed at public ignorance of the suffering and economic loss caused by such illnesses'.[52] 'They want the public to know more about rheumatic diseases';[53] to 'show'[54] or to 'inform the public of'[55] their seriousness. 'The aim is to dispel public ignorance',[56] '[t]o make the public aware'.[57] Yet the nature of the public's ignorance had changed since the 1930s. Not only was the public ignorant of the nature of the rheumatic diseases and what could be done about them. Not only was it largely unaware of the huge cost of the rheumatic diseases to industry. It was also unaware of who might be affected by them. 'These are diseases which are normally associated in the public mind,' commented one paper, highlighting the error, 'with the old and with those working in damp and cold conditions.'[58] Nothing could be further from the truth. Thus as it broadened its appeal, the ERC/ARC also began to suggest that virtually everybody in the country was at risk from the disease. Statistics produced in the 1960s suggested that only one person in fifty would escape the affliction during their lifetime. '[I]f the public realised the disease could strike down anyone overnight, and was not just a disease of the elderly,' claimed one ARC official in 1971, pointing out the charitable implications of such enlightenment (and simultaneously also contradicting the idea of giving as investing for retirement), 'they would be more generous.'[59]

If the public was still ignorant, it was still apathetic – in part, as the Secretary of the ARC in Scotland put it, because rheumatism lacked 'the emotional appeal of other diseases which the public hear about'.[60] Repeatedly, the ARC revived the old comment that rheumatism did not 'conjure up the horror of diseases like cancer'.[61] It was not dramatic or fatal, and so failed to attract money.[62] The decline of mortality from acute rheumatism meant that the 'masked-killer' imagery of the 1930s was increasingly unavailable to the ARC.[63] As David Hall, Chairman of the Newcastle branch of the ARC put it, 'it's not a killer disease, it's not like cancer, it's one of those things which people just suffer from, and suffer silently quite often'.[64] And if the disease was not dramatic, nor were the treatments. In an age of heart transplants, the ARC lamented that they had no 'tremendously dramatic breakthroughs'[65] in treating the rheumatic diseases, which consequently remained under-resourced. So the drama tended to focus on revelations about the prevalence of the rheumatic diseases in the population, revealed by what the papers called 'shock reports' or 'shock figures'.[66] As the Sheffield fund-raiser, Mary Trevena, put it, it could happen to anyone.[67]

If the ERC/ARC employed the older notion of an ignorant and apathetic public, it also occasionally employed a very different image. After all it was a tricky thing to harp on about the public's ignorance, apathy and lack of generosity at the same time that it sought to broaden its support among the public. The public gave and gave again at countless fund-raising events. So alongside this image of an ungenerous, ignorant public, fund-raisers also began to highlight instances of the public's munificence, publicly thanking 'the public who had given so generously.'[68] The 'public's response and generosity,' according to Mrs John Whitehurst, a delegate to an ARC conference in 1968, 'was tremendously inspiring.'[69] Indeed, very occasionally the public was more than generous. It sometimes attained a modicum of enlightenment, as when one fund-raiser noted that 'the public are becoming increasingly aware of the problems involved'.[70] It also sometimes engaged in a political action of sorts, as when 'public support' worked against Corporation bureaucrats who tried to move the ARC's 'Noddy Wishing Well' in York.[71] But if the ARC sometimes applauded the triumphs of the public, it did so only rarely. The dominant image of the public remained that of ignorance and apathy.

Rather than represent the ARC's sectional interests in terms of a universalistic 'public opinion', the ARC now introduced new groups concerned about the public. In the 1930s concerns about an ignorant and apathetic public were largely represented as those of doctors and their rich supporters. During the 1950s and 1960s these concerns were increasingly put into the mouths of volunteers and those with the disease who took part in the campaign.[72] As Rona Cragoe, a fund-raiser successfully treated for rheumatoid arthritis, put it in 1965: 'If members of the public could see the look of delight on the faces of those who can, after years of disability, perform some trifling act without help, they would be hard indeed to begrudge a contribution towards research funds.'[73] Then again in 1971 another arthritic, Mrs Beatrice Hall of Uppingham, was reported as surprised by the 'little that is known by the public about the prevalence of the disease'.[74] And in the same year John Clark abandoned a 900 miles sponsored walk (in which he was to have pushed an empty wheelchair) explaining, 'I was relying too much on the good will of the public – but it appears they are just not interested.'[75]

By putting such words into the mouths of lay volunteers, the ARC and the newspapers that reported them began to imagine a new sense of community among those with or at risk of the disease – virtually everyone in the country. This was to be a community united against the ignorance and apathy that promoted the indifference and misunderstanding that many rheumatics experienced in their daily lives, which perpetuated a lack of NHS resources for this group of diseases, and which encouraged the neglect of rheumatology as a speciality. It was to be a community in which doctors, patients and others affected by the disease were united in a fight against both the disease and the attitudes that promoted and protected it. Unfortunately, little correspondence by patients has survived from the 1950s and 1960s to evaluate how they responded to such an imagined community, or to the portrayal of the public it was often set against. Nevertheless, there were differences between doctors and other members of this 'community'. Many people with rheumatism enclosed, with their financial donations, advice on how to deal with the disease, which they hoped would be passed on to others in need. Needless to say, the ERC/ARC took the money, but rarely the advice.

Donors and volunteers had other differences with doctors. One such difference was over the common distinction between 'friends' and 'the public', as when one volunteer noted that 'We find our friends are very good but we personally try to interest the public in our fund raising.'[76] Yet to physicians such 'friends' could be quite subversive. They complained of the ways in which 'friends' provided advice and care that tended to undermine medically sanctioned programmes of treatment. And they worried that 'friends' were the gateway to all sorts of alternative therapies that challenged medicine in this area. But physicians too differentiated between their own 'friends' and the public. The 'public men' of the 1930s were themselves described by the founding physicians as their 'friends',[77] and as we have seen their 'public' status was quite distinct from that ignorant entity, 'the public'. These 'friends' had their counterparts in the 1960s and 1970s, a source of power and influence for successful fund-raisers within the organization, and quite distinct from the allegedly subversive friends of the volunteers.[78] To the extent that the 'public' was defined in relation to such 'friends', it also began to develop different meanings for volunteers and doctors. The 'friends' of patients and lay volunteers were often also part of that entity that doctors identified as 'the public'.

If volunteers challenged the ARC's use of the public, so too did others. As the ARC began to exploit the consumer boom of the 1960s, it found itself in competition with commercial companies that differed with them over what the public was ignorant of, and introduced an uneasy concept for many doctors, that of 'public choice'. For example, threatened by the competition from growing sales of charity cards, in 1964 Valentines of Dundee Ltd – the commercial manufacturers of greetings cards – began to produce its own charity cards. Hitherto charity cards had been available almost exclusively through the charities themselves, and Valentines promised both to make them more widely available and to provide the charities with a significant source of income. 'Contrary to what so many of the public believe,'[79] Valentines argued that most of the cost of existing charity cards went on production and administration, a sensitive point for charities always anxious to demonstrate how little went on such costs. For Valentines the solution to this problem was 'to offer the public a wide choice'[80] of cards, and, without consulting the organizations, it selected the ARC and five other charities to receive a percentage of the income from the sales of its cards, perhaps hoping to stifle dissent. The ruse did not work, for the ARC and the other five rejected the offer, and Valentines dropped them and substituted some other charities.[81] But it did force the ARC to identify its own position with that of the public. 'The public want these sort of cards,' it claimed with reference to its own cards; 'We are satisfying a public demand.'[82] As in the case of the Noddy wishing well, the ARC was very willing to represent itself as the voice of the public when fund-raising was at risk.

The ARC's concept of the public also seems to have changed in other ways. Increasingly, it seems to have come to be associated not only with the masses and the crowd, but also with notions of 'community' and 'people'. Thus during the 1960s and 1970s, when a radio or television interviewer asked what the 'public' should do about rheumatism, ARC officials sometimes answered that the 'community' or 'people' should do this or that.[83] Many newspapers edited ARC press releases, using the terms 'the public', 'people' and 'the community' quite interchangeably. Both the alternative terms – 'people' and 'the community' – seem to have reflected a shift away from viewing the public as an undifferentiated mass, to seeing it as associated with particular localities and groups. This shift took place against a growing academic interest in the 1950s and 1960s in 'community studies' and 'community medicine' (both of which, in different ways, focused on local studies) and also in fiction that sought to recreate allegedly disappearing working-class communities.[84] Such a focus on local community dovetailed nicely with the ARC's increasing use of local groups for fund-raising, as well as its increasing use of epidemiological studies to highlight the prevalence of rheumatic disease among certain communities, in the Rhondda Valley, in Leigh, in the mining village of Walkden near Manchester, and elsewhere.[85]

Conclusion

Representations of the public, it is clear from the foregoing, changed substantially between 1936 and 1970. In 1936 the public was portrayed as a largely undifferentiated entity in which individuality was submerged in the mass. It was also an emotionally vulnerable entity, easily swayed by the power of the press and by advertisers and quacks. And it was an ignorant entity, apathetic towards the rheumatic diseases, just as it was terrified of cancer. All such portrayals allowed organizations such as the ERC to depict the public as untrustworthy.

They also allowed such organizations to both differentiate themselves from the public, and to elevate themselves above it. These portrayals thus vested hopes of progress in disease charities and their allies within business and industry: a small group of enlightened elites, akin to the small, cultivated minority that F.R. Leavis and others envisaged as defenders of culture and taste.[86] They also allowed these charities to ally themselves with attempts to sustain social order. At a time of concern about economic, industrial and social discord, this vision of the public served to assert a leadership role for the ERC in efforts to restore harmony, bringing all sides together against a common enemy, the rheumatic diseases. It also allowed the ERC to imagine itself as a leader in attempts to improve national unity and efficiency as the country prepared for war against Germany.

By 1970, such a distrust of the mass general public had been seriously challenged.[87] The public was no longer seen as a relatively undifferentiated mass. Instead it comprised a diverse range of groups, some perhaps with competing interests. Moreover, the public was not as manipulable as it once had been. Portrayals of the public suggested that there were signs of (albeit limited) enlightenment and rationality among its members, who were also increasingly individuated and emotionally contained. Emotionality, which once had worked on an undifferentiated mass public, now worked in different ways on different groups within the public, so highlighting a need for targeted education and appeals that had not been perceived thirty-four years before. Such a fracturing of the public was signalled by its increasing association with 'community'. If critics of mass culture in the 1930s had posited the breakdown of community ties in modern societies, by the 1970s such notions had less influence.

The breakdown in the notion of an undifferentiated public was fed by full employment, a booming consumer market in the 1960s, the declining significance of industry to philanthropy and by the welfare state. Under these circumstances, philanthropic organizations such as the ERC/ARC began to see opportunities for appealing for support to a diverse range of groups. This process was aided by the appointment in the late 1950s and early 1960s of marketing experts who began to divide up the public into a vast number of groups to whom particular appeals could be directed. It was also aided by the increased use of epidemiological techniques to study the impact of the rheumatic diseases in particular communities and groups, and to assess the effect of variations across the country in the range and quality of health services provided to these communities and groups. For these reasons the notion of an undifferentiated public was much harder to sustain, and differences, which might once have been portrayed as variations within the mass general public, came to be marks of different publics. For example, in 1936 different public responses to cancer and arthritis were often portrayed as within a spectrum of emotionality exhibited by the mass general public; more often, that is, than as the emotional characteristics of different publics. By 1970 the equation seems to have reversed. Such differences were still portrayed as within a spectrum of emotionality displayed by the mass general public. But this portrayal was increasingly subordinated to one in which different emotional responses came to define different publics.

This is not to say that the ERC/ARC of the 1960s and 1970s made no attempt to universalize the characteristics of the public(s) to which it appealed. On the contrary, it continued to write of the public – singular – as if it was an undifferentiated mass characterized by apathy and ignorance. But if the public in general exhibited ignorance and apathy, in the ERC/ARC's view it did so for a multitude of reasons, all of which had to be targeted individually to ensure that they were overcome. It was because of this that, at the same time that the ERC/ARC complained about a general public indifference and apathy, it also sought to divide up the public so as to appeal for support to specific factions. Thus the vision of an undifferentiated public was constantly in danger of succumbing to pressures that encouraged division and dissection. The mass general public was a much more unstable entity in 1970 than the one that had existed thirty-six years before.

Finally, if the ERC/ARC's mass general public was unstable because it was constantly being divided and dissected by the disease charities, it was also unstable because the disease charities served much narrower professional ends in 1970 than in 1936. Whereas the ERC's founders had been general physicians with an interest not just in the rheumatic diseases but also many other diseases and health issues, their successors were more specialized. The former tended to see public ignorance and emotionality as general threats to the broad range of disease campaigns with which they were involved, as well as specific threats to each particular disease campaign. By contrast, their successors tended to focus on ignorance and emotionality mainly as threats to the particular disease with which they were involved. Thus, despite a booming consumer market in the 1960s, they found themselves in competition (in ways their forebears had not) with other disease campaigns to define public ignorance and apathy in a manner that favoured their special interests. Thus, if rheumatologists used the vision of an undifferentiated public to explain the low status of their field and the poor quality of provision for this group of diseases; if scientists used it to explain problems in funding basic or clinical research into the rheumatic diseases; if volunteers used it to explain the problems of arousing interest in this group of diseases: it was not necessarily true that others saw it this way. While many doctors and scientists shared with the ERC/ARC a vision of the public as ignorant and, if not apathetic, at least emotionally suspect, they often used such a vision for very different and sometimes contradictory purposes.[88] They might portray themselves as representing the public and its interests, but they also represented their own interests through the public.[89]

Acknowledgements

Earlier versions of this chapter were given at the Department of the History of Science, Harvard University; the Department of the History of Science, Medicine and Technology, Johns Hopkins University; the History Department, Sheffield Hallam University; the Science Studies Unit, Edinburgh University; the Department of History and Economic History, Manchester Metropolitan

University; and the 1998 Annual Meeting of the Society for the Social History of Medicine. The chapter is stronger for the comments of participants at these seminars, meetings and colloquia. Its weaknesses, of course, are my own.

Notes

1 For an outline of the conventional view see A. Irwin, 'Science and its publics: continuity and change in the risk society', *Social Studies of Science*, 1994, vol. 24, pp. 168–84, especially 170–2. See also A. Irwin and B. Wynne (eds), *Misunderstanding Science? The Public Reconstruction of Science and Technology*, Cambridge: Cambridge University Press, 1996.

2 Hereafter the acronym ERC will refer to the period before 1964, ARC to 1964 and after, and ERC/ARC to periods that cross the 1964 divide.

3 D. Cantor, *Medicine, Philanthropy and the Rheumatic Diseases in Britain, 1920–1970*, forthcoming. D. Cantor, 'The aches of industry: philanthropy and rheumatism in inter-war Britain', in J. Barry and C. Jones (eds), *Medicine and Charity before the Welfare State*, London and New York: Routledge, 1991, pp. 225–45.

4 R. Williams, 'Culture is ordinary', in R. Gable (ed.), *Resources of Hope*, London and New York: Verso, 1989, pp. 3–18, at p. 11. Williams refers not to the 'public', but to the 'masses': 'there are in fact no masses, but only ways of seeing people as masses'.

5 D.L. LeMahieu, *A Culture for Democracy. Mass Communication and the Cultivated Mind in Britain between the Wars*, Oxford: Clarendon Press, 1988. See also J. Carey, *The Intellectuals and the Masses. Pride and Prejudice among the Literary Intelligentsia, 1880–1939*, London: Faber & Faber, 1992. For an account of how American advertising executives distanced themselves from the masses see Jackson Lears, *Fables of Abundance. A Cultural History of Advertising in America*, New York: Basic Books, 1994, p. 233. However, for more optimistic accounts by American theorists of mass society see G.W. Bush, *Lord of Attention: Gerald Stanley Lee and the Crowd Metaphor in Industrializing America*, Amherst, MA: University of Massachusetts Press, 1991, pp. 90–172; E. Leach, 'Mastering the crowd: collective behavior and mass society in American social thought, 1917–1939', *American Studies*, 1986, vol. 27, pp. 99–114, at p. 105ff.

6 In this view they differed from American commentators such as Floyd Alport who argued that the public was an imagined crowd and that what caused collective behaviour was not an irrational suggestibility, but rather the impression of universality. See Leach, 'Mastering the crowd', p. 106.

7 'Obey these rules! Or – another 25,000 will die next year!', *Daily Mirror*, 1 October 1937, p. 14. For other aspects of the *Mirror* campaign see 'I write of pain', *Daily Mirror*, 29 September 1937, p. 10; 'Sir Frank Fox backs the campaign', *Daily Mirror*, 5 October 1937, p. 2; 'FOOD!', *Daily Mirror*, 6 October 1937, p. 3; 'Godfrey Winn's personality parade', *Daily Mirror*, 27 October 1937, p. 11. All newspaper references come from the ARC's cuttings books. They have all been checked for accuracy in the British Library's (BL) newspaper collections. All references *with* page numbers have been located in the BL. All those *without* page numbers (n.p.) were not in the BL collections, and these 'erroneous' citations refer only to the ARC's cutting books. The ARC's references seem particularly inaccurate in the late 1960s, especially 1967.

8 'Devonshire Royal Hospital. £30,000 needed for extensions', *Buxton Advertiser*, 7 August 1937, p. 3.

9 'Devonshire Royal Hospital'.

10 See Lord Horder's comments in 'Work of the Empire Rheumatism Council', *The National Insurance Gazette*, 27 January 1938, pp. 58–9, 64, especially p. 58.

11 J. Fenton in 'Doctor wants rheumatism "unmasked"', *The Star* (London), 13 July 1938, p. 6.

12 Fenton, 'Doctor wants rheumatism "unmasked"'.

13 Lady Snowden quoted in 'Great Bath Appeal launched in London', *Bath and Wilts Chronicle and Herald*, 28 January 1937, p. 3.

14 Lord Horder in 'Town and country', *The Tablet* (London), 13 November 1937, vol. 170, no. 5088, p. 67.

15 'Rheumatic disease. "Degree of its killing is masked"', *Edinburgh Evening News*, 28 May 1937, p. 9; 'The ravages of rheumatism. "Degree of its killing is masked"', *Liverpool Daily Post*, 29 May 1937, p. 8; 'The masked killer', *Harrogate Herald*, 2 June 1937, p. 9.

16 'At least a million rheumatic sufferers', *Bath Weekly Chronicle and Herald*, 2 April 1938, p. 23.

17 W.S.C. Copeman, 'A few "Great Thoughts" on the E.R.C. for 1937', 3 January 1937, Arthritis Research Council (hereafter ARC) archives: 'Organisation and minutes of R.C.P. Committee on Rheumatic Diseases'. The Arthritis Research Council is the current title of the former Empire Rheumatism Council and its successor the Arthritis and Rheumatism Council for Research. Its archives are located at its head office in Chesterfield, England.

18 Ministry of Health, *Reports on Public Health and Medical Subjects*. No. 23: *The Incidence of Rheumatic Diseases*, London: HMSO, 1924.

19 'Fifth column rheumatism?', *Yorkshire Evening Post* (Leeds), 10 September 1940, p. 2. The reference was to police powers to confiscate diathermy apparatus that could be used to signal to enemy aircraft.

20 F. Fox, 'The Empire campaign against rheumatism', *Journal of the Royal Institute of Public Health and Hygiene*, 1937/8, vol. 1, pp. 165–70, at p. 165.

21 J. Fenton, 'Presidential address on propaganda in relation to rheumatism', *Journal of the Royal Sanitary Institute*, 1938, vol. 59, pp. 349–355, at p. 351.

22 Fenton, 'Presidential address', p. 351.

23 E.S. Turner, *The Shocking History of Advertising!*, London: Michael Joseph, 1952, p. 168. For a discussion of the relations between 'Truth in Advertising' and rheumatism see D. Cantor, 'Cortisone and the politics of drama, 1949–55', in J.V. Pickstone (ed.), *Medical Innovations in Historical Perspective*, Basingstoke and London: Macmillan, 1992, pp. 165–84, at pp. 172–3.

24 '"Ruthless War" on rheumatism', *Times* (London), 2 November 1937, p. 13; 'Ruthless war on rheumatism', *North Western Daily Mail* (Barrow-in-Furness), 2 November 1937, p. 8; 'Ruthless war on rheumatism', *Liverpool Daily Post*, 2 November 1937, p. 13; '"Ruthless War" on rheumatism', *Halifax Daily Courier and Guardian*, 2 November 1937, p. 3; 'Ruthless war on rheumatism', *Nottingham Evening Post*, 2 November 1937, p. 3; 'Campaign against rheumatism. Ruthless war needed, says Lord Horder', *Aberdeen Press and Journal*, 3 November 1937, p. 9; 'No quarter to rheumatism', *Yorkshire Post* (Leeds), 2 November 1937, p. 5; 'Rheumatism. "No quarter war on savage enemy"', *Scotsman* (Edinburgh), 2 November 1937, p. 7; 'Rheumatism. "No quarter war on savage enemy," says Lord Horder', *Paisley Daily Express*, 2 November 1937, p. 5.

25 Thus one planning document suggested that 'Certain "key" men might be recognised...who being "individualists" (& ambitious successful men) might be encouraged to decentralise & virtually run little "corners" of the campaign.' W.S.C. Copeman, 'A few "Great Thoughts"'.

26 'Progress report of the organising secretary. December 1, 1938 to February 28, 1939', ARC archives: Executive Committee minute book, No 1.

27 LeMahieu, *A Culture for Democracy*; Carey, *The Intellectuals and the Masses*; V. Cunningham, *British Writers of the Thirties*, Oxford and New York: Oxford University Press, 1989.

28 See Cantor, *Medicine, Philanthropy and the Rheumatic Diseases*.

29 On the attitudes of such physicians see C. Lawrence, 'Incommunicable knowledge: science, technology and the clinical art in Britain 1850–1914', *Journal of Contemporary History*, 1985, vol. 20, pp. 503–20; C. Lawrence, 'Still incommunicable: clinical holists and medical knowledge in interwar Britain', in C. Lawrence and G. Weisz (eds),

Greater than the Parts. Holism in Biomedicine, 1920–1950, New York and London: Oxford University Press, 1998, pp. 94–111.

30   Lord Horder to Lord Leverhulme, 1 October 1935. ARC archives: 'Organisation and Minutes of R.C.P. Committee on Rheumatic Diseases'.

31   Memorandum, 'Appeals and publicity policy. A note by the assistant secretary', n.d. [?]1955/6, ARC archives: 'Appeal and publicity file'.

32   Inquisitor, 'Industry should help pay for medical research', *The Advertising World* (London), December 1936, vol. 68, no. 12, p. 136.

33   Cantor, *Medicine, Philanthropy and the Rheumatic Diseases*.

34   These were the Nuffield Foundation (1943), which had a special interest in rheumatism research; the welfare organization, the British Rheumatism Association (1947); and the Horder Centres (1953), which provided homes for people with arthritis.

35   Memorandum, 'Appeals and publicity policy'.

36   'Proposal for new fund raising activities', memorandum attached to minutes of meeting of Appeals Committee, 18 January 1967. See also J. Pellow, 'Proposals for new fund-raising activities', 6 July 1966, ARC archives: Appeals Committee minute book.

37   Memorandum, 'Proposal for new fund raising activities'.

38   P.L. Stobo to M.C.G. Andrews, 17 July 1959, ARC archives: 'Messrs. S.H. Benson Ltd. Advertising'.

39   This and the following paragraph are derived from Cantor, *Medicine, Philanthropy and the Rheumatic Diseases*, chapter 9.

40   For example one ARC proposal was to create an investment club. The idea of this club was to pass on savings to its members by bulk-buying things like holidays and wines, arranging insurance for its members, offering weekly cash prizes to members through a raffle and acting as an investment club for its members. Under this scheme, one shilling of the half-crown membership fee would be loaned to the club at 2½ per cent interest, and reinvested by the club at 7 per cent interest. The club would thus make 4½ per cent interest on investments, and 'give the clubs the added incentive of the familiar working-class savings club'. Pellow, 'Proposals for new fund-raising activities'.

41   Interview between S. MacGregor and Dr M. Mason on BBC Radio 4's *World at One* programme, broadcast 1.00 p.m., 31 August 1971. ARC archives: 'ARC radio and TV broadcasts 1971', Report No. RH.100, continuation p. 1.

42   The ERC/ARC had always attempted to use public opinion for its own purposes. As Horder put it in 1944, 'Our part is to stimulate; to keep up the pressure of public opinion for action': ERC, *Eighth Annual Report of the Empire Rheumatism Council, 1943–44*, London: ERC, 1944, p. 5. See also 'Treatment of rheumatism', *Times* (London), 2 January 1945, p. 2. But such comments tended to refer to a generalized public, rather than the divided public of the 1960s and 1970s.
       For an example of a later attempt to get the public to form a pressure group to overcome long NHS waiting lists see the comments by the consultant orthopaedic surgeon M.B. Devas, 'Pressure group wanted to overcome treatment delay', *Hastings and St Leonard's Observer*, 24 June 1972, p. 6. See also J. Laming, 'The Cinderella disease', *Kentish Gazette* (Canterbury), 17 August 1973, p. 26.

43   B. Mackie, '"Cinderella" disease. But it seldom has fairy tale ending...', *Evening Express* (Aberdeen), 28 May 1968, p. 4. For other descriptions of the rheumatic diseases as 'Cinderella diseases' see Interview between S. Duffy and Lt. Col. Harcourt-Rae on Scottish ITA's *Dateline* programme, broadcast 6.00 p.m., 31 May 1971, ARC archives: 'ARC radio and TV broadcasts 1971', Report No. RH.71, continuation p. 1. Anon., 'What happened during Arthritis Month', *ARC. Newsletter of the Arthritis and Rheumatism Council for Research*, 1967, no. 8, p. 3. I. Duthie, 'Rheumatism on radio (2)', *ARC. Newsletter of the Arthritis and Rheumatism Council for Research*, 1971, no. 21, pp. 9–11, at p. 11.

44 'Services available for rheumatism sufferers', *Annals of the Rheumatic Diseases*, 1971, vol. 30, pp. 428–43; *Services Available for Rheumatism Sufferers (Second Report)*, London: ARC, 1973. A four-page article in 1970 anticipated the 1971 report, bringing its findings to the attention of ARC supporters. 'Facilities for sufferers', *ARC. Newsletter of the Arthritis and Rheumatism Council for Research*, 1970, no. 18, pp. 3–6.

45 On the nineteenth-century origins of charity shops and charity cards see F. Prochaska, *The Voluntary Impulse. Philanthropy in Modern Britain*, London: Faber & Faber, 1988, p. 61.

46 M. Trevena, 'Compassion can seep away along the hard path of the fund-raiser', *Morning Telegraph* (Sheffield), 11 November 1966, p. 4.

47 M. Clapson, *A Bit of A Flutter. Popular Gambling and English Society, c.1823–1961*, Manchester and New York: Manchester University Press, 1992.

48 However, responses to gambling were not consistent. If the ERC encouraged gambling, others saw it as 'corrupting', for instance Trevena, 'Compassion'. One report deprecated the £915 million spent on gambling in 1965, compared to the 'pitiful' £300,000 spent on research into the rheumatic diseases. Article beginning 'Do people as a rule...', *She*, June 1967 (n.p.).

49 'Arthritis – ten million victims', *Bath and Wilts Evening Chronicle* (Bath), 19 January 1972, p. 7.

50 Trevena, 'Compassion'.

51 Ibid.

52 'Arthritis publicity campaign', *Guardian* (London), 20 February 1967 (n.p.). See also similar reports in 'Joint war on arthritis', *Yorkshire Post* (Leeds), 20 February 1967, p. 8; 'Societies sponsor "Arthritis Month"', *Scotsman* (Edinburgh), 20 February 1967 (n.p.); 'Rheumatic diseases campaign', *Morning Telegraph* (Sheffield), 20 February 1967, p. 3; 'Arthritis month', *Nursing Mirror and Midwives Journal*, 31 March 1967, vol. 123, p. 596.

53 'Aid for disabled', *Evening Standard* (London), 14 April 1967 (n.p.); Vigilant, 'Two out of five suffer these pains', *Express and Star* (Wolverhampton), 17 April 1967, p. 10.

54 'Fighting pain', *Evening News* (London), 13 May 1967, (n.p.).

55 'Arthritis month planned', *Coventry Evening Telegraph*, 3 April 1967, p. 7.

56 'Arthritics at Abbey service', *Daily Telegraph* (London), 20 February 1967 (n.p.).

57 'Spotlight on disease problem', *Birmingham Evening Mail*, 20 February 1967 (n.p.); 'Drive to publicise "National Problem"', *Birmingham Post*, 20 February 1967, p. 7.

58 'Fighters who need more aid', *South Wales Echo* (Cardiff), 31 May 1967, p. 6.

59 H. Brooking, the ARC's South East Organizing Secretary in 'Only cash can beat scourge of rheumatism', *Leatherhead Advertiser*, 8 April 1971, p. 13.

60 Interview between Duffy and Harcourt-Rae, *Dateline* programme, continuation p. 1.

61 S. Douglas, 'Ordeal of a mother', *Yorkshire Evening Post* (Leeds), 16 May 1968, p. 4.

62 'The "undramatic" disease that costs £120m. a year', *Glasgow Herald*, 14 May 1968, p. 10. For another comparison of cancer and the rheumatic diseases see the 1971 article that reported that Stoke Rotarians were told that cancer and rheumatic diseases had a very different 'public image', and that '[c]ancer and some other diseases have a dramatic appeal which rheumatoid and arthritic diseases lack'. See '"Wallflower" diseases', *Staffordshire Weekly Sentinel* (Hanley, Stoke-on-Trent, Staffs), 2 July 1971, p. 6. For other suggestions that, unlike rheumatism, 'cancer appeals more to the popular imagination, it's such a terrible thing and it kills people', see Mrs Gardiner's comments in Interview between J. Warmsley and Mrs Gardiner on BBC Radio Brighton's *News Desk* programme, broadcast 6.15 p.m., 20 May 1968, ARC archives: 'Arthritis week 1968. Publicity', Report No. RH.4, continuation p. 1. See also the comments of I. Duthie that 'It's not a dramatic disease; it has no great emotional appeal and it's been rather [a] cinderella': 'Rheumatism on radio (2)', p. 11.

63 P.C. English, *Rheumatic Fever in America and Britain. A Biological, Epidemiological and Medical History*, New Brunswick and London: Rutgers University Press, 1999.

64 Interview between P. MacDonald and D. Hall on BBC Television's *Look North Newcastle* programme, broadcast 6.00 p.m., 1 September 1971, ARC archives: 'ARC Radio and TV Broadcasts 1971', Report No. RH.103, continuation p. 2.

65 Comments of Hugh Brooking in interview between V. McKecknie and H. Brooking on Radio Brighton's *Coffee Break* programme, broadcast 10.30 a.m., 11 June 1971, ARC archives: 'ARC Radio and TV Broadcasts 1971', Report No. RH.94, continuation p. 1.

66 B. Mackie, '"Cinderella" disease'. See also Anon., 'What happened during Arthritis Month', p. 3. This was a reference to a 'shock report' produced by John Lawrence for the World Health Organization on occupation and the rheumatic diseases summarised in 'Occupation and the rheumatic diseases. ARC researcher prepares report for the World Health Organisation', *ARC. Newsletter of the Arthritis and Rheumatism Council for Research*, 1967, no. 8, p. 4.

   If the ERC relied on 'shock' figures, it also sometimes jumped on the cancer bandwagon. In one example it emphasized the ways in which techniques developed to study aspects of rheumatic disease might also benefit its more dramatic brother, cancer. Interview between J. Newall and L. Bitensky on BBC World Service's *Science in Action* programme, broadcast 11.30 GMT, 3 June 1968, ARC archives: 'Arthritis Week 1968. Publicity', Report No. RH.15, especially continuation p. 2.

67 Trevena, 'Compassion'.

68 'Lymington's "Nearly New" shop opens', *Evening Echo* (Bournemouth), 25 February 1972, p. 14. See also 'Flag Day', *Carmarthenshire*, 28 May 1971 (n.p.). See also for the public's 'magnificent' response, '3,000 see big charity match at Wokingham', *Bracknell News*, 4 May 1972, p. 7; and, for its 'tremendous support', J. Hurst, 'More help sought', *Windsor, Slough and Eton Express*, 22 October 1971, p. 9.

69 'Arthritis research', *Harrogate Herald*, 12 June 1968, p. 9. Indeed appeals began to use the encouragement provided by public support as a reason for supporting the ARC. 'Good support by the public would so encourage my committee members who work hard for A.R.C.' noted one fund-raiser in an appeal to the public. 'To help sufferers', *Littlehampton Gazette* (Sussex), 5 June 1971 (n.p.).

70 E. Jeffcock, 'Arthritis Council branch', *Northumberland Gazette* (Alnwick), 30 June 1972, p. 8.

71 'Kicked out Noddy finds new home at Theatre Royal', *Northern Echo* (Darlington), 17 November 1971, p. 4.

72 Fund-raisers themselves occasionally reported back to ARC critical remarks about public ignorance by prominent individuals. Thus according to Colonel G.E. Mott, the Lord Mayor of Birmingham, Alderman E.W. Apps, whose wife suffered from chronic rheumatism, was critical of rheumatism research, saying that the general public and general practitioners know little about the results. Colonel G.E. Mott, 'Report on visit to Newcastle and Birmingham', [?]December 1956, ARC archives: 'Newcastle (£250,000 appeal, 1957)'.

73 R. Cragoe, 'Experience', *ARC. Newsletter of the Arthritis and Rheumatism Council for Research*, 1965, no. 3, p. 17.

74 S. Helstrip, 'Mrs Hall's efforts will help arthritis research', *Lincoln, Rutland and Stamford Mercury* (Stamford, Lincolnshire), 5 November 1971, p. 10.

75 'The push off. Apathy kills wheelchair walk plan', *Windsor, Slough and Eton Express*, 6 August 1971 (n.p.).

76 Interview between K. Adie and Mrs I. Brown on BBC Radio Bristol's *Women Wise* programme, broadcast 11.03 a.m. on 5 July 1971, ARC archives: 'Recipe collection. Press and radio. 1971', Report No. RH.98, continuation p. 2.

77 See for example the comments by W.S.C. Copeman regarding Lord Horder's unhappiness that the ERC was over-reliant on his 'friends' to launch the campaign. W.S.C. Copeman to F. Fox, 1 February 1937, ARC archives: 'Organisation & minutes of R.C.P. Committee on Rheumatic Diseases'.

78 The term 'friend' was a common phrase used by ARC physicians I interviewed in the 1980s to describe some of the people to whom they turned for philanthropic donations in the 1960s and 1970s. Of course such clinicians were also fearful of the 'friends' of competing physicians, since their donations provided the latter with power and influence within the organization.

79 Anon., 'Six good causes will profit', *British Stationer Weekly* (London), 11 September 1964, no. 106, p. 1. Charity card sales boomed during the early 1960s: Save the Children sold nearly 5 million in 1963, and the ERC/ARC's own sales rose from 10,000 in 1961 to 30,000 in 1963, and they ordered 200,000 for 1964. R. Burbeck, 'Best wishes, but...', *Daily Sketch* (London), 11 September 1964, p. 6.

80 Anon., 'Six good causes will profit'.

81 'Charities dropped from card plan', *Times* (London), 29 September 1964, p. 6. Those dropped were the ARC, OXFAM, the Imperial Cancer Research Fund, the National Society for the Prevention of Cruelty to Children, the Royal National Life-Boat Institution and the British Limbless Ex-Servicemen's Association. They were replaced by Mr Pastry's Swimming Pool Fund, the Widow's Friend Society and the Printers' Pension, Almshouse and Orphan Asylum Corporation, none of which printed their own cards.

82 Burbeck, 'Best wishes, but...'.

83 People: When the Secretary of the ARC in Scotland was asked about whether 'people' were interested in the disease, his response concerned the 'public'. Interview between Duffy and Harcourt-Rae, *Dateline*, continuation p. 1. See also one physician's widely reported slippage from 'people' to 'public': 'It is alarming how people continue to underestimate the rheumatic diseases. We want the public to realize that they constitute an urgent, national problem.' 'Societies to sponsor "Arthritis Month"', *Times* (London), 20 February 1967, p. 14. The physician was Dr Michael Mason. See also S.J.S. Boordman and K. Needham, 'Arthritis month', *West Sussex Gazette* (Arundel), 30 March 1967, p. 6; K. Needham and S.J.S. Boordman, 'Rheumatism', *The News* (Portsmouth), 30 March 1967, p. 2; S.J.S. Boordman, 'Arthritis month', *Chichester Observer*, 23 March 1967, p. 6. For a similar slippage by the Public Relations Officer for Arthritis Month see P. Barron, letter beginning 'Your readers...', *Medical News*, 7 April 1967, p. 10.

   Community: When in 1971 the epidemiologist, Philip Wood, was asked on Radio Brighton 'is there any way in which we, the public, can help?' he responded with accounts of how the 'community' tended to be more impressed with fatal disease like cancer, stroke and heart disease than chronic disease due to arthritis and rheumatism. Interview between J. Russell and P. Wood on Radio Brighton's *Coffee Break* programme, broadcast 10.30 a.m., 8 June 1971, ARC archives: 'ARC radio and TV broadcasts 1971', Report No. RH.87, continuation p. 4. Also when Philip Wood was asked on Southern Television's *Day by Day* programme, 'If it's as dreadful a thing as you're making it sound then why is it that as a public we seem to be relatively unaware of it and unsympathetic towards it,' he responded slipping from public to community: 'The public you say is unaware, this is the public's judgment, the community as a whole views with horror fatal disease but crippling disease that is chronic it seems to accept.' Interview between B. Westwood and P. Wood on Southern Television's *Day by Day* programme, broadcast 6 p.m., 7 June 1971, ARC archives: 'ARC radio and TV broadcasts 1971', Report No. RH.79, pp. 2–3.

84 On fiction see S. Laing, *Representations of Working-Class Life 1957–1964*, Basingstoke: Macmillan, 1986, chapter 3. On 'community studies' see Laing, *Representations of Working-Class Life*, chapter 2; C. Critcher, 'Sociology, cultural studies and the post-war working class', in J. Clarke, C. Critcher and R. Johnson (eds), *Working Class Culture. Studies in History and Theory*, London: Hutchinson, 1979, pp. 13–40, especially pp. 21–4; R.A. Kent, *A History of British Empirical Sociology*, Aldershot: Gower, 1981, pp. 133–9, 143–4.

On 'community medicine' see J. Lewis, *What Price Community Medicine? The Philosophy, Practice and Politics of Public Health Since 1919*, Brighton: Wheatsheaf Books, 1986.

85 Miner's Welfare Commission, 'Rheumatism among miners. First report on a survey of rheumatic complaints and a clinic and x-ray study conducted from an experimental treatment clinic at Walkden in Lancashire', prepared by J.S. Lawrence and J. Aitken-Swan, 1950, Public Record Office, Kew (PRO): POWER 8/278. Published reports included J.S. Lawrence and J. Aitken-Swan, 'Rheumatism in miners – I: rheumatic complaints', *British Journal of Industrial Medicine*, 1952, vol. 9, pp. 1–18; J.H. Kellgren and J.S. Lawrence, 'Rheumatism in miners – II: X-ray study', *British Journal of Industrial Medicine*, 1952, vol. 9, pp. 197–207; J.S. Lawrence, 'Rheumatism in coal miners – III: occupational factors', *British Journal of Industrial Medicine*, 1955, vol. 12, pp. 249–61; J.H. Kellgren and J.S. Lawrence, 'Osteo-arthrosis and disk degeneration in an urban population', *Annals of the Rheumatic Diseases*, 1958, vol. 17, pp. 388–97; J.S. Lawrence and P.H. Bennett, 'Benign polyarthritis', *Annals of the Rheumatic Diseases*, 1960, vol. 19, pp. 20–30; J.S. Lawrence, 'Prevalence of rheumatoid arthritis', *Annals of the Rheumatic Diseases*, 1961, vol. 20, pp. 11–17; J.S. Lawrence and M. Molyneux, 'Degenerative joint disease among populations in Wensleydale, England, and Jamaica', *International Journal of Biometeorology*, 1968, vol. 12, pp. 163–75; W.E. Mial, J. Ball, and J.H. Kellgren, 'Prevalence of rheumatoid arthritis in urban and rural populations in South Wales', *Annals of the Rheumatic Diseases*, 1958, vol. 17, pp. 263–72; B.M. Ansell and J.S. Lawrence, 'Fluoridation and the rheumatic diseases', *Annals of the Rheumatic Diseases*, 1966, vol. 25, pp. 67–75.

86 LeMahieu, *A Culture for Democracy*; Carey, *The Intellectuals and the Masses*; F. Mulhern, *The Moment of Scrutiny*, London: New Left Books, 1979; I. MacKillip, *F.R. Leavis. A Life in Criticism*, London: Allen Lane, 1995.

87 For a critique of the notion of mass culture see A. Swingewood, *The Myth of Mass Culture*, London: Macmillan, 1977.

88 Indeed, 'rheumatologists' themselves may have used this vision for contradictory purposes since it was itself deeply divided. From the 1930s to the 1970s, the speciality of 'rheumatology' was divided between orthopaedists, academic rheumatologists, specialists in physical medicine (themselves divided between those with the diploma and those with membership of the Royal College of Physicians), specialists in rehabilitation and the combined specialty of rheumatology/physical medicine or rheumatology/rehabilitation. The ERC/ARC's involvement in complex struggle between these various groups is discussed in Cantor, *Medicine, Philanthropy and the Rheumatic Diseases*.

89 The point can also be made of the emergence in the mid-1980s of interest in 'the public understanding of science'. Against a background of concern about the Thatcher government's cutbacks in spending, the growth since the 1960s and 1970s of a popular distrust of science and the increasing willingness of lay activists to challenge scientific practices, scientists sought to represent their own interests through an allegedly ignorant public that needed to be educated about science and educated to support it. Irwin and Wynne, *Misunderstanding Science?*. See also Royal Society, *The Public Understanding of Science. Report of a Royal Society ad hoc Group Endorsed by the Council of the Royal Society*, London: Royal Society, 1985; W.F. Bodmer, *The Public Understanding of Science*, London: Royal Society. 1986.

Part III

The state and the public sphere

8 Policy, powers and practice

The public response to public health in the Scottish city

Deborah Brunton

Sanitary reform, pursued in the name of public health, was one of the most significant means by which the state intervened in the life of private citizens during the nineteenth century – so much so, that it is often seen as the archetype of expanding and increasingly intrusive Victorian government. In *The Structural Transformation of the Public Sphere*, Habermas pays little attention to the nitty-gritty of state administrative practice, but provides us with a theoretical model of the workings of the public sphere that informed legislation. Habermas identifies the public sphere as a sphere of discourse, originating among the eighteenth-century bourgeoisie, which was aimed at shaping the role and function of the state, but was largely detached from the institutions of the state. Through debate in print and face-to-face discussion, the middle orders of society set aside their private interests to arrive at a consensus as to the universal laws that best governed the whole population.[1] This literary sphere was the main mechanism through which the bourgeoisie accomplished its 'political task of…the regulation of civil society'.[2] Habermas sees the growth of state intervention from the mid-nineteenth century as a consequence of the disintegration of this disinterested public sphere following the growth of class and sectional interests. Within urban and industrial societies, governments were faced by lobbying from increasingly consolidated interest groups voicing conflicting appeals for legislation to advance or protect their own particular interests. With no public consensus as to the ideal body of laws, politics increasingly became a matter of state mediation between corporate interests, while individual participation in the public sphere was replaced by passive consumption of state benefits and mass-produced cultural goods.[3]

This chapter re-examines Habermas's model of the public sphere in a specific historical context. Whereas Habermas is concerned with the formation and degradation of a universalistic public sphere concerned with shaping the work of central government, this study looks at public debates at the local level: the mid-nineteenth-century discourse on public health policy in four major cities of Scotland – Edinburgh, Glasgow, Aberdeen and Leith.[4] My purpose is to ask whether, seen from this perspective, there is any evidence of the systematic distortion of public politics by class interests or state welfare measures that Habermas sees as characteristic of the later nineteenth century.

The results of this study support those critics of Habermas who argue that his analysis of the public sphere is overly simplistic and idealized. It has been argued, for instance, that the public sphere was never the unified and universalistic entity that Habermas envisages, but rather comprised from the beginning a multiplicity of more-or-less local publics pursuing their own collective interests.[5] This is confirmed in the case of the Scottish cities, where, by the 1840s, there existed an open and inclusive sphere of diverse local publics conducting a variety of vigorous discourses dealing with different aspects of local government activities – the setting of policy, the drafting of legislation and public health practice. They did so not just through the literary sphere of the popular press, but through private letters, public meetings, deputations and private face-to-face encounters.[6]

Moreover, Habermas assumes that the separation of state and public was a necessary precondition for an active debate over the proper role of government. However, the Scottish experience suggests that the public sphere developed in response to the creation of new forms of government, and that the involvement of local government agencies in such discourse actually fostered rather than undermined the vigour of the public sphere. The lively Scottish exchanges documented here took place against a background of close connections between civic institutions and the urban population. Local government bodies were composed of private citizens, elected by their fellow residents to part-time and temporary public office, and directly answerable to a large section of urban society. Given this common identity of citizen and legislator, it is not surprising that the institutions of civic government participated in, and helped to shape, the various public discourses around sanitary reform.

Finally, whereas Habermas supposes that public debate involved a suspension of private interests in favour of the pursuit of the public good, the Scottish experience indicates that no such neat dichotomy of private versus public interest can be drawn. Public debate around sanitary measures always involved a measure of private as well as public interest, while the resolution of such debates involved not simply weighing the relative costs and benefit to individuals and to the population, but also the likely advantage and disadvantage accruing to the participants in the discourse. However, this should not be equated with the large-scale alignment of class interests that Habermas ultimately holds responsible for the fragmentation of the public sphere and the growth of state intervention. Rather, the Scottish discourses over public health were constituted by individuals and small, loose groups sharing a common locale or occupation and often crossing class boundaries. At this local level, the pursuit and negotiation of private interests, far from distorting public discourse, was an important factor in motivating and sustaining participation across a wide social spectrum.

Civic government and the urban public

In the mid-nineteenth-century Scottish city, the institutions of government were inseparable from the wider public: the private world of the citizen and the public realm of governance flowed into one another. The large burghs were governed by police commissions, a uniquely Scottish institution. These bodies were created by the old institutions of burgh government, the town councils, to take on the ever-increasing range of tasks associated with managing the urban environment.[7] The commissions were relatively large institutions – numbering between eighteen and thirty-six members – with powers to raise funds through rates on local property. The police commissioners themselves were drawn from the ranks of the upper middle classes. Male householders owning property of value equivalent to £15 to £30 annual rental (the qualification varied between cities) were entitled to stand for election as commissioners in the wards in which they lived. The commissions were therefore geographically if not socially representative of the city populations. Most commissoners were small manufacturers and traders – drapers, bakers, quill-makers, and publicans – but a handful were professional men, mainly lawyers and doctors. Commissioners combined the role of public official and private citizen. The post of police commissioner was a temporary one, usually held for a three-year period, and part-time. Elected officials spent most of their days functioning as private citizens, formulating and exchanging ideas with other inhabitants as to the proper work of local and central government. These they brought to the council chamber in their roles as public officials. Thus, to borrow Habermas's terminology, *citoyen, homme* and legislator were joined in the same person.

The commissioners may have belonged to the upper middle classes, but they answered to a much wider section of urban society. The commissioners directly represented a middle- and lower middle-class electorate. The franchise was based on property ownership of a third of the value required of the commissioners themselves – just £5 to £10 annual rental. Women, however wealthy, were excluded from voting. The commissioners were also accountable to the cities' ratepayers, who funded their work. Property of £5 rental value in Edinburgh and of just £3 annual rental in Aberdeen qualified for assessment for the rates, and both male and female proprietors were liable to pay the tax.[8] Even tenants, who did not directly pay rates, were clearly aware that they contributed to local taxation through their rent, and saw themselves as citizens with a right to voice their opinions on the work of local government. Electors could express their opinion of the work of the police commissioners directly to their representatives at ward meetings. Ratepayers – and indeed any citizen – made their views known at public meetings and through the popular press, deputations, letters, and petitions sent to the commissioners.

The urban public had plenty to comment on. The police commissioners undertook a broad range of work; policing, in the modern sense, was just a small part of their duties. They were responsible for paving, cleaning and lighting the streets, and providing drainage, water and gas. In addition the commissioners took on a huge range of miscellaneous tasks as varied as the provision of slaughterhouses and fire engines, controlling the sale of gunpowder, preventing the obstruction of thoroughfares and regulating lodging houses and hackney cabs.[9] These apparently disparate responsibilities were informed by the common goal of bringing the archetypal bourgeois virtues of order and cleanliness to the public spaces of the city.

Public health reform fitted seamlessly into the police commissioners' remit.[10] Sanitary reform was fundamentally a local issue in Scotland. With only weak central government, civic authorities were responsible for all aspects of public health policy and practice. The Scottish authorities implemented a wide range of Victorian sanitary practices. Alongside programmes to provide amenities – water, drainage and cleansing – all of which were believed to contribute towards protecting the health of inhabitants, the police commissioners took control of the environment using extensive powers against all forms of dirt but especially disease-inducing 'nuisances'. During fever epidemics they controlled the spread of infection by isolating victims and fumigating their homes. By the 1860s, Scottish police authorities had specialist committees dedicated to public health work and had begun to appoint medical officers of health. This broad regime of sanitary reforms was initiated, shaped and approved by a variety of publics constituted through multiple spheres of discourse.

Sanitary reform and the literary sphere

The middle and later decades of the nineteenth century saw a flourishing literary sphere of discourse on sanitary reform. In the Scottish cities and across the country sections of the population used the popular press to express their views on the proper role of government in maintaining and promoting the public health. In Edinburgh, Aberdeen and Glasgow, residents voiced their opinions on public health through newspaper articles and letters, books and pamphlets.[11] Participation was limited to the middle classes: only the bourgeoisie had the leisure and skills to enter the literary sphere. The authors of works on sanitary reform were mainly doctors, lawyers and journalists. Only occasionally did the social boundaries of the genre expand to include builders and members of the aristocracy.[12]

Clearly, a nineteenth-century public was willing to undertake the duty of considering the proper role of government in public health reform. However, this Victorian literary sphere was not concerned with establishing a consensus as to whether local government should or should not be engaged in sanitary reform. With the sole exception of Lord Cockburn, who mourned the improvement of the picturesque slums of Edinburgh's Old Town, every author was agreed as to the merits of sanitary reform and the need for government intervention to improve the health of city populations. Rather, contributors considered the detailed role of their own local government in sanitary reform, the adequacy of their existing efforts and the need for further intervention. Each author put forward their own favoured agenda of practice for their own city, but made no effort to engage in debate over the relative merits of their own and earlier proposals.[13] Even where there were two clear sides to a question – such as whether civic authorities or private enterprise should be responsible for building working-class housing in the wake of wholesale slum demolition – the debate failed to ignite.[14]

Pamphlets and articles argued that local police commissioners should make ever greater efforts to control epidemic disease among the poorer classes, and to improve the unhealthy areas of the city inhabited by the lower orders, where the urban environment threatened the physical and moral health of the inhabitants. The charmingly titled *A Monster Growl at Some Black Spots on the Face, Body and Extremities of Auld Reekie. By a Northern Bear – but not the Czar* (1854), for example, identified specific areas of Edinburgh ripe for sanitary improvement.[15] During the fever epidemics of the 1840s, authors demanded that the local authorities provide free medical services to the poor and accommodation for fever victims.[16] A handful of authors called on other agencies, notably the Church, to help improve the moral and physical health of the poor.[17]

This nineteenth-century literary discourse on public health appears to fit Habermas's democratic ideal of disinterested eighteenth-century bourgeois debate. Both sets of contributors appeared to set aside their class interests to proffer disinterested advice on the appropriate role and activities of government. Such government action would not directly benefit the middle-class contributors to this literary sphere. They lived in districts that were already clean, well serviced and healthy. Bourgeois commentators – along with all other inhabitants – would benefit only indirectly from such sanitary reforms by living and working in a clean, civilized city, which prospered through its large and healthy population of productive workers.

However, this literary sphere simultaneously provided a vehicle for authors to disinterestedly champion the public good and to advance their private ends. Participation in the literary sphere brought dividends. A few authors made money through their efforts. Lurid accounts of slums and slum dwellers by Scottish journalists such as George Bell enjoyed healthy sales, satisfying a voyeuristic bent among the reformist middle classes.[18] Medical men, who were prominent among the contributors to the literature, pursued their professional ambitions by publishing analyses of the need for sanitary reform in medical journals, thus increasing their status among their peers.[19] Other citizens stood to gain simply by the act of taking up a pen. Assessing the rights and wrongs of the work of the guardians of the public health demonstrated one's status as a public-spirited citizen and brought kudos within middle-class circles.

Institutions as well as individuals pursued their interests through the literary sphere. Pamphlets on public health ostensibly intended to draw the attention of public-minded citizens and the civic government to the need for action also promoted the work of voluntary organizations. Robert Deuchar's *Observations on the Prevalence of Epidemic Fever in Edinburgh and Glasgow* (1844), for example, celebrated the work of the charitable Fever Board. At the same time, it called for the police commissioners to support the work of the charity by joining the fight to control epidemics through improvements to the city's cleansing services, systematic fumigation of homes and better fever hospital accommodation.[20] Such appeals for local authority action in line with the objectives of particular charities brought a quasi-official sanction of their aims and achievements.[21]

These nineteenth-century local discourses over sanitary policy and practice were remarkable for the involvement of civic government within the debates. The police commissioners contributed a substantial number of pamphlets to the discussion of public health reforms, both collectively and as individuals. The Glasgow Police Commissioners issued a pamphlet in 1842.[22] Employees of the police commissioners also contributed to the literary sphere. Alexander Murray, the Edinburgh Police Commissioners' Inspector of Cleansing and Lighting, published *Nuisances in Edinburgh, with Suggestions for the Removal Thereof; Addressed to the General Commissioners of Police* in 1847.[23] Urban police authorities also regularly commissioned reports from independent experts, many of which were subsequently published. The police commissioners were not the only local government institutions to participate in this public sphere. Adam Black, Lord Provost of Edinburgh and a member of the Town Council, not of the police commissioners, wrote a pamphlet explaining the need for the extension of powers of the two bodies in 1848.[24]

Civic government used the public sphere in exactly the same way as did voluntary bodies. Ostensibly, the literature produced by the commissioners and their employees presented disinterested discussions as to the best means of advancing the public good by determining the best and most economical methods of improving public health among the population. However, pamphlets also advertised the civic authorities' existing public health work, and, more importantly, sought to persuade the public of the need for the police commissioners to extend their powers over the urban environment in the name of protecting the public health. In *Nuisances in Edinburgh*, for example, Alexander Murray pointed to deficiencies in the existing Police Act and presented the case for new and stronger powers to tackle existing problems such as drainage and lodging houses, and to pursue new policies such as the provision of public conveniences.[25] Civic government also used the literary sphere to set the sanitary reform agenda, to test the views of the public on possible new initiatives and to shape opinion on the direction of future public health policy. The commissioners sponsored the publication of pamphlets by experts on issues such as water quality and methods of sewage disposal, and even on bills of mortality, even though they had no immediate practical recommendations.[26]

Discourse and the legislative process

Within Scottish cities, there was a second, separate sphere of discourse concerning public health around attempts by the civic authorities to acquire new legislative powers. This was an important forum for debate: procuring new local acts of Parliament was a regular feature of urban life. The Edinburgh civic authorities, for example, obtained no less than fifteen local acts on government and city improvement between 1830 and 1867. Such acts of Parliament were the engines of nineteenth-century local government action, required to launch major construction projects such as building harbours and bringing in water supplies, to create new administrative bodies and to extend the powers of the local authorities, including the right to institute public health reforms. The process of acquiring local legislation was in the hands of the police commissioners. They drafted the bill (occasionally copying clauses from other acts) and sent the proposed measure to Westminster, under the care of a deputation of the police commissioners and a group of legal advisers. There the bill would be polished before being submitted to Parliament.

Before being sent to London, the draft bills became the subject of public scrutiny and public debate. Members of the population expressed their views on the proposed legislation not through the literary sphere, but through a variety of forms of communication – public meetings, letters, deputations and petitions directly addressed to the police commissioners. Such scrutiny was a valued right: there were vigorous protests in 1834 when Edinburgh's commissioners tried to cut short public consultation.[27] The subject of this sphere of debate was very narrow. Where the authors of pamphlets were concerned with sketching the broad role of the police commissioners in sanitary reform, the discourse around draft legislation was directed at defining in details the limits of government action. The discourse around new legislation was concerned only with economic issues – contributors were prompted to act by fears that specific clauses of the draft measure would damage their economic interests. The restricted content of the discourse was dictated not by any narrow-mindedness among the urban population, but the practicalities of the legislative process. If any member of the public could show that a bill affected their financial interests, then the measure would be referred to a select committee, or, if the objections were deemed sufficiently serious, the entire bill would be thrown out.

This sphere of debate involved a quite different public to those engaged in the literary discourse over sanitary policy. Objections came not just from members of the bourgeoisie, but also from a cross-section of urban society, from the upper classes to the lower middle classes. Ratepayers, businessmen and the owners of resources that the police commissioners wished to exploit for the public good, all protested against draft legislation. The Aberdeen police commissioners, for example, had a long battle with local anglers and landowners over the likely effects of extracting water from the River Dee.[28] In 1837, the Edinburgh police commissioners had a fierce tussle with the Earl of Moray over his irrigated meadows. These fields, which lay within the expanding city, were fertilized with sewage, and yielded large and valuable crops of grass but were also believed to produce a miasma that was detrimental to health.[29] The imposition of rates predictably proved a subject for protests. In 1848, Edinburgh's teachers rose up when the police commissioners decided that buildings used for education – previously exempt – should be subject to rates.[30] Most frequently, disputes arose over attempts to regulate urban trade. Companies, artisans and small shopkeepers protested against new regulations. The Union Canal Company fought against the requirement to use police steelyards to weigh coal, Edinburgh's butchers protested against regulations on the slaughtering of cattle, and the city's pawnbrokers opposed police powers to search their premises for stolen goods.[31]

The police commissioners played a crucial role in initiating and fostering public debate about the appropriateness of the powers sought in new legislation. By circulating the draft legislation as widely as possible, they encouraged members of the urban population to express their views on the proposed measures. Citizens were alerted to the authorities' intention to bring forward a local bill by the old-fashioned method of notices on church doors, and the more modern form of newspaper advertisements.[32] Copies of draft legislation were circulated to trade institutions and professional associations, they were reprinted in newspapers and the Glasgow police bills were sent to the city's public reading rooms.[33]

This was not simply an act of courtesy by the civic authorities towards the public who were the intended beneficiaries of the bill, but an attempt to protect the interests of the body of police commissioners. Opposition to any aspect of the legislation during its passage through Westminster slowed the progress of the bill. This added to the police commissioners' outlay, as deputations and their legal advisers had to spend longer in London rallying support for their proposed legislation. If the measure was thrown out of Parliament, the police commissioners were left with nothing to show for their efforts except large legal bills. Individual police commissioners did not suffer financially when draft legislation did not become law – the ratepayers ultimately had to foot the bill. However, the reputation of the body of commissioners suffered, and they became the objects of public censure. Consequently, it was in the interests of the institution to root out all objections to proposed legislation before it was sent to Westminster, and to deal with controversial clauses that might threaten the success of the whole bill.

The interests of the institutions of civic government, rather than the relative gains and losses to the public at large and to private individuals, determined the police commissioners' response to lobbying over legislation. The commissioners would pursue contentious clauses if they felt that the objectors were unlikely to take their case to Parliament. When confronted by objections from small traders or ratepayers, the civic authorities stood firm or attempted to find a compromise. However, if faced by determined protest from wealthy individuals or large companies, the commissioners would give in: the risks to the public finances and to their collective reputation were too high. Such considerations outweighed even an apparently strong case for pursuing the public interest. The case against the Earl of Moray's irrigated meadows, for example, seemed conclusive. There was a wide discussion over the threat to health posed by the meadows, with letters, pamphlets and even a public petition urging the authorities to act. However, the Edinburgh police commissioners abandoned attempts at regulation when the Earl announced his intention of opposing the bill in Westminster and boasted that he could have any clause he wished altered by the House of Lords.[34]

Debating public health practice

Habermas assumes that the function of the public sphere is to shape legislation. However, in Scottish cities, the debate over the role of government extended beyond matters of policy to include administrative practice. A third sphere of

discourse was concerned not with prescribing the appropriate sphere of government action, but with debating the appropriate exercise of those powers. Such
discourse was not confined to Scottish cities. Historians of medicine have shown
that large infrastructure projects to provide water and sewerage were frequently
the subject of local disputes throughout Britain.[35] However, the Scottish police
commissioners' minutes show that sustained controversy was also aroused by
small-scale, routine sanitary reform. By far the most common subject of
comment by the citizenry was the provision of public conveniences, a very minor
element of public health practice compared to cleaning, paving and drainage.

The police authorities acquired powers to provide public conveniences for
their populations in the 1840s. There were multiple motives for their actions.
Unregulated defecation and urination left 'accumulations of filth' in the public
spaces of cities that residents found aesthetically unacceptable.[36] These posed a
danger to the health of other inhabitants and the dirt was designated a nuisance
likely to induce disease.[37] Excretion in the public streets was also perceived as an
uncivilized and uncontrolled behaviour, showing a lack of restraint and consideration for one's fellow citizens.[38] The act of relieving oneself in public
necessitated the exposure of those parts of the anatomy that were increasingly
prescribed as 'private'. Persons urinating or defecating in public areas indulged
in an 'indecent practice' that resulted in 'indelicate exposure' and thus undermined the moral order of the city.[39] The public convenience simultaneously
tackled all these problems of disease, dirt and immorality, bringing 'cleanliness
and decency as well as [improving] the public health', not only for the users of
these facilities but for all inhabitants passing through the streets.[40]

The public convenience exemplifies the bourgeois ideals that informed much
of the police commissioners' work.[41] In place of the dark, dirty, smelly yet public
corners in which the atavistic citizen might relieve himself – areas which repli-
cated the vices of the slum within the respectable city street – were facilities that
embodied the goals of sanitary reform. Under the police authorities, conveniences were regularly emptied, cleaned and disinfected,[42] they were lit[43] (later
models had huge gas lamps) and they were ventilated through openings or
special tubes.[44] Conveniences had screens to 'conceal the interior from the view
of passers-by', thus ensuring that upright citizens were not confronted with the
unsettling sight of exposed genitalia.[45] The authorities were only concerned that
inhabitants should not observe adult male anatomy: until the late 1870s all
public conveniences were for men.

While the public convenience embodied middle-class values, the civic authorities did not foist their use on the working classes. The geographical distribution
of public conveniences strongly suggests that they were not directed to the lowest
social ranks: in all the Scottish cities, slum areas were notable for their lack of
facilities right through to the 1880s.[46] Nor did the authorities make much effort
to enforce or regulate the use of conveniences. Rather than coercing citizens, the
commissioners' approach was one of passive benevolence: providing facilities in
the expectation that the public, sharing their social and moral values, would use
them.[47] Conveniences were positioned piecemeal, according to need. Some were

sited to serve local inhabitants, but most were positioned for the use of 'passengers'.[48] They were placed close to areas routinely traversed by large numbers of pedestrians – docks, railway stations, major thoroughfares, parks, markets, monuments and even temporary exhibitions.[49] Alternatively, conveniences were sited in locations where citizens habitually relieved themselves, to deal with the resulting environmental and sanitary disorder.[50]

Long after the police commissioners had established their authority to mount programmes of providing conveniences, the implementation of these powers prompted a series of dialogues between civic governments and groups of inhabitants. The discourse took a less public form than debates over policy or legislation – discussions on public conveniences never reached the popular press or provoked inhabitants to call public meetings. Instead, residents sent letters, formal petitions and deputations to the police commissioners. During the 1850s the Glasgow authorities received no less than fifty submissions regarding public conveniences, while Edinburgh's police commissioners were sent a further twenty-two. The discourse was concerned not with matters of principle – whether providing public conveniences was an appropriate sphere of action for civic government – but with the specifics of siting individual facilities. Ultimately, the dispute was over the right to determine the use of public space. In the case of public conveniences, private citizens clearly perceived that they had some say in the use and condition of the areas of public space immediately around their homes and business, areas which could be observed from private spaces, which they traversed frequently.

Submissions to the police commissioners fell into two roughly equal groups. On one side stood residents who requested that the police commissioners establish conveniences, believing that such a facility would improve the health and the aesthetic and moral condition of their neighbourhood, and fulfil both the public good and their own private interest in the space. For example, the residents of Saxe-Coburg Place, on the edge of Edinburgh's New Town, requested a convenience to deal with a neighbouring street that was 'made a public necessary [i.e. was used as a lavatory], at all times of the day, as well as at other periods'. They feared the 'consequent disease' arising from the resulting nuisance, and emphasized the detrimental effect on the morals of both local residents and the wider community from offenders 'exposing their persons not only to the neighbourhood, but to passengers'.[51] The second set of submissions came from inhabitants who objected to the erection of particular conveniences and requested their removal. It was not the principle that rankled. The Glasgow Police Commissioners noted that petitioners against one privy agreed 'that the conveniences referred to were very necessary and much required'.[52] Rather, while conveniences ensured moral and environmental order in the street, they focused dirt and immoral behaviour within their structure. For residents who perceived that the area immediately around their homes and businesses was in an acceptable condition, the arrival of a public convenience had a deleterious effect on their surroundings. Petitioners complained that excrement contained within a public convenience was offensive, unpleasant and that it smelt.[53] As a result conveniences constituted a nuisance which was 'detrimental to health'.[54] Public conveniences also posed an ill-defined sexual threat. The trustees of a Leith school felt that the erection of a privy so near to an establishment attended by children of 'tender years' and of both sexes was unseemly.[55] In addition, inhabitants felt a generalized sense of revulsion against public conveniences that was expressed in a consistent if less than rational refusal to place them close to statues and thus allow citizens to relieve themselves in front of statesmen in effigy.[56]

Participation in this public sphere was not, therefore, dictated by class but by locale. Police commissioners received submissions from groups of residents of particular areas or specific streets, church congregations, shop and hotel proprietors, and even the owners of Glasgow's Southern Necropolis.[57] Although care is always needed when relating the geographical location of residents to their social status, it is clear that a wider range of social classes participated in this public sphere than those concerned with policy or legislation. Comment came not only from members of the middle-class electorate but also from working-class ratepayers and tenants (who complained through their landlords). The two camps of residents – those requesting conveniences and those objecting to facilities – were not dictated by social class. Requests for conveniences did not always come from the poorer areas of the city, while protests were not made exclusively by the residents of respectable districts. Each type of submission came from a range of addresses. In Leith, for example, the residents of St Bernard's Street – a wide, highly respectable Georgian thoroughfare – and those living in closes on Storrie's Alley – a narrow, poor street in the over-crowded centre of the burgh – protested about the impact of conveniences on their local environment.[58]

Such direct approaches to the police commissioners were a highly effective form of comment: all submissions were duly considered by the civic authorities and usually resulted in prompt action. The authorities' response – as when dealing with objections to draft legislation – was dictated by a need to protect the interests of the body of police commissioners. Determined opponents of a particular public lavatory could go to court to demand that the law require the commissioners to suspend the building of or to alter or remove conveniences. Losing such a case incurred financial penalties – the ratepayers had to meet the legal fees plus the cost of altering or demolishing conveniences – and was embarrassing to the whole body of police commissioners, who were left open to criticism for their lack of judgement. The police commissioners therefore had to tread warily. Such court cases were a regular, if infrequent, feature of civic life, and cases were brought not just by wealthy and powerful inhabitants but also by the residents of lower middle-class areas. On the other hand, the courts did not invariably uphold complaints: plaintiffs had to prove some real damage to their private interests before a judge would decide against the civic authorities.

The police commissioners therefore pursued the public interest unless convinced that the residents' objections were sufficiently serious to carry the day in court. Requests for conveniences were granted routinely by the commissioners so long as an appropriate site was available, thus satisfying both the public and private interests. When faced with objections to facilities, the commissioners would enter into dialogue with the protestors. If the objections to a convenience were moral or aesthetic, the police commissioners offered to take remedial action by repairing, cleaning, whitewashing and otherwise improving the facility to obviate the grounds of complaint.[59] In response to public protest, for example, the Aberdeen authorities promised to 'deodorise' a convenience and keep it in an 'unobjectionable' state, and to 'scour' out another with water.[60] To defuse any threat to morals, the police commissioners added screens to urinals, or agreed to reorient conveniences so that the entrance faced away from houses and towards the street.[61] The commissioners would give in to protestors and remove conveniences only if they agreed that the facility in question did constitute a nuisance, and was thus a genuine threat to the health of the local population.[62] Rather than abandoning provision, however, the commissioners would often seek an alternative site for the facility within the same area.[63] Local authorities would ignore protests if they were convinced that there were no real medical or moral grounds for the objection. If it could be argued that the convenience was appropriately sited, well used and did not formally constitute a nuisance, then the courts were unlikely to uphold a complaint.[64]

Conclusion

The public spheres that emerged in Scottish cities during the mid-nineteenth century suggest that the model of state–public interaction offered by Habermas in *The Structural Transformation of the Public Sphere* is too simple. A single subject, such as public health, produced multiple and inter-related spheres of discourse. These spheres discussed not only broad issues of policy – the fundamental role of local government – but also the details of legislation and practice, thus setting precise limits to the police commissioners' actions. Such multiple spheres of discourse allowed the public to debate a range of issues: the discourse on sanitary reform, for example, went beyond matters of health to address economic and moral considerations. The variety of public spheres also permitted a wide range of participation. While only the middle classes felt obliged to debate the broad thrust of public health policy, every citizen – elector, ratepayer and tenant – was roused to comment on the implementation of that policy when translated into concrete form, such as a public lavatory placed (metaphorically) on their doorstep.

The interests represented in these public spheres were equally more complex than Habermas suggests. Public and private interests did not always conflict, and individuals advanced their interests by allying themselves with the public good, thus achieving goals as disparate as the abstract satisfaction of going into print and the practical comfort of a neighbourhood public convenience. When left to judge between conflicting interests, the local state could not stand as a wholly disinterested party. The police commissioners as an institution also had its own agenda – to be seen to promote the public good but also to exercise care and judgement in that pursuit, so that the public interest did not founder in the courts or in Parliament, leaving citizens to foot the bills.

The Scottish records also show the close involvement of the state in the public sphere. Habermas sees a separation of the state and public as a necessary context for the constitution of the public sphere. He does identify a blurring of the boundary between state and society in the nineteenth century, but attributes it to the expansion of government powers, by which the state acquired an increasing influence over the sphere of private life. This was a reflection of the increasingly politicized nature of debates within the public sphere. In the Scottish city, the state did intervene in private life in the fashion described by Habermas – for example, through the provision of public conveniences or regulations on the isolation of fever cases. However, the public and the institutions of government were connected in other ways. The police commissions were made up of private citizens, elected to public office on a temporary and part-time basis, who continued to think and act as citizens. There was no inherent conflict between the two roles. This close connection between government and public was not inimical to discourse. Scottish urban governments encouraged public discourse by creating the spaces – such as ward meetings – where members of the public could comment on the work of civic authorities. By circulating draft legislation they invited comment through public media – such as meetings, or the columns of newspapers – as well as direct communication with the body of commissioners through letters and face-to-face interactions. Through such actions, the commissioners fostered the creation of a range of public spheres where all aspects of public health policy and practice were discussed.

The state also took part in public discourses. In the literary discourse over sanitary reform, the commissioners sought to legitimate their existing programme of work and to drive the agenda for future debate. By entering into dialogue with inhabitants objecting to proposed legislation or practice, the police commissioners themselves negotiated the boundaries of their own sphere of responsibilities, justifying their action by appeal to the public good. The presence of the state in the public sphere encapsulates the intricate relations between the public and the private realms, and the impossibility of separating the two. Late nineteenth-century civic government did not extend its powers simply as a response to the politicization of the public sphere and in a form extraneous to local society. The public and the local state, through spheres of discourse that crossed the public/private boundary, jointly built the institutions of government and set the agenda of, and limits to, its praxis.

Acknowledgements

I would like to thank the staff of the Edinburgh, Glasgow and Aberdeen City Archives for all their help in researching this chapter. This work was conducted as part of my post as Wellcome Trust University Award Holder at Huddersfield University.

Notes

1 J. Habermas, *The Structural Transformation of the Public Sphere*, trans. T. Burger, Cambridge, MA: MIT Press, 1989, pp. 51–88. Habermas's work has been criticized for the circularity of his argument as to the criteria for participation in the public sphere. See B.H. Smith, *Belief and Resistance: Dynamics of Contemporary Intellectual Controversy*, London: Harvard University Press, 1997, pp. 88–124.

2 Habermas, *Structural Transformation*, p. 52.

3 Ibid., pp. 145–7.

4 Dundee, the other obvious candidate for study, was excluded simply because sufficiently detailed records have not survived.

5 Cf. M. Ryan, 'Gender and public access: women's politics in nineteenth-century America', in C. Calhoun (ed.), *Habermas and the Public Sphere*, London: MIT Press, 1994, pp. 259–88.

6 H.C. Boyte, 'The pragmatic ends of popular politics', in Calhoun (ed.), *Habermas and the Public Sphere*, pp. 340–54.

7 K. Carson and H. Idzikowska, 'The social production of Scottish policing', in D. Hay and F. Snyder (eds), *Policing and Prosecution in Britain 1750–1850*, Oxford: Clarendon Press, 1989, pp. 271, 283–8; R. Tyzack, '"No mean city"? The growth of civic consciousness in Aberdeen with particular reference to the work of the Police Commissioners', in T. Brotherstone and D.J. Withrington (eds), *The City and its Worlds. Aspects of Aberdeen's History since 1794*, Glasgow: Cruithne Press, 1996, pp. 150–67, at p. 151.

8 Carson and Idzikowska, 'The social production of Scottish policing', p. 285; Tyzack, '"No mean city"?', p. 151.

9 Tyzack, '"No mean city"?', pp. 150–67, provides a detailed account of the developing work of the Aberdeen Police Commissioners. There is still no comprehensive study of the work of Scottish police commissioners – perhaps because they took on such an enormous quantity of work.

10 There are a number of accounts of sanitary progress in Scotland. See for example I. Adams, *The Making of Urban Scotland*, London: Croom Helm, 1978, pp. 13–53; S. Blackden, 'The development of public health administration in Glasgow, 1842–1872', PhD thesis, University of Edinburgh, 1976; H. MacDonald, 'Public health legislation and problems in Victorian Edinburgh, with special reference to the work of Dr. Littlejohn as Medical Officer of Health', PhD thesis, University of Edinburgh, 1971.

11 There is a huge and surprisingly underused Scottish popular literature on public health, an honourable exception being C. Hamlin, 'Environmental sensibility in Edinburgh, 1839–1840: the "fetid irrigation" controversy', *Journal of Urban History*, 1994, vol. 20, pp. 311–39.

12 Although this literature is dominated by middle-class authors in Scotland, Sigsworth and Worboys suggest that in some English towns working-class groups also lobbied for sanitary reform through the press. See M. Sigsworth and M. Worboys, 'The public's view of public health in mid-Victorian Britain', *Urban History*, 1994, vol. 21, pp. 237–50.

13 Lord Cockburn, *A letter to the Lord Provost on the Best Ways of Spoiling the Beauty of Edinburgh*, 3rd edn, Edinburgh: Adam & Charles Black, 1849.

14 *A letter to the Lord Provost Containing Suggestions for Improving the City of Edinburgh. By a Citizen*, Edinburgh: M. Walker & Co., 1855; H. Johnston, *Letter to the Lord Provost, Magistrates and Council of the City of Edinburgh on the State of the Closes in the Lawnmarket, High Street, Canongate and Cowgate*, n.p., 1856.

15 *A Monster Growl at Some Black Spots on the Face, Body and Extremities of Auld Reekie. By a Northern Bear – but not the Czar*, Edinburgh: Thomas Grant, 1854.

16 See for example R. Cowan, *Vital statistics of Glasgow, Illustrating the Sanatory [sic] Condition of the Population*, Glasgow: n.p., 1840; A. Hunter, *To the Public of Edinburgh*, Edinburgh: for the author, 1847.

17 Rev. W. Tasker, *The Territorial Visitors Manual*, Edinburgh: John Johnstone, 1849.

18 G. Bell, *Blackfriar's Wynd Analysed*, Edinburgh: Johnstone & Hunter, 1850.

19 W. Tait, *Observations on the Health of the Edinburgh Police Read before the Medico-Chirurgical Society*, n.p., 1846; R. Cowan, *Vital statistics of Glasgow. Read before the Statistical Society of Glasgow*, Glasgow: David Robertson, 1838.

20 R. Deuchar, *Observations on the Prevalence of Epidemic Fever in Edinburgh and Glasgow; And Means Suggested for Improving the Sanitary Condition of the Poor*, Edinburgh: William Whyte & Co, 1844.

21 *Annual Report of the Glasgow Association for Establishing Lodging-Houses for the Working Classes*, Glasgow: W.G. Blackie & Co., 1857.

22 *Notes Explanatory of the Heads of the New Police Bill for Glasgow, Promoted by the Present Police Board*, Glasgow: W. Lang, 1842.

23 A. Murray, *Nuisances in Edinburgh, with Suggestions for the Removal Thereof; Addressed to the General Commissioners of Police*, Edinburgh: Adam & Charles Black, 1847.

24 A. Black, *A Vindication of the Municipality Extension and Police and Sanitary Bills Proposed by the Town Council*, Edinburgh: Adam & Charles Black, 1848. Black exemplifies the complex public and private roles pursued by individuals. He served for many years as a city official, and was a leader publisher in Edinburgh, producing many of the pamphlets discussing the work of the civic authorities.

25 Murray, *Nuisances in Edinburgh*.

26 See for example A. Watt, *The Glasgow Bills of Mortality for 1841 and 1842* [drawn up for the Town Council], Glasgow: Edward Khull, 1844; *The Public Wells of Glasgow with Analytical Reports by R.D. Thomson & Dr. Penney*, Glasgow: James Hedderwick, 1848; T. Thorburn, *Statistical Analysis of the Census of the City of Edinburgh, 1851, Compiled by Order of the Lord Provost, Magistrates and Council*, Edinburgh: Adam & Charles Black, 1851.

27 Edinburgh Police Commissioners Minutes (hereafter Edinburgh PCM), 10 March 1834, Edinburgh City Archives, General Commissioners Minutes, 1832–4, p. 511.

28 Aberdeen Police Commissioners Minutes (hereafter PCM), 3 March 1862, 30 June 1862, Aberdeen City Archives, Commissioners Minutes, vol. 9, pp. 545, 568.

29 Edinburgh Police Commissioners, Bills Committee (hereafter Edinburgh BC), 6 May 1834, Edinburgh City Archives, ED 9/15/1, pp. 65–9, 83.

30 Edinburgh BC, 12 January 1848, 24 July 1848, Edinburgh City Archives, ED 9/15/2, pp. 67, 120–3.

31 Edinburgh BC, 4 April 1834, 6 May 1834, Edinburgh City Archives, ED 9/15/1, pp. 65–9, 83; ibid., 16 February 1848, 24 July 1848, Edinburgh City Archives, ED 9/15/2, pp. 75–7, 124–6.

32 Glasgow Police Commissioners Minutes (hereafter Glasgow PCM), 4 November 1841, Glasgow City Archives, E 1.1.19, pp. 111–12; ibid., 3 November 1842, Glasgow City Archives, E 1.1.20, p. 294.

33 Aberdeen PCM, 19 November 1861, Aberdeen City Archives, Commissioners Minutes, vol. 9, pp. 517–19; Glasgow PCM, 20 February 1843, Glasgow City Archives, E 1.1.20, pp. 351–2.

34 Edinburgh PCM, 16 April 1834, Edinburgh City Archives, General Commissioners Minutes, 1832–4, p. 641.

35 C. Hamlin, 'Muddling in Bumbledom: on the enormity of large sanitary improvement in four British towns, 1855–1885', *Victorian Studies*, 1988, vol. 32, pp. 55–83; G. Kearns, 'Private property and public health reform in England 1830–1870', *Social Science and Medicine*, 1988, vol. 26, pp. 187–99.

36 Glasgow Police and Statute Labour Committee (hereafter Glasgow PSLC), 1 July 1850, Glasgow City Archives, E.1.2.4, p. 61.

37 Glasgow PCM, 31 August 1846, Glasgow City Archives, E 1.1.22, n.p.

38 The connections between dirt, vice and disorder have a long history. See for example N. Elias, *The Civilising Process*, trans. E. Jephcott, Oxford: Blackwell Publishers, 1994, pp. 110–17; K. Thomas, 'Cleanliness and godliness in early modern England', in A.

Fletcher and P. Roberts (eds), *Religion, Culture and Society in Early Modern Britain*, Cambridge: Cambridge University Press, 1994, pp. 80–2.

39 Glasgow PCM, 31 August 1846, Glasgow City Archives, E 1.1.22, n.p.; Edinburgh Town Council Minutes, Cleaning and Lighting Committee Minutes (hereafter Edinburgh CLCM), 25 December 1863, Edinburgh City Archives, SL 46/1/2, n.p.

40 Glasgow PCM, 31 August 1846, Glasgow City Archives, E 1.1.22, n.p.

41 Mary Poovey convincingly argues that much of public sanitary reform was based on ideals of domestic hygiene. M. Poovey, *Making a Social Body: British Cultural Formation, 1830–1864*, London: University of Chicago Press, 1995, pp. 115–31.

42 Leith Police Commissioners, Cleaning Committee Minutes (hereafter Leith CCM), 24 October 1865, Edinburgh City Archives, SL 80/4/14, p. 406; Edinburgh CCM, 21 July 1843, Edinburgh City Archives, ED 9/3/4, p. 149.

43 Edinburgh CCM, 21 September 1852, Edinburgh City Archives, ED 9/3/6, p. 142; Glasgow PSLC, 17 October 1853, Glasgow City Archives, E 1.2.5, p. 301; Aberdeen PCM, 15 November 1847, Aberdeen City Archives, Commissioners Minutes, vol. 8, p. 190.

44 Edinburgh CCM, 20 September 1850, 22 January 1852, 9 March 1852, Edinburgh City Archives, ED 9/3/6, pp. 40, 89, 100; Edinburgh CLCM, 18 June 1861, Edinburgh City Archives, SL 46/1/1, n.p.; P. Kearney, *The Glasgow Cludgie: A History of Glasgow's Public Conveniences*, Newcastle upon Tyne: People's Publications, 1985, p. 19.

45 Edinburgh CCM, 27 September 1853, Edinburgh City Archives, ED 9/3/6, p. 275.

46 Cf. P. Stallybrass and A. White in *The Poetics and Politics of Transgression*, London: Methuen, 1986, pp. 125–48. Stallybrass and White rightly point to the conflation of slums and slum dwellers, but much sanitary reform while placed in opposition to the slum actually took place in areas less poor and therefore not irredeemably bad.

47 A.P. Donajgrodzki, '"Social police" and the bureaucratic elite: a vision of order in the age of reform', in A.P. Donajgrodzki, *Social Control in Nineteenth Century Britain*, London: Croom Helm, 1977, pp. 51–76.

48 Glasgow PSLC, 18 December 1848, Glasgow City Archives, E 1.2.3, p. 224; ibid., 23 August 1852, Glasgow City Archives, E 1.2.5, pp. 48–9; Leith CCM, 13 March 1844, Edinburgh City Archives, SL 80/4/10, p. 137; Edinburgh CCM, 7 October 1840, Edinburgh City Archives, ED 9/3/4, p. 6.

49 See for example Edinburgh CCM, 19 January 1863, Edinburgh City Archives, SL 46/1/1, n.p.; Edinburgh CLCM, 20 March 1873, Edinburgh City Archives, SL 46/1/2, n.p.; ibid., 21 June 1886, Edinburgh City Archives, SL 46/1/4, p. 141; Leith CCM, 3 June 1868, 13 July 1868, Edinburgh City Archives, SL 80/4/17, pp. 279, 323; Glasgow PSLC, 24 November 1856, Glasgow City Archives, E 1.2.6, p. 128.

50 Edinburgh CCM, 16 December 1842, 1 September 1843, 30 March 1844, Edinburgh City Archives, ED 9/3/4, pp. 107, 166, 251; ibid., 1 June 1854, Edinburgh City Archives, ED 9/3/7, p. 71; Leith Police Commissioners Minutes (hereafter Leith PCM), 26 September 1853, Edinburgh City Archives, SL 80/1/12, pp. 240–1; Glasgow PSLC, 7 October 1850, Glasgow City Archives, E 1.2.4, p. 109.

51 Edinburgh PCM, 8 January 1849, Edinburgh City Archives, ED 9/1/11, p. 527.

52 Glasgow PSLC, 23 August 1852, Glasgow City Archives, E 1.2.5, p. 49.

53 Glasgow PSLC, 8 June 1857, Glasgow City Archives, E 1.2.7, p. 89; Edinburgh CCM, 17 September 1845, 3 February 1847, Edinburgh City Archives, ED 9/3/5, pp. 85, 178; Edinburgh CLCM, 2 July 1866, Edinburgh City Archives, SL 46/1/2, n.p.; Aberdeen PCM, 19 April 1847, Aberdeen City Archives, Commissioners Minutes, vol. 8, p. 161; ibid., 15 October 1860, Aberdeen City Archives, Commissioners Minutes, vol. 9, p. 459.

54 Leith CCM, 16 September 1853, Edinburgh City Archives, SL 80/4/11, p. 380; ibid., 8 February 1855, Edinburgh City Archives, SL 80/4/12, p. 62; Glasgow Police Board Minutes (hereafter Glasgow PBM), 23 January 1865, Glasgow City Archives, E

1.3.2, p. 337; Edinburgh PCM, 3 February 1847, Edinburgh City Archives, ED 9/3/5, p. 178; ibid., 29 April 1851, 1 November 1853, Edinburgh City Archives, ED 9/3/6, pp. 54, 295.

55 Leith PCM, 27 November 1851, Edinburgh City Archives, SL 80/1/11, pp. 208–9.

56 Glasgow PSLC, 28 March 1859, 11 April 1859, Edinburgh City Archives, E 1.2.8, pp. 235, 242–3; Edinburgh CCM, 12 May 1875, Edinburgh City Archives SL 46/1/3, n.p.

57 See for example Glasgow PSLC, 27 February 1852, 10 January 1853, 7 February 1853, 28 November 1853, 12 December 1853, Glasgow City Archives, E 1.2.5, pp. 140–1, 162, 167, 335, 348; ibid., 14 May 1855, Glasgow City Archives, E 1.2.6, p. 90; ibid., 1 March 1858, Glasgow City Archives, E 1.2.7, p. 323; ibid., 23 September 1861, Glasgow City Archives, E 1.2.10, p. 169; Glasgow Police Board, Statute Labour and Cleaning Committee, 11 March 1870, Glasgow City Archives, E 1.7.7, p. 131; Leith PCM, 2 July 1850, 13 January 1851, 2 March 1852, SL 80/1/12, pp. 114, 157, 184; Leith CCM, 6 June 1861, Edinburgh City Archives, SL 80/4/13, p. 60; ibid., 6 February 1866, Edinburgh City Archives, SL 80/4/15, p. 47; Edinburgh CCM, 9 October 1845, Edinburgh City Archives, ED 9/3/5, pp. 99–100; ibid., 5 September 1854, 1 December 1855, Edinburgh City Archives, ED 9/3/7, pp. 100, 200–1; Edinburgh CLCM, 16 October 1871, Edinburgh City Archives, SL 46/1/2, n.p.; ibid., 15 August 1887, Edinburgh City Archives, SL 46/1/4, p. 184; Aberdeen PCM, 19 April 1847, 19 January 1852, Aberdeen City Archives, Commissioners Minutes, vol. 8, pp. 161, 440; ibid., 15 October 1860, Aberdeen City Archives, Commissioners Minutes, vol. 9, p. 459.

58 Leith CCM, 20 April 1863, Edinburgh City Archives, SL 80/4/13, pp. 193–4; ibid., 20 June 1865, Edinburgh City Archives, SL 80/4/14, p. 290.

59 Edinburgh CCM, 3 February 1847, Edinburgh City Archives, ED 9/3/5, p. 178; ibid., 5 October 1852, Edinburgh City Archives, ED 9/3/6, p. 152; ibid., 7 June 1855, 21 February 1856, Edinburgh City Archives, ED 9/3/7, pp. 164, 218; Edinburgh CLCM, 9 September 1861, Edinburgh City Archives, SL 46/1/1, n.p.; ibid., 22 February 1864, 13 August 1867, Edinburgh City Archives, SL 46/1/2, n.p.; ibid., 1 October 1883, 4 March 1884, Edinburgh City Archives, SL 46/1/4, pp. 40, 58; Leith CCM, 8 May 1863, Edinburgh City Archives, SL 80/4/13, p. 204; Glasgow PBM, 6 October 1862, Glasgow City Archives, E 1.3.1, p. 41.

60 Aberdeen PCM, 19 April 1847, Aberdeen City Archives, Commissioners Minutes, vol. 8, p. 161; ibid., 15 October 1860, Aberdeen City Archives, Commissioners Minutes, vol. 9, p. 459.

61 Aberdeen PCM, 2 February 1846, Aberdeen City Archives, Commissioners Minutes, vol. 8, p. 101; Glasgow PSLC, 7 April 1862, Glasgow City Archives, E 1.2.10, p. 375; Edinburgh CCM, 9 March 1852, 27 April 1852, Edinburgh City Archives, ED 9/3/6, pp. 100, 106; ibid., 18 November 1854, 21 February 1856, Edinburgh City Archives, ED 9/3/7, pp. 119, 218; Edinburgh CLCM, 23 August 1871, Edinburgh City Archives, SL 46/1/2, n.p.

62 Glasgow PSLC, 18 October 1852, Glasgow City Archives, E 1.2.5, pp. 86–7; ibid., 30 October 1854, Glasgow City Archives, E 1.2.6, p. 6; ibid., 18 November 1861, Glasgow City Archives, E 1.2.10, p. 212; Aberdeen PCM, 16 August 1847, Aberdeen City Archives, Commissioners Minutes, p. 117.

63 Edinburgh CCM, 5 October 1852, 28 September 1853, Edinburgh City Archives, ED 9/3/6, pp. 151, 279; ibid., 5 October 1854, 22 October 1856, Edinburgh City Archives, ED 9/3/7, pp. 104, 280–1; Edinburgh CLCM, 11 February 1861, 30 September 1861, 15 October 1861, Edinburgh City Archives, SL 46/1/1, n.p.; ibid., 2 July 1866, 12 June 1871, 23 August 1871, 10 July 1872, 20 March 1873, 29 August 1873, Edinburgh City Archives, SL 46/1/2, n.p.; ibid., 27 September 1875, Edinburgh City Archives, SL 46/1/3, n.p.; ibid., 30 January 1888, Edinburgh City Archives, SL 46/1/4, p. 200; Glasgow PSLC, 14 February 1859, Glasgow City

Archives, E 1.2.8, p. 203; ibid., 29 July 1861, Glasgow City Archives, E 1.2.10, p.130; Glasgow PBM, 20 October 1862, 29 June 1863, Glasgow City Archives, E 1.3.1, pp. 57, 288; ibid., 8 June 1868, Glasgow City Archives, E 1.3.5, p. 79; Leith CCM, 2 January 1845, Edinburgh City Archives, SL 80/4/10, p. 192.

64 Glasgow PSLC, 29 November 1852, 4 April 1853, Glasgow City Archives, E 1.2.5, pp. 110, 197; ibid., 27 August 1860, Glasgow City Archives, E 1.2.9, p. 277, ibid., 26 August 1861, 13 January 1862, 7 April 1862, 21 April 1862, E 1.2.10, pp. 151, 279, 375, 387; Glasgow PBM, 9 March 1863, Glasgow City Archives, E 1.3.1, p. 188; ibid., 23 January 1865, Glasgow City Archives, E 1.3.2, p. 337; Edinburgh CCM, 17 September 1845, Edinburgh City Archives, ED 9/3/5, p. 88; ibid., 21 August 1865, 2 July 1866, 11 May 1869, 16 December 1870, 5 May 1873, Edinburgh City Archives, SL 46/1/2, n.p.; ibid., 11 September 1874, 1 April 1876, Edinburgh City Archives, SL 46/1/3, n.p.; Leith CCM, 6 February 1866, Edinburgh City Archives, SL 80/4/15, p. 48.

9 Public sphere to public health

The transformation of 'nuisance'

Christopher Hamlin

The subject of this chapter is the Habermasian tragedy of the transformation of public sphere into administrative bureaucratic state.[1] The case I explore is local environmental management with regard to matters affecting comfort and health. I am interested in a public sphere rooted in the materiality of urban life. Mundane matters of living safely in communities have not figured much in histories of political philosophy or civil society. Instead, the Habermasian public sphere blooms in salons and coffee houses, and in an explosion of publication. There, eighteenth-century citizens engage in rational and critical discussion of the gamut of grave and grand issues of public life.

We do not think of those citizens dealing with such matters as how near Y's privy can be to Z's windows. Yet these too concern life, liberty and property, not to mention truth and beauty. Such issues too are essential to, perhaps exemplary of, civil society; it is about such issues that a public *modus vivendi* must be somehow manufactured. My exploration of these issues here develops perspectives of a pre-Habermasian scholarly enterprise, the efforts of nineteenth-century political archaeologists to discover, primarily in English common law, the foundations of an organic constitution. In reviewing the efforts of ordinary people to grapple collectively with the unavoidable material problems of community, these scholars felt they were closing in on the origins of the habits and skills of a rational and critical conversation that is at once democratic and authoritative, concrete and abstract, in short, something analogous to the idealized public sphere of Habermas. They saw the communal problems that produced such a public discourse exemplified in the dung, offal, trash and smoke of the early modern town. The biological imperative of their production and the physical imperative of their diffusion gave such materials a publicity that existed independently of anyone's choice. They were continually produced; were vital to the town's life; were valuable (at least at some times and in some places); pervaded air, water and soil; were disgusting to many, an injury to comfort and health and even an active cause of disease for some. Concentration of population necessitated institutions for the resolution of conflict over their management, so this argument went; these institutions, emerging as the fora for reconciling liberty, property, health and sensibility might take the sort of form Habermas describes.[2]

I am concerned here neither with the validity of these characterizations of early modern urban governance nor with how satisfactorily those institutions met Habermasian canons of democracy and rationality. Rather, I use the case to suggest that, historically and necessarily, matters of local environment do have a prominent place at the Habermasian table and to consider the wonderfully amorphous and ambiguous concept of health as a key vehicle in that rational and critical conversation. The chapter moves, then, in two directions: on the one hand towards bringing urban environmental management into discussion of the transformation of the public sphere, on the other towards illuminating the rise of public health with the ideas of Habermas.

Public health, equality, liberty, property

The idea that something like a public sphere could (and should) emerge organically from the tackling of communal problems by communities of free persons was a theme of a number of mid- to late nineteenth-century English and German historians and political writers, the most notorious of whom was the antiquarian Joshua Toulmin Smith and the most famous, the Fabian social theorists Beatrice and Sidney Webb. These 'romantic constitutionalists' had no common political philosophy or identity, and were never a group. They shared a fascination with the evolution of government through the management by ordinary people of the regular conflicts of communal life.[3] The unwritten English constitution was the purest form of this evolution.[4] In their organic vision of government, the folk mote and the court leet reflected first-order modes of communal decision-making. Gradually, the record of resolution of conflict had ossified into custom, common law and constitution, which, in true public sphere spirit, was seen as the apotheosis of rigorous and rational conversation over every issue of human relations. Such a record precipitated also the particular institutions of parish vestry, county bench, Parliament and monarch (the relative importance of the latter two being a major issue of disagreement among such writers). In this view the bureaucratic state was recent and derivative. For some it was a perversion of tradition, for others a necessary extension of it.[5]

While these ancient and local institutions embraced all conflict, environmental management had some claim as the *ur*-problem of that praxis. Living together demanded working concepts of property and its antitheses, theft, trespass and violation.[6] Out of the adjudication of conflicts evolved concepts of rights. The manorial courts leet, for example, had expanded from an initial concern with nuisance, to become general units of government in Birmingham and Manchester.[7] Political philosophy, from this vantage point, arose not in the 'world of letters', but on the wings of dung – and party walls, gutters and drains, and nuisance trades in the street.[8] In medieval England, noted the author of an 1881 *Practical Guide for Inspectors of Nuisances*, urban environmental nuisances had been labelled 'oppressions'.[9]

Prior to the mid-nineteenth century health was not privileged in discussions of urban environmental management. The Webbs note that the eighteenth-century improvers who drained and widened streets improved health too, but more commonly they acted in the name of safety, commerce and amenity.[10] And yet the language of public complaint often gravitated towards health. In his manual for justices of the peace, Richard Burn provided sample indictments of public nuisances. That for bone boiling, for example, suggests the intermingling of health and sensibility. The complaint was that:

> divers large quantities of tripe and other entrails and offal of beasts in the said boiler unlawfully and injuriously did boil, whereby divers noisome and unwholesome smokes and smells did then, and on the said other days and times, from thence there arise, so that the air there was greatly corrupted and infected; to the great damage and common nuisance of all the liege subjects of our said lady the Queen.

The term 'noisome', noted Burn, implied harm as well as disagreeability; 'infection' meant only that a malign capacity had been communicated to the air; it did not yet imply any specific disease.[11]

By the mid-nineteenth century health had become the rationale for urban improvement projects as local boards of health evolved into general-purpose local government entities. To make pathology the central way to understand conflicts among neighbours was to mobilize a general model of transmissible harm. The permeability of streets, dwellings, bodies, even minds, to air, water, occult emanations and perhaps even to what could be seen or imagined, meant that the condition of any space affected spaces and bodies around it.[12] One did not need to think of specific diseases; a model of transmissible harm simply suggested more, and more serious ways that one person's doings trespassed on others, and was therefore a public problem. By the end of the century the public 'health' had become the most powerful justification for urban public action, and on many matters; increasingly, the central state was translating it into imperatives. 'Health' added immediacy: to label whatever seemed objectionable as harmful to health was to play a trump card.

In the process 'public health' became a secular cosmology. Not all would have equal access to the declaration of health threat, however: public health would represent middle-class standards.[13] Even earlier, an appeal to the quality of the environment had been a means of the imposition of the will of some citizens on others, like pig-keepers or others who worked 'offensive trades' in the streets. In such efforts 'public health' became a banner of solidarity. Like citizenship, region, religion, ethnicity or class, it was a discursive means to build a public, discipline a community, impose an identity stronger and more inescapable than the continued assent of free people.[14] In matters that would otherwise be impossibly conflictual, the seductive dualism of 'pollution' or 'purity' could authorize immediate action. Following Mary Douglas and Norbert Elias, one might even say that 'public health' was developed to do public work: we continue to use it regularly as the hallmark of rational public action.[15] Public health, then, was not only a function of the new state, but one means of its emergence.

Nuisances and common law

The primary legal and cultural means by which activities and conditions of environment, like keeping heaps of dung in and around one's dwelling, came to have such signification was the transformation of the concept of nuisance in the 1840s and 1850s. Cholera effected this transformation, giving dung management a higher medical rationality that obscured the fact that regulating such matters was a longstanding problem of reconciling conflicting rights. The transformation is manifest in a series of acts bearing on nuisance regulation passed by the British Parliament between 1846 and 1875. This legislation changed radically the way a thing or activity became a nuisance. It opened the possibility of *categorical* nuisances and substituted designation for debate, the authority of the bureaucrat for the ongoing working out of community standards. From the viewpoint of pre-1846 traditions of nuisance law, the designated nuisance was anathema. The changes both reflect the power the state had already achieved and were also one of the means by which that state came to seem the obvious locus of environmental regulation.

Before considering that new approach, it is necessary to look at what it replaced. Early nineteenth-century nuisance law was mainly a division of common law, sometimes supplemented by local statutes administered by improvement or sewers commissions, courts leet or municipal corporations. In theory, the common law of nuisances, because it was made by local judges, magistrates or juries on a case-by-case basis, represented local sensibilities. Through it, communities determined the extent of property rights, the degrees of environmental amenity to be enforced and the compensation to be given for damages suffered. A common feature of such resolution was a visit or tour by a large jury that could impose community standards. While generic cases, like building construction, might be resolved formulaically, many cases involved negotiating fairness and justice, civic virtue and individual rights.[16]

In the mid-nineteenth century Blackstone's *Commentaries* from the 1760s remained the magisterium of common law.[17] Blackstone explained that nuisances were either common or private. A common nuisance was 'the doing of a thing to the annoyance of all the king's subjects, or the neglecting to do a thing which the common good requires' or 'inconvenient and troublesome offences that annoy the community in general' (IV, 166–7). A private nuisance was 'whatsoever annoys or doth damage to another' (III, 5). Annoyance was 'anything that worketh hurt, inconvenience, or damage' (III, 216). Public authorities were responsible for acting against common nuisances; the sufferer acted against a private nuisance. In either case, a nuisance action was an accusation about the effects of another's behaviour. Dung etc. was not automatically a nuisance; it became so when someone claimed annoyance and customary modes of community determination upheld the claim.

The nuisance law Blackstone summarized had little to do with health. Of the seven categories of common nuisances Blackstone lists, four – conducting a disorderly inn, running a lottery, eavesdropping or being a 'public scold' – have nothing to do with environment at all. Three do: firecracker manufacture and sales; obstruction of or failure to repair highways or waterways; and offensive trades, particularly hog-keeping.[18] Blackstone does not mention dung-keeping, which by the 1860s would be the archetypal public nuisance whose removal was the job of the new inspectors of nuisances. Private nuisances included damage to enjoyment of property, such as deterioration of a landowner's riparian rights (from contamination or abstraction of water) or deterioration of customary air and light. Damages to health were not excluded, but there was no need to demonstrate such damage since the annoyance of bad smell, for example, was sufficient grounds for action. Objections to water contamination were more likely to be concerned with sight, smell, fisheries or cattle watering than with disease.

Public and private nuisances were often not different in kind from one another: at issue, in theory, was the generality of the injury, and, in practice, whether or not a public authority was willing to take action. But, in either case, such actions formed an important part of the praxis of civil society.

The records of the London Assizes of Nuisance and of Building from the early fourteenth to the late sixteenth centuries give us a sense of such environmental management.[19] Neighbours brought charges against new construction that blocked light or allowed eavesdropping, gutters that emptied on to their property, dung heaps that encroached against their walls or privies that contaminated a cellar. These were resolved by a site visit from a large jury, who would order alteration or decide compensation. Eighteenth-century records of courts leet and early nineteenth-century records of London sewer commissions (commonly known as sewers courts) give a similar impression: visits by large numbers of stakeholders, and attempts to translate into a compensation award the multiple expressions and trespasses on rights, the needs of the public and the likely costs and benefits.[20]

Champions of common law made much of its efficiency and expediency. The sufferer from a nuisance, common or private, could abate it immediately, notes Blackstone, 'so long as he commits no riot'. If a neighbour erects a wall 'so near to me that it stops my ancient lights' I would have the right to 'enter…and peaceably pull it down' (III, 5–6). Or one could tear down a gate across a public road.

The vision of a community of property-enjoying equals, in which even the poor, who had but to announce their annoyance, were protected, was probably always an illusion.[21] This was clearly a bourgeois public sphere in which access to the debate might well require substantial resources. It would be naïve to think that these legal means lessened conflict, protected health or represented an ideal civil society in any sense.[22] One person's annoyance did not automatically trump another's property rights; common law blocked action at least as much it facilitated it; the peaceable intrusion to tear down the wall might well cause riot; and whoever would take summary action ran the risk that the matter would not be judged a nuisance.[23] Where large capital was at stake, the intricacies of common law made action lengthy, expensive and uncertain. Although, as the Corporation of Birmingham and the alum manufacturer Peter Spence found to their cost, the nuisance law had teeth,[24] it was an unreliable means to protect the health of a community. In 1854 a group of London offensive tradesmen argued that the difficulty of common law action was appropriate; the burden of expense discouraged trivial or malicious legal action.[25]

But, at least ideally, in this pre-1846 mode of decision-making, a wide section of the community were to become amateur political philosophers in articulating concepts of rights and public good. Decisions were local, because each alleged nuisance had to be dealt with individually, and the full range of issues had to be considered in each case. The balancing doctrine that would become prominent in late nineteenth-century American nuisance law did not triumph in a similar way in England, and somehow courts had to reconcile rights with broader social utility.[26] Toulmin Smith, the great defender of common law, concluded that "'Nuisance,"...includes whatever is, or threatens to be, more injurious to the health, comfort, property, or general welfare, of whoever may be touched by it, than is compensated for by any amount of general good produced by its existence.'[27]

Nuisances in the bureaucratic state

Already by the mid-eighteenth century, towns were shifting to summary adjudication of many common nuisances. Through by-laws, towns dictated exactly what encroachments on common sensibility were to be construed as categorical nuisances within their borders.[28] A key stage in this process was the Towns Improvement Clauses Act of 1847 (10 & 11 Vict. C. 34), a compilation of approved clauses for use in local acts. It addressed indecent exposure, the leashing of dogs, over-street clothes lines, stone throwing, doorbell ringing and kite-flying, and indicated how far Parliament would, in principle, allow towns to go in statutorily defining nuisances.[29] Such summary process could be justified on the grounds that rights of property had been waived in the legislative processes that led to the framing and passage of a local act.[30]

All the while that nuisance law was evolving from plaints of annoyance to local codes, the sanitarians were elevating decomposing dung to the pinnacle of pathology. The Nuisances Removal Acts mark the union of these traditions. The 1846 Act was an emergency measure in the face of cholera. Renewed in 1847, it became permanent in 1848, was amended in 1855 and 1860, and incorporated into general legislation in 1875. Unlike the 1848 Public Health Act, it was not adoptive: all designated local authorities acquired powers for removing nuisances, understood as faulty drains, faulty or overcrowded dwellings, and accumulations of filth.[31] With the exception of the 1855 amendment, nuisances legislation was uncontroversial.

The new sanitary expediency did not end contests over rights in offensive or dangerous materials. The acts allowed summary removal of such stuff, but those who would do so should expect trouble, warned a commentator: 'the provisions of the statute are in some respects an infringement of the rights of property'; '[a] hasty and unexpected intrusion,...may create serious irritation,...painful collisions and probably riots and tumults'.[32] Resistance to the new sanitary order is evident both in changing provisions in the amendments for disposing of seized filth and for designating how, and by whom, 'nuisance' was to be determined.

Edwin Chadwick's 1848 Public Health Act recognized the worth of dung, but allowed the sanitary state to take it without compensation. Upon finding 'any accumulation of manure, dung, soil, or filth, or other offensive or noxious matter' that 'ought to be removed', the inspector was to give notice, and, if the material remained twenty-four hours later, to dispose of it, with the local authority keeping any profits from the sale.[33] Under the universal Nuisances Removal Act, procedures were more gradual, with room for appeal. The authority was to act only upon receiving notice from two householders of a 'filthy and unwholesome condition' or one that is a 'nuisance or injurious to the health'. Having given twenty-four hours notice, members of the local authority or two medical men were to inspect. If they found grounds, they would request a summons to the responsible parties to appear before two justices, who might then make an abatement order. Proceeds from the sale of seized filth were to go to the poor fund.[34] The 1855 Act (18 & 19 Vict. C 121, sect 8) included caveats, however. 'So long as the...[filth] be necessary for business or manufacture', was not kept longer than necessary, and 'best available means' were used to prevent 'injury to health', no action could be taken. And if action were taken, the profits from sale, less costs of removal, were to go to the owner (sect.18).[35] The reconciling 1875 Act combined rapidity of removal with protection of property. So long as the filth was for sale or private use and did not constitute a public nuisance, its owner was not subject to penalty, though nothing was said of how to determine 'nuisance'. Yet urban sanitary districts retained the summary powers of 1848.[36] If one could no longer so readily maintain that one's filth was innocent until proven otherwise, the owner's entitlement to the proceeds of its sale might make the bureaucratic state a bit more palatable.

All this minute legalism, noted the Webbs, marked a profound change in public administration over the course of a century. Expert in the labyrinthine regulations of the Local Government Board and his authority's by-laws, a clerk to one of the new urban district councils would have been baffled by an eighteenth-century vestry, utterly at a loss to respond to a leet jury, who would inform him 'that their right to declare the customs of the Manor, to make presentments and to give verdicts,...came down from "time out of mind", and that there were no Acts of Parliament which affected them'.[37]

Ostensibly what impelled the transformation of 'nuisance' from a contestable accusation in a community of civic equals to an ontological status to be detected by some low form of scientific authority was the threat of disease, particularly zymotic disease, an internal rotting generated by contact with exogenous material undergoing a similar form of rot, and specifically cholera. While injury to health had always been one form of injury that a 'nuisance' *might* cause, here the question now was of deadly disease that such nuisances *did* cause; disease that threatened not a few neighbours, but all of society. As the traditional means of dealing with such materials, the common law of nuisances might remain the foundation for a new and powerful public health legislation, but the local democracy of the parish or leet court or the slow working out of rights were inappropriate when cholera threatened. If lives mattered, sensibility must yield to epidemiology: unlike nuisances, disease and mortality were matters for measurement not debate.[38]

The authority of epidemiology and pathology account for *the passage* of nuisance legislation in the late 1840s and the corresponding disappearance of a public sphere approach, but they do not help us understand *the use* of the new laws. It is in examining that use that we get a better sense of why that authority was so valuable. For what developed after 1848 was not an epidemiologically driven nuisances administration but a regime in which local bureaucrats took responsibility for designating things, acts and conditions nuisances in a manner that, as far as we can see, was largely arbitrary or categorical, informed neither by high science nor by thorough and open debate.

The medicalization of nuisances was part of their absorption by the growing public health bureaucracy. The 1848 Public Health Act required appointment of an inspector of nuisances who was to report to a medical officer of health if there were one, or, failing that, directly to the local board of health. The Nuisances Removal Acts gave special authority to the views of two properly qualified medical practitioners who could designate a nuisance.[39]

Oddly, this medicalization was favoured both by those who supported expansion of the sanitary state and those who opposed it. The former believed medicine would authorize actions not being taken, the latter that it would constrain actions that might be. Despite Chadwick's misgivings, most sanitarians saw a central role for medical public officials in fighting epidemics and in preventive medicine more generally. Initially, however, the authority given to medical men in the Nuisances Removal Acts was as much a matter of their ubiquity. Few medical men had any public appointment that would make them responsible for nuisances – W.H. Duncan, the first proper medical officer, was appointed in Liverpool only in 1847. But qualified practitioners were widespread, far more so than officials charged with policing public nuisances. Regardless of whether they held a public appointment, medical men, it was hoped, would act scrupulously against dangerous practices, such as urban pig-keeping. As the medical profession gained power following the reform legislation of 1858, it became more successful in bringing nuisances into the domain of public medical practice. The 1875 Public Health Act required appointment of a medical officer of health in each district, with nuisance prevention as one duty. The inspector of nuisances, whose office had evolved from eighteenth-century developments in urban police and turnpike administration, then became a member of the public health staff – the eyes and nose of the medical officer.[40] Well staffed and medically informed, the local public health authority was then set to go forth and abolish nuisances.

To those like the bone boilers and fat renderers who might be accused of causing nuisances, this medicalization was attractive because it promised to protect them from capricious prosecution. Expertise was now not embodied in a busybody medical officer of health but in the austere epidemiology of

John Snow. The implications of Snow's work in the second (1854) edition of *The Mode of Communication of Cholera* had been quickly evident to South London industrialists. In the 1855 Select Committee on the Nuisances Removal Acts, Snow appeared on their behalf, the only medical witness the Committee heard. His message was clear. In epidemiology the bar had been raised. The so-called nuisance trades did not cause specific diseases. 'I am not aware,' Snow concluded, 'that occasional sickness is produced in any useful trade or manufacture.'[41] A doctor could be trusted to know this, insisted bone boiler Alexander Kintrea; an ordinary police inspector might be swayed by the untrustworthy senses.[42] Medicine, then, would focus on the truly dangerous nuisances, and away from the harmless effluvia of useful trades.

Both sides were wrong. Local public health administrators, though authorized by the ethos of scientific medicine, continued for most of the rest of the century to focus on traditional environmental nuisances, whether or not these could be linked to disease. Doubtless, in many cases action was taken against conditions that threatened health, but that did not have to be demonstrated: none of the sanitary acts made action dependent on epidemiology, either in the specific case at hand, or more generally. Though the 1855 Act sought to clarify it, the relationship between nuisances and injury to health remained ambiguous: in defining nuisances, the act used the phrase 'nuisance or injurious to health'. William Glen, chief contemporary authority on public health law, explained that a nuisance need not injure health:

> but inasmuch as it is scarcely possible to define what is a nuisance under the Act apart from its being injurious to health, it would hardly be safe for the justices to act unless...the particular thing complained of is...likely to injure the health.[43]

The 1875 Act, following the 1848, made an inspector's view that something 'ought to be removed' sufficient grounds for action.

There were good reasons for such peremptory action – the difficulty of epidemiological demonstration, coupled with the unacceptability of waiting for disease to strike before taking action against known causes. But the effect of the creation of that authority (coupled with the fact that the Chadwickian boards of health had evolved into general-purpose local government boards) was to make medicine the readiest rationale for any public action of environmental or social regulation. The medicalization of nuisances needs, then, to be understood in terms of a crisis of public authority created by the failure of those critical and rational means of the local state to adapt to urbanization and industrialization. We can infer that crisis from what little is known of the application of those laws.

The grand problem of statutory nuisance law was how to determine a nuisance. That problem had troubled witnesses from industrial towns testifying to the 1855 select committee. Manchester's clerk Joseph Heron worried that 'almost anything may be declared to be a nuisance'. The engineer Thomas

Hawksley complained that nuisance might 'mean anything which any person who resides in the neighbourhood may consider to be disagreeable'.[44] What Hawksley and Heron neglected to add was that common law privileged exactly that disagreeability as the 'annoyance' that was to require action. How much annoyance, how measured, to whom, and under what circumstances constituted a nuisance was precisely what was at issue.

The pressure to narrow the concept of nuisance and to invest it in rule-bound authority was a product of urbanization and industrialization. The grand common law principles of personal and property rights reflected evolution in a community of leisured equals. But what of a complex industrial community of unleisured unequals? Blackstone defined injuries affecting health as occurring where, 'by any unwholesome practice of another, a man sustains any apparent damage to his vigour or constitution' (III, 122). In the industrial town almost everyone's activities annoyed, and many damaged vigour. Heron of Manchester noted that there were trades which no 'chemical or engineering skill could...make otherwise than offensive and dangerous to the health'.[45] The evolution of nuisance statutes reflects that new context. Compensation clauses or those absolving manufacturers, while they did not forestall common law action, protected industrialists from capricious prosecution. By-laws defining categorical nuisances prevented endless mutual accusation of neighbours, all of whom were committing some objectionable act. Medicalization might seem the means for prioritizing the few really serious complaints with which a public can deal.

But in whose name would those statutes be enforced? All the parties seemed to have assumed that the ethos of epidemiology would be a sufficient guide in every matter with which a nuisances inspector might have to deal, that placing power in the hands of medicine was tantamount to creating a perfect system of decision rules. We know in retrospect that it cannot have been so. Although we know too little of their actual doings, it would appear that in many cases nuisance inspectors became enforcers of the bourgeois standards of the Victorian suburb quite as much as assailants of epidemic disease – though the categories overlapped and mutually reinforced one another. The medical officers of health and the inspectors were tied less closely to the central medical state than to local government authorities of broad purview. Often their appointments were at the pleasure of the board, and if the defence of local standards of appearance and amenity occupied them as much as combating deadly disease that is not surprising. The author of one handbook for inspectors of nuisances broached the delicate question of how to avoid becoming 'the dupe of ill-will or idle rumor'; neighbours might enlist the inspector in their battles against one another. It was better to look than to speak; essential to strike a balance – that 'whilst nothing important may escape his attention, he shall not be too prying or too much of the busybody'.[46]

An 1874 return shows a magnitude of activity hard to reconcile with any notion of narrowly medical applications, the more so given the great variability of nuisances reported in towns of similar size and make-up: in Bradford, there were over 3,000 official nuisances, in Liverpool 45,000, while in rural market towns there were often several hundred.[47] Minute books confirm this impression. The inspector of nuisances at Garston near Liverpool was concerned with such issues as an overhanging bush and unfilled puddles, and, more importantly, was being led in his inquiries, at least partly, by the complaints of neighbours.[48] The 1903 Annual Report of the Gateshead Inspector, William Jours, reflects the broadening range of public health administration, but many of the same concerns. About a fifth of Jours's more than 3,000 cases dealt with domestic waste removal; another fifth with the dilapidation of buildings and grounds.[49]

The 1874 return also shows also that designations of nuisance were rarely contested. This is striking. Viewed in light of the heritage of common law, the nuisance inspectors were, after all, committing grave impositions on rights of property. And the designations were being made not by a gentleman bred to govern, or even by a learned professional, but by a rather low-level municipal official whose whole task was to go about designating nuisances. The explanation, I believe, is the compound authority created by the marriage of public health, with its links to high science as a means to prevent deadly disease, and the old heritage of nuisances, with its links to the rights of the property owner to live free of annoyance. Notwithstanding John Snow's demonstrations, new knowledge of specific acute diseases with single causes did not quickly drive out old ideas of sensible annoyances that injured the constitution. Concepts like predisposition made it possible to take seriously insults to sight, smell or imagination – like the queasiness felt by some persons in walking next to a cemetery – as harmful to health, and therefore as public nuisances, well into the era of bacteriology.[50] Indeed one may argue that concepts of environmentally caused illness had so long coevolved with common law rights that they could not be disentangled. Thus the inspector's authority derived from an accretion of symbols: the presumption of an annoyance to all the monarch's subjects and thereby to the monarchy itself (Burn's indictments ended by alleging that the acts in question were 'against the peace of our said lady the Queen, her crown and dignity'), the common good, and an ability to root out the disease that would surely spring out if the strict standards of the newly house-proud were not meticulously met. And, of course, to yield to the inspector's genteel standards was proof of one's own gentility.

Conclusion

In terms of the history of public health, it is surely true that the new standards, at least with regard to dung keeping, helped prevent disease. But that is not the only history at stake. Political life at its most local level is also implicated. The conception of public life sketched here is of people using 'health' to argue about whether they had gone to sufficient lengths to clean up their own messes. In the switch from annoyance to disease, profound changes occurred: 'community' became medicalized; not only was disease causation the *best* vehicle for complaining about our neighbours, it became the *main* one. Nuisance became a matter of coercion rather than adjudication. An approach that recognized potential conflict in any social setting, and provided a remedy in community resolution, gave way to one in which nuisance was no longer a refutable accusation, but an abstraction defined by an official. Community standards need no longer be continually worked out; they were assumed and enforced. Thus Toulmin Smith's contrast of common law and empirical legislation foreshadows Foucault:

> The one system [under common law] is founded on a trusting faith in the intelligence and honesty of the average of men. The other...can rest on nothing else than – the assumption that all men, except central functionaries, are dishonest, and that none but such functionaries have any intelligence.[51]

Yet the state was not to blame: it was communities themselves that found the power of summary action so tantalizingly delicious, so easy a way of imposing the presumed public will on everyone. The victims remained the poor: in general the sanitary legislation was much more aggressive and arbitrary about conditions within houses than it was with large nuisance-producing industries.

There are ironies here. One might expect science, that purified form of communicative action, to facilitate the workings of the public sphere and render public discourse more critical and more rational. Yet at the same time as medical science was gaining access to specific causes of disease it was becoming increasingly unnecessary actually to demonstrate harm. One would not expect to find this science providing the symbolic authority for a tautology-perpetrating functionary who can condense the grave process of determining rights into an arbitrary utterance of designation – 'I know a nuisance when I see it.' Health had been successfully fetishized – but only because 'nuisance' had been fetishized before it.[52]

The call to make public health again truly public, to reconnect it with community, has been frequent in recent years.[53] It reflects demands for social services that are local and gentle, flexible and responsive, but also the bewilderment of states and professions with a new set of public health problems that seem troublesomely philosophical – issues related to smoking or life-style regulation for example. However sceptical we may be about the idealized public sphere, we would be well to include in this conversation a fuller understanding of the experiences of local publics in the past in creating their own defensible forms of public administration.

Acknowledgements

I would like to thank the Editor and my colleague David Waldstreicher for their comments on earlier drafts of this chapter.

Notes

1 J. Habermas, *The Structural Transformation of the Public Sphere*, trans. T. Burger with F. Lawrence, Cambridge, MA: MIT Press, 1989.
2 See for example C. Baskerville, 'Sanitation and the city', in Baskerville (ed.), *Municipal Chemistry*, New York: McGraw Hill, 1910, p. 3: 'The growth of a city causes it to assume, willingly or no, corresponding obligations. The inhabitants must breathe, they must be fed and watered, its wastes must be got rid of, facilities for the safe coming and going of its people at all times must be provided, as well as protection from fire and other adventitious circumstances'; A. Shaw, *Municipal Government in Great Britain*, New York: Century, 1895, p. 7.
3 J. Redlich and F.W. Hirst, *The History of Local Government in England, Being a Reissue of Book 1 of Local Government in England*, 2nd edn, with an Introduction and Epilogue by B. Keith-Lucas, New York: Augustus Kelley, 1970, pp. xi, 151.
4 Habermas's scenario is mainly appropriate to the experience of continental countries; his discussion of legal traditions leaves out common law entirely, for example (cf. Habermas, *Structural Transformation*, pp. 53, 76).
5 Such forms of government drew forth a great deal of interest from nineteenth-century German political theorists who in some way were Habermas's predecessors both in recognizing something like a public sphere and accounting for its disappearance. For both the Prussian Rudolph von Gneist and the Austrian Josef Redlich the English constitutional tradition exemplified the organic evolution of government. But while von Gneist located the epitome of this tradition in the eighteenth century (coincidentally with Habermas's public sphere), and saw it thereafter succumbing to the bureaucracies, professions and statutes of the resurgent state, Redlich regarded state growth in the nineteenth century as the maturation of local problem-solving not its repudiation. B. Keith-Lucas, 'Introduction', in Redlich and Hirst, *History of Local Government in England*, pp. ix–xv. For another view see H. Finer, *English Local Government*, London: Methuen, 1933, pp. 8–20.
6 J. Redlich, *Local Government in England*, edited with additions by F.W. Hirst, 2 vols, London: Macmillan, 1903. More recently, see D. Eastwood, *Governing Rural England: Tradition and Transformation in Local Government, 1780–1840*, Oxford: Clarendon Press, 1994.
7 B. Keith-Lucas, *The Unreformed Local Government System*, London: Croom Helm, 1980, pp. 29–30; B. Webb and S. Webb, *English Local Government from the Revolution to the Municipal Corporations Act: Statutory Authorities for Special Purposes*, London: Longmans, Green, 1922, pp. 254–8; W. Sheppard, *The Court Keeper's Guide for the Keeping of Courts Leet and Courts Baron*, 7th edn, London: Atkins, 1685, pp. 13, 44–6. Some recent historians who have looked closely at the leet and similar courts find them problematic in various ways as institutions of broad public will. For a recent defence see W. King, 'Leet jurors and the search for law and order in seventeenth-century England: "galling persecution" or reasonable justice', *Histoire Sociale – Social History*, 1980, vol. 13, pp. 305–23; *idem*, 'Early Stuart courts leet still needful and useful', in ibid., 1990, vol. 23, pp. 271–99.
8 Habermas, *Structural Transformation*, pp. 30–1, 51, 54–5. This list is urban. One could make a similar list of fishing, hunting and pannage rights. The centrality of environmental issues in Magna Carta and the associated Charter of the Forest is noteworthy in this regard.
9 F.R. Wilson, *A Practical Guide for Inspectors of Nuisances*, London: Knight, 1881, pp. 4–5.
10 Webb and Webb, *English Local Government*, pp. 274, 314–5, 343; Keith-Lucas, *The Unreformed Local Government System*, pp. 113, 120–1. The first historian of this legislation, F.H. Spencer, writes that 'this mass of legislation represents the first efforts of a community undergoing a very rapid economic development to provide itself with local institutions suitable to its changing industrial organisation': *Municipal Origins: An Account of English Private Bill Legislation Relating to Local Government, 1740–1835; with a Chapter on Private Bill Procedure*, London: Constable and Co, 1911, p. 309.

11 *Burn's Justice of the Peace*, 29th edn, 7 vols, London: Sweet, Maxwell, & Son, 1845, vol. 5, s.v. 'Nuisance, Public', p. 242.

12 E. Garrett, *The Law of Nuisances*, London: Clowes, 1890, p. 118. See the key case of Fletcher v. Rylands, on the pervasive permeability of actions on one property, whether it be 'beast or water, or filth or stenches', affecting others.

13 For various treatments of this question cf. G. Kearns, 'Cholera, nuisances, and environmental management in Islington, 1830–1855', in W.F. Bynum and R. Porter (eds), *Living and Dying in London*, London: Wellcome Institute for the History of Medicine, 1991, pp. 94–125; *idem*, 'Private property and public health reform in England, 1830–1870', *Social Science and Medicine*, 1988, vol. 26, pp. 187–99; C. Hamlin, 'Muddling in Bumbledom: local governments and large sanitary improvements: the cases of four British Towns, 1855–1885', *Victorian Studies*, 1988, vol. 32, pp. 55–83; J. Prest, *Liberty and Locality: Parliament, Permissive Legislation, and Ratepayers' Democracies in the Nineteenth Century*, Oxford: Clarendon Press, 1990, pp. 66, 178.

14 Following Mary Poovey, it acts as a means of cultural formation: M. Poovey, *Making a Social Body: British Cultural Formation, 1830–1864*, Chicago: University of Chicago Press, 1995.

15 M. Douglas, 'Environments at risk', in B. Barnes and D. Edge (eds), *Science in Context*, Cambridge, MA: MIT Press; 1982, pp. 260–75; *idem*, *Purity and Danger: An Analysis of the Concepts of Pollution and Taboo*, London: Routledge & Kegan Paul, 1966.

16 F.M.L. Thomson, *Chartered Surveyors: The Growth of a Profession*, London: Routledge, 1968, pp. 140–2.

17 W. Blackstone, *Commentaries on the Laws of England*, 4 vols, New York: Strouse, 1892.

18 An anonymous contemporary suggests that Blackstone's conception of the domain of public nuisances was typical of the eighteenth century. He includes insolent servants as well as street butchers. See 'A Gentleman of the Temple', *Public Nuisance Considered under the Several Heads of Bad Pavements, Butchers Infesting the Streets, the Inconveniences to the Publick, Occasioned by the Present Method of Billitting the Foot-Guards, and the Insolence of Household Servants, with Some Hints Towards Remedy and Amendment*, London: E. Withers, 1750. On the development of street conditions as a common nuisance and of a public response see Webb and Webb, *English Local Government*, pp. 316–17. With regard to health nuisances, in particular, another contemporary authority, Richard Burn, in *Justice of the Peace*, does include a child inoculated with smallpox as a category of public nuisance: 'Nuisance, public', p. 236.

19 *London Viewers and Their Certificates, 1508–1558: Certificates of the Sworn Viewers of the City of London*, ed. J.S. Loengard, London: London Record Society, 1989, esp. pp. i–li; *London Assize of Nuisance, 1301–1431: A Calendar*, ed. H. Chew, and W. Kellaway, London: London Record Society, 1973.

20 M.D. Harris, *The Coventry Leet Book: Or Mayor's Register, Containing the Records of the City Court Leet or View of Frankpledge, A.D. 1420–1555, with Divers Other Matters*, London: Early English Text Society/Kegan Paul, 1907–11; J. Ritson, *A Digest of the Proceedings of the Court Leet of the Manor and Liberty of Savoy, Parcel of the Duchy of Lancaster, in the County of Middlesex, from the Year 1682 to the Present Time*, London, 1789, pp. 20–6; Westminster Sewers Commission Archives, 1809, Greater London Records Office WCS 169. For a recent vindication of these institutions see D. Sunderland, '"A monument to defective administration"? The London Commissions of Sewers in the Early Nineteenth Century', *Urban History*, 1999, vol. 26, pp. 348–72.

21 'These Institutions provide, at every man's door, a regular, unevadable, and simple tribunal, in whose action all men from time to time have to bear a part; which is costless in its procedure and equitable in its practice; before which every man's voice shall be heard': J.T. Smith, *Practical Proceedings for the Removal of Nuisances to health and Safety: and for the Execution of Sewerage Works, in Towns and in Rural Parishes, under the common law and Under Recent Statutes*, 4th ed., London: H. Sweet, Stevens & Sons, and W. Maxwell, 1867, p. 4.

22 The American historian William Novak has given the combination of common law, environmental regulation and local by-laws considerable credit for successful regulation of nuisances in nineteenth-century American cities: *The People's Welfare: Law and Regulation in Nineteenth-Century America*, Chapel Hill: University of North Carolina Press, 1996, esp. chapter 6. Novak is focusing more on the evolution of law than on the fabric of cities, however, and it is unclear how representative are the legal decisions he examines, nor what were their practical effects.

23 Garrett, *The Law of Nuisances*, pp. 146–7. A superb and balanced analysis of the strengths and weaknesses of common law in dealing with one form of environmental problem is C. Higgins, *A Treatise on the Law Relating to the Pollution and Obstruction of Watercourses; Together with a Brief Summary of the Various Sources of River Pollution*, London: Stevens and Haynes, 1877.

24 Smith, *Practical Proceedings for the Removal of Nuisances*, pp. 16–18.

25 Modern legal historians have been puzzled at how little the common law was invoked to deal with offensive trades in the industrial revolution – though, in fairness, their attention has focused mostly on jurisdiction at the highest levels, where there is regular reporting of cases, and neglected the resolution of disputes within the parish, the manor or the municipal corporation. See D.R. Coquillete, 'Mosses from an old manse: another look at some historic property cases about the environment', *Cornell University Law Review*, 1979, vol. 64, pp. 761–822, esp. pp. 761–81; P.S. McLaren, 'Nuisance law and the Industrial Revolution – some lessons from social history', *Oxford Journal of Legal Studies*, 1983, vol. 3, pp. 155–221.

26 C. Rosen, 'Differing perceptions of the value of pollution abatement across time and place: balancing doctrine in pollution nuisance law, 1840–1906', *Law and History Review*, 1993, vol. 11, pp. 303–85.

27 Smith, *Practical Proceedings for the Removal of Nuisances*, p. 97.

28 Initially most of these by-laws required Parliamentary approval; after the middle of the nineteenth century they frequently required only the approval of bureaucrats in the Home Office or Local Government Board. F.H. Spencer, *Municipal Origins: An Account of English Private Bill Legislation Relating to Local Government, 1740–1835; with a Chapter on Private Bill Procedure*, London: Constable & Co., 1911, p. 275; Webb and Webb, *English Local Government*, pp. 300–1, 318–9.

29 W.C. Glen, *The Law Relating to the Public Health and Local Government, in Relation to Sanitary and other Matters, Together with the Public Health Act, 1848, the Local Government Act 1858, and the Other Incorporated Acts*, London: Butterworths, 1858, p. 335. It is important to note that the great age of municipal improvement acts that began in the mid-eighteenth century continued throughout the nineteenth, despite availability of general legislation.

30 It is also crucial to note that such legislation supplemented rather than replaced common law: what was legal under statute might be a nuisance in common law; equally, even if no one complained, an action might be criminal if it had been designated a nuisance. On the adoption of the Public Health Act, see C. Hamlin, *Public Health and Social Justice in the Age of Chadwick: Britain, 1800–1854*, Cambridge: Cambridge University Press, 1998, chapter 9.

31 The 1855 Act was celebrated by Toulmin Smith, the great and controversial champion of common law, as embodying the principles of common law in requiring all local authorities to enforce environmental standards of health and safety: Smith, *Practical Proceedings for the Removal of Nuisances*, pp. 3, 22–5, 96–8. Yet he doubted it gave them any powers that they did not already hold under common law.

32 W.G. Lumley, *The Act for the More Speedy Removal of Nuisances, and the Prevention of Contagious Diseases, 9 & 10 Vic. c. 96…and the Poor Law Commissioners' Circular Letter*, London: Charles Knight, 1846, p. 11.

33 W.C. Glen, *The Law Relating to the Removal of Nuisances Injurious to Health, and to the Prevention of Epidemic, Endemic, and Contagious Diseases, with the Statutes, Including the Public Health Act, 1858*, London: Butterworths, 1858, pp. 80–1, 140.

34 J. Archbold, *The Parish Officer, Comprising the Whole of the Present Law Relating to the Several Parish and Union Officers, as well as of the Guardians of the Poor in England; Comprising also the Law as to Church Rates, Highway Rates, Vestries, Watching and Lighting, etc.*, 2nd ed. *by William Cunningham Glen*, London: Shaw & Sons, 1855, pp. 202–4. Reference is to the 1848 version (11 & 12 Vict c 123 s 1).

35 Glen, *The Law Relating to the Removal of Nuisances*, pp. 12, 27.

36 W.G. Lumley, *Lumley's Public Health Act of 1875*, London: Shaw & Sons, 1876.

37 Webb and Webb, *English Local Government*, p. 390.

38 For this view of the evolution of local government see Finer, *English Local Government*, p. 11.

39 Glen, *The Law Relating to the Removal of Nuisances*, p. 131. The Improvement Clauses Act of 1847 had allowed appointment of an inspector of nuisances.

40 The Webbs suggest an evolution also from the office of turnpike surveyor: *English Local Government*, pp. 166–7.

41 Select Committee on the Public Health Bill and the Nuisances Removal Amendment Bill, P.P., 1854–5, vol. 13, qq. 119–139. 'From my printed publication they have learnt that my opinion is, that measures necessary to protect the public health would not interfere with useful trades' (q. 119).

42 Ibid., qq. 291, 317.

43 Glen, *The Law Relating to the Removal of Nuisances*, p. 13.

44 Select Committee on the Public Health Bill and the Nuisances Removal Amendment Bill, qq. 1503, 1517, 530–32.

45 Ibid., q. 1510.

46 'Return showing the appointments of...Medical Officers of Health and Inspectors of Nuisances now operating under the General Sanitary Acts, or any Local Act', P.P, 1873, vol. 55, p. 359; E. Smith, *Handbook for Inspectors of Nuisances*, London: Knight, 1873, pp. 29–31.

47 'Return from urban and rural sanitary authorities in England and Wales of nuisances reported and dealt with, and estimated cost of sanitary structural works...for 1874', P.P., 1875, vol. 64, p. 434.

48 See the notebooks of James Standing, inspector of nuisances of Garston, in Liverpool Public Library, GAR. See also Prest, *Liberty and Locality*, p. 178; H.J. Dyos, *Victorian Suburb: A Study in the Growth of Camberwell*, Leicester: Leicester University Press, 1961, pp. 82–3.

49 W. Jours, *County Borough of Gateshead. The Annual Report of the Gateshead Inspector of Nuisances for the Year 1903*, Gateshead: Howe Bros, 1903.

50 C. Hamlin, 'Predisposing causes and public health in the early nineteenth century public health movement', *Social History of Medicine*, 1992, vol. 5, pp. 43–70; *idem*, *Public Health and Social Justice in the Age of Chadwick*; W. Eassie, *Cremation of the Dead: Its History and Bearings upon Public Health*, London: Smith, Elder, 1875, p. 60.

51 Smith, *Practical Proceedings for the Removal of Nuisances*, p. 35.

52 M. Edelstein, *Contaminated Communities: Social and Psychological Impacts of Residential Toxic Exposure*, Boulder: Westview, 1988; B. Wynne, 'Misunderstood misunderstandings: social identities and the public uptake of science', in A. Irwin and B. Wynne (eds), *Misunderstanding Science? The Public Reconstruction of Science and Technology*, Cambridge: Cambridge University Press, 1996, pp. 19–46; D. Collingridge and C. Reeve, *Science Speaks to Power: the Role of Experts in Policy-Making*, New York: St Martin's, 1986; R. Sclove, *Democracy and Technology*, New York: Guilford Press, 1995.

53 J. Ashton (ed.), *Healthy Cities*, Milton Keynes: Open University Press, 1992; A. Petersen and D. Lupton, *The New Public Health: Health and Self in the Age of Risk*, London: Sage, 1996; S. Tesh, *Hidden Arguments: Political Ideology and Disease Prevention*, New Brunswick: Rutgers University Press, 1987.

10 In the beginning was the lymph

The hollowing of stational vaccination in England and Wales, 1840–98

Logie Barrow

In mid-June of 1871, the *Lancet* reported a court case that it considered to have disturbing implications.[1] A man named apparently no more than 'Jones' who 'had not a farthing of money, [had been] removed in [a] prison van' from Islington police court after saying that 'he and his family were often without food'. He had broken the 1853 and 1867 Vaccination Acts that required all parents to have their children vaccinated against smallpox. An epidemic was currently raging in Islington and indeed in Europe.

Jones had initially complied with the law by taking two of his children to a local 'vaccination station' to be immunized. But his legal responsibilities did not end there. He was also required by Clause 9 of the 1853 Act and Clause 17 of the 1867 Act to take his children back to the 'station' one week later for inspection, to confirm the operation's success. If successful, the children instantly became available for giving lymph to the next vaccinees, who were likely during epidemics to be plentiful and (if parents or adults) clamorous. However, as Jones informed the bench, the local Medical Officer had told him not to take his children out 'because there was smallpox in the house, and a child lying dead of it in the next room'. For the Medical Officer, surely, the recentness of the vaccination made Jones's children a public health risk, as they might themselves infect others on the way to the 'station', let alone in it. The *Lancet* endorsed the Medical Officer's judgement, and condemned 'the length' to which 'the idea of stational vaccination...[could be] carried' – in this case, to 'being made the means of propagating smallpox'. Jones – who now himself 'appeared very ill, and who had risen from his bed to obey the summons' – had simply followed what seemed to be well-founded medical advice (empowered, incidentally, under broader and even more recent legislation). Nevertheless, the bench concluded that he was in breach of the Acts, and fined him (with fingers in Clause 29 of 1867) a total of £2 or two weeks' jail.

It is easy to ironize with the *Lancet* that 'the authorities of Islington must [have been] wishing to make vaccination unpopular'. Presumably, they were seeking to make Jones into an example. That this misfired so badly – not least for the *Lancet* – is indicative of profound tensions inherent in the Vaccination Acts' administration.

Partly as a result of these tensions, many anxious people were goaded into non-vaccination or even anti-vaccinationism. Moreover, some public authorities (including many Poor Law Guardians and, by the 1890s, even some magistrates) became lax to the extent that compulsion often became unworkable. Finally, in 1898 new legislation was enacted allowing parents to register a 'conscientious objection' before the bench (assuming the latter would accept it), and thereby exempt their children from compulsory vaccination, inspection and extraction. Until a deadline of mid-December of that year, this 'conscience clause' was retrospective for all children under fourteen. In many towns and some villages around England, its passage was in effect celebrated with huge and sometimes fractious queues of parents seeking exemption. Elsewhere, anti-vaccination agitators seem to have persuaded indeterminate numbers that even a 'conscientious' declaration before magistrates was an unnecessary insult to individual liberty.[2]

The important point to note is that parents – aside from their own (in many cases) fluctuating balance of decision between the risks of vaccination and of smallpox – objected to what they saw as the confusing and unfair workings of the state machinery of compulsion that so often over-rode their own or their doctors' judgements of what might be best for their families and for public health. These qualities, I shall argue, boosted opposition to compulsory vaccination, and especially to the practice of stational operations.

Underlying these qualities, moreover, were divisions between different sectors of the state itself. The growth of public vaccination represents an important Victorian attempt to expand the sphere of statutory authority to include aspects of private lives. It was resisted, not always necessarily because of objections to compulsory vaccination – though these were undoubtedly a growing factor – but also because the public vaccination facilities set up to provide for the poor proved deeply objectionable to many parents and doctors alike. The tension between universal compulsion and a discriminatory system of public provision was indicative of incoherence within the sphere of public authority.

Public policy and the growth of stational vaccination

In 1840 legislation had been passed allowing vaccination freely but not compulsorily at public expense to anyone demanding it. The assumption had been that no one except 'the poor' would take advantage of this, as the operation was to be provided by their local Poor Law Guardians. Thus, from the very start, public vaccination was snarled up with the 1834 Poor Law – that is, with an apparatus which at that time (whatever later complexities and ironies) was widely and viscerally hated for degrading the powerless before the more-or-less powerful. True, in 1841, Parliament had tried to draw that sting by means of a one-clause Act declaring public vaccination to be non-pauperizing. But mere words could hardly erase impressions left by much weekly practice through nearly six ensuing decades.

Public vaccination exacerbated a second set of post-1834 tensions: between local and central. Whitehall's often all-too-justified distrust of virtually any operation performed outside its supervision (privately, but also often 'publicly' too) deepened over nearly two generations. A third set of tensions added to the general misery: locally and often nationally, the Anglo-British state often stood out in Europe for its amateurishness. Not that this necessarily lessened its effectiveness. But orthodox medics were struggling for respect as professionals and often felt degraded by supervision, whether local or from Whitehall.

Into these often mutually aggravating tensions came the 1853 Act making vaccination compulsory for everyone within three months of birth. Or rather, it made compulsory the possession of a certificate of successful vaccination: an unknowable number of private medicators, however qualified, were happy – for fees – to sign the officially stipulated certificate after almost any 'vaccination' as slight as some parent might wish. Those parents who lacked access to such lax practitioners had no alternative to public vaccination – seen as all too near the Poor Law. Not only was it administered by the Guardians, but also many public vaccinators were Workhouse or local Medical Officers, seizing on additional duties to boost their profile and earning power.

Probably the greatest insult to parents, however, was the practice of arm-to-arm vaccination. This practice, which involved injecting 'lymph' from the sores on the arm of a baby vaccinated a week earlier, encouraged everyone on the official side, from operators to Whitehall, to view babies as inconvenient extensions of arms, not vice versa. Parents seem often to have sensed this priority. But until 1898, English (including Welsh) vaccination authorities privileged the practice of arm-to-arm vaccination over the use of preserved lymph – whether derived from humans or animals.

They did so for reasons of public health and safety: recently extracted human lymph was widely held to be purer than preserved lymph, which was understandably though not universally seen as liable to contamination.[3] In England (unlike, usually, Scotland or Ireland), this preference for fresh lymph on a mass scale implied another for what we have heard the *Lancet* calling 'stational vaccination' – in other words, the establishment of official centres where numbers of children could be brought to be vaccinated at set times, preferably every week. Thus in the early 1860s John Snow (famed for his researches on cholera and general hygiene) argued that 'operators who visit the patients at their homes must use stored lymph',[4] which for him meant inferior material. Thirty years later, one *Lancet* editorialist was still 'fail[ing] to see how' vaccination could 'be carried to every man's door' except with preserved lymph.[5] The argument was a trifle artificial: for decades, vaccinifers (those children used as the source of lymph) for babies of at any rate better-off parents had often been trundled around in a carriage. Nevertheless, from the early 1860s, central authorities increasingly pressured public vaccinators to concentrate all such work exclusively in stations, for the express purpose of ensuring reliable supplies of fresh lymph. So strong was Whitehall's suspicion of home vaccination, that public vaccinators were sometimes penalized for resorting to it – or even for setting foot in parents' homes for the purpose of convincing them to come to the station. (By contrast, in Ireland and even more in Scotland, home vaccination was routine.) Further, where population in England was sparse, Whitehall increasingly preferred to ignore the law's insistence on the three-month maximum age: better, once or twice a year, to arrange the more or less recently-born arms into chains of fresh human vaccination, than to leave each arm to be vaccinated with stored lymph on random dates. The only governmentally endorsed use of such lymph was for operating on the first vaccinifer in a series. (This was the purpose of that oldest of official vaccinal institutions, the National Vaccine Establishment.)

Some vaccinators, at least, agreed that stations represented an effective means of fulfilling this aim. At times like Christmas, for instance, busy parents might be all the less inclined to shoulder the extra burden of having their children vaccinated and nursing them through the indisposition or illness that often followed. At such times, stations provided a useful means of bringing together the few children who were presented for vaccination, and hence of maintaining the continuity of lymph supply from one week to the next. Even when attendance fell so low as to undermine arm-to-arm continuity, stations could still prove a useful resource. Thus at one in Inner London, around 'the day of the marriage of the Prince of Wales' in 1863, one long-prominent vaccinator, J.F. Marson, was reduced to using stored lymph. Results reportedly confirmed its untrustworthiness: even after arm-to-arm service had resumed, '[t]he effect...was that the lymph for some time afterwards...did not produce such fair vesicles [i.e. pustules regarded as indicators of how well the vaccination had "taken"] as before the interruption'. Nevertheless, the large numbers normally attending here helped redress the situation: 'the interesting fact...[was] that by selecting the best arm of the day to vaccinate from, Mr Marson has now worked...[the lymph] back again to as good a state as before'.[6] Thus stations could serve as miniature stockfarms, with babies as incubators for the production of vaccines thought to be of high quality.

There was another reason why the authorities favoured stational vaccination, namely ease of surveillance. During the debates over the framing of what was to become the 1853 Act, some elite lobbyists newly gathered in the Epidemiological Society had feared that large numbers of unsuccessful vaccinations were being recorded as successful, and that Whitehall was consequently working with gross overestimates of the extent of immunity among the population.[7] This was why Clause 9 of the 1853 Vaccination Act – one of those we have seen ensnaring Jones – required parents of public vaccinees to bring their children back to the public vaccinator for confirmation that the operation had been successful. The status of such confirmation remained insecure, however. Orthodox medics continued at sixes and sevens as to what constituted effective vaccination: the preferred angle, depth and number of insertions; the type of lymph used and its origins; the number and appearance of vesicles; severity of post-vaccinal symptoms; the question whether more lymph conferred more immunity; the duration of that immunity; definitions of hygiene; and much else – even whether blood and lymph should mix. Consequently, from about 1860, a missionary handful of medical 'policemen' – many of them founding Epidemiologicals now swaying on a succession of saplings of state we can dignify as Whitehall – tried to cut through all this by enforcing a code of practice via inspection.

The inspectors, employed as civil servants, reported to Whitehall after visiting any public vaccinator. Such visits occurred every two years or so and seem to have been more-or-less pre-announced. For any but the most part-time vacci-nator, they were crucial: payment came not only from the Guardians as a fee for every 'successful' operation (as defined usually by the vaccinator) but also, in addition, as a top-up or 'grant' recommended by Whitehall. This too was paid via the Guardians, sometimes grudgingly. Whitehall's recommendation was supposed to follow that of its inspector. If he disliked those operations or vesicles he happened to see, or regarded a vaccinator as in any way sloppy – medically or even bureaucratically – then no grant would come for the work of the previous two or so years. As an ultimate sanction, Whitehall could withdraw approval of the vaccinator's appointment and demand that the Guardians sack him. Not surprisingly, we hear public vaccinators louder in complaint against inspection than in praise of it, and louder still when they felt mistreated than when the grant came through. But whether the complaints were representative or not, they underlined where power ultimately lay, and also perhaps how cursory some or perhaps most inspections were.

Concentration of vaccination in stations was seen as an important means of facilitating the enforcement of official standards of practice. Thus A.E. Steele of Liverpool, one of the system's keenest provincial supporters, reasoned that it was 'only when a sufficient number of arms can be gathered together that vaccina-tion can be carried out in the best and most efficient manner'. His notion of how stations contributed to efficiency – informed perhaps by the fact that his own was designated 'Educational' (i.e. for medical students) – is revealing: it was here, he observed, 'that the largest proportion of typical vesicles and the rarest deviations therefrom [were] to be seen'.[8] Stations, in other words, provided a valuable means of making vaccination practices and procedures visible, for purposes both of inspection and regulation. 'Educational' stations (about twenty around the country, all sited near medical schools) were seen as vital for disseminating best practice to fresh medics. But stational vaccination more generally shared this virtue of making vaccinational practices more readily visible, in particular to the inspecting authorities.

Thus, with the growing insistence on stations, public vaccination was being made increasingly public. First, it was carried out under the auspices – and considerably at the expense – of the public authorities: Guardians in the first instance. Second, it was increasingly concentrated in designated public spaces – stations – rather than dispersed in the private spaces of vaccinees' homes. And third, these officially new spaces were the sites of supervision by the central public authorities.

Vaccinators' objections to public vaccination

Central surveillance of their work was a cause of mounting annoyance to vaccinators. It was not just that medicators private or public saw government inspection as weakening the authority of their expertise. They also had to contend with growing official interference in their practice, and – most annoyingly – with a growing burden of paperwork. From 1840, a little pen-pushing had obviously been one precondition for any public vaccinator claiming his fee for every operation he judged 'successful'. This onus of bureaucratic labour was increased from 1853 with additional certificates to be filled in for contingencies such as unfitness for vaccination (perhaps many times per child) or insusceptibility (after many attempts). The hope was that all this state labour (entirely unpaid when an operation was private) would help trace individuals or even generate epidemiological data.

All too often, though, it opened a floodgate of informational garbage, fed on alienation. One Essex practitioner even proposed collecting the various blank forms 'to make a bonfire of' – an idea that the *Lancet* found tempting. More strategically, the *Lancet* suggested, vaccinators might refuse to fill in the forms so as to impale masses of parents on a fine of up to £1 per child. In the end, the journal calmed down and advised compliance so that '*all the imperfections of the Act will come out*'.[9] Certainly the bureaucratic requirements of the 1853 Act proved imperfect in practice. By 1867, William Farr, Treasurer and soon to be Vice-President of the Statistical Society, and Superintendent of Statistics at the General Register Office, could be heard lengthily detailing the imperfections to London BMA members:

> An average book...of one of the most diligent London registrars, contains, in 500 entries, only 65 complete....If you name any half-dozen sub-districts at random, I will...get the books, and prove...that the [1853 Act]...has been a complete failure.

The fault, for Farr, lay in 'the amount of clerical labour which is thrust upon the surgeon'. This was not so much a matter of snobbery or even of habit, as of stress: 'What hindrance these certificates throw in the way of a man whose station is full of children, and who wants to get away to other patients, or to a woman at a distance in labour, we can easily conceive'. Farr considered the 1853 Act to be 'a piece of amateur legislation'. But its 1867 and partial successors hardly lessened vaccinators' 'amount of clerical labour'.[10]

Central government interference was only one source of annoyance to public vaccinators. They also harboured deep-seated resentment at the conditions imposed on them by their local employers, the Guardians. Public vaccinators had to bear often quite heavy costs, both emotional and financial, during their work. True, the substitution of stational for home (the jargon-word was 'domiciliary') operations was in one way a relief: it threw an onus on parents to come to the station or risk a fine. But whether in home or station, operators sometimes had to brave 'insults and injuries on the spur of the moment' from parents.[11] The remuneration for such onerous service was often insultingly light. Guardians were anxious to minimise costs of vaccination to ratepayers, and so endeavoured to keep fees as low as possible. In the few instances where stational vaccination was adopted before the 1860s, Guardians even occasionally quibbled about paying rent for rooms.[12] Indeed, the Epidemiologists claimed that 'the exertion of the public vaccinators [was] not infrequently discouraged by...Boards [of Guardians]...whenever any large number of vaccinations had been reported'.[13]

Advocates of Poor Law attitudes sought to influence central policy too. At one stage, legislators considered inserting into the 1853 Act a clause that would have imposed yet further burdens on vaccinators: if, 'in consequence of vaccination' (as if 'consequence' were never controversial!), the vaccinee were to become 'sick or indisposed' (again, such precision!), 'then...it shall be the vaccinator's duty...to attend...and furnish [the vaccinee] with such needs as may be necessary...without additional fee or reward'.[14] Mercifully, this clause did not survive, but its very words underlined how some legislators regarded public vaccinators as little more than an unwarranted burden on ratepayers.

If Poor Law meanness did not altogether triumph centrally, it loomed locally. Guardians were able to impose unfavourable conditions of service because public vaccinators' appointments were keenly sought, particularly by young practitioners newly arrived on the scene. Consequently, Guardians were able to exploit competition for such appointments to cut fees. Occasionally, they even switched to vaccinal 'amateurs' – who might include 'unqualified' as well as more or less heterodox practitioners and neighbours of all kinds. So far as some Guardians were concerned, there was evidently little to choose between qualified and unqualified practitioners – another fact that rankled with the former, who objected that the Guardians' practice of requiring them to register an operation as 'successful' before paying them their fee brusquely degraded them to the level of 'no-cure-no-pay' quacks. Thus public vaccination threatened a still tender professionalism.[15]

Doctors had few means of fighting such exploitation. Poor Law medicators in many localities from Lancashire to Cornwall to London were, from the 1840s, increasingly taking action along trade union lines: in 1856, a Poor Law Medical Reform Association was set up that soon seems to have represented more than half the publicly employed practitioners in England. One anonymous 'M.D.' claimed in 1852 to know of 'many large districts' where the medical men 'one and all' refused Poor Law work, and where as a result 'the poor were left to the mercy of men without any qualification whatsoever, save extreme poverty'.[16] But there is little evidence that such attempts at collective action were successful in securing more favourable terms for vaccinators. On a local and individual basis, at least into the 1850s, doctors might undertake to vaccinate the poor gratis, thus hoping to shame the Poor Law authorities by refusing their paltry fee. But such refusals often only enraged brother-practitioners: free vaccination reeked of the kind of competition between practitioners that some Guardians already exploited. On the other hand, it might sometimes be unavoidable for repelling yet worse competitors, such as chemists or even the heterodox.[17] Ultimately, though, practitioners' favoured strategy was to seek to eliminate competition for vaccinators' posts altogether, by eliminating the posts themselves. Thus from the 1840s to the 1890s the commonest demand from many of their representative bodies was that all qualified local medical men be recognized as public vaccinators.

Central initiatives to improve standards of practice did little to improve the lot of the vaccinator. In important respects they actually worsened it. From the late 1860s, significant cuts were made in the number of public vaccinators, while increasingly rigid restrictions were imposed on the geographical areas within which they could practice. This concentration was partly intended to increase inspectability. Significantly, though, it also targeted one peculiarly 'malign' type of competition between vaccinators. They were remunerated on a fees-for-service basis, but their areas had often been defined rather loosely. For Whitehall, the resulting competition encouraged vaccinators to heed best practice less than the preferences of parents. Parents, unlike Whitehall and its Epidemiologicals, were generally seen to prefer the fewest insertions of lymph per child, and might play vaccinators off against each other to secure this. 'There is,' as Edward Cator Seaton (quintessential Whitehall Epidemiological) reminded the 1871 House of Commons Select Committee on Vaccination, 'such a thing as competition down-wards....a public vaccinator would say "Mr So and So will vaccinate in four places; I will do in two".' This 'serious difficulty',[18] as Seaton saw it, spurred both Whitehall and soon many Boards of Guardians to refuse any kind of payment for vaccination of anyone from outside the operator's strictly defined area.

The problem, so far as vaccinators were concerned, was that such measures played into Guardians' hands. Obviously, 'reducing' competition by cutting jobs actually increased it between candidates for these, enabling Guardians to slash pay yet further. Thus during the period of contraction, Guardians sometimes added insult to injury by not re-employing the more expensive of their former vaccinators – usually the older or more experienced ones. Public vaccinators thus found themselves caught in contradictions between the expectations of the central and local vaccination authorities: the desire of the central authority to promote high standards was inherently in conflict with the Guardians' desire to limit rate-borne expenditure. In such circumstances, vaccinators were among the losers.

Thus vaccinators were bedevilled by contradictions between central demands to improve the quality of public vaccination – including an increasingly heavy admin-istrative burden – and Guardians' efforts to minimize the cost of such a service. Little wonder that these contradictions led to increasing dissatisfaction among vaccinators with the requirements of the Vaccination Acts. In matters vaccinal at least, the sphere of public authority was riddled with divisions and tensions.

Parents' problems with stational vaccination

If medics were dissatisfied with the terms of the Vaccination Acts, many parents were more so. The practice of vaccination itself was often considered objection-able, particularly by parents who feared that the introduction of foreign material into their children's bodies involved some kind of contamination: some parents were known to suck the lymph out of their children's arms, once out of sight of the vaccinator.

Often extraction, too, was seen as endangering children's health. Ten years after the introduction of compulsory vaccination, the *British Medical Journal* observed in 'many districts' a belief among 'parents...that mischief will result to their children from the taking of lymph from their arms; and...[thus] they not only refuse to present them for inspection...but frequently hide them to prevent the vaccinator from getting at them'.[19] Indeed, stations exposed vaccinifers as much as vaccinees to risks of infection and contamination, particularly where pressure of numbers encouraged a vaccinator to zigzag with the same implement between the two groups. But parental fears about extraction were often very complex. The passage of a week between vaccination and inspection apparently encouraged a view of lymph as melded with a child's bodily fluids and thus perhaps as more or less inalienable without consent. One early public vaccinator told the 1833 Commons Select Committee that mothers 'particularly' objected to extraction 'from a female':[20] why, he never explained, but we may speculate on feelings about female feebleness and inviolability.

The fact that parents were compelled from 1853 to subject their children to operations that they might otherwise avoid provoked widespread feelings of outrage: 'the parent', as 'king upon the family throne', was usurped.[21] Where, as so often, those operations were performed under the auspices of the Poor Law authorities, they fuelled deeper anxieties about the consequences of such usurpation. Within the workhouse itself, parents' fears were routinely ignored. As early as about 1840, the Poor Law Commissioners had vaguely interpreted existing obligations as allowing Guardians 'without permission of the parent, the right to vaccinate any child in their custody, during any danger of contagion from smallpox'.[22] When, during 1840, Thomas Wakley of Finsbury and the *Lancet* 'had no hesitation' in telling his fellow MPs 'that the poor would be inclined to believe the operation was designed not to protect but to destroy their offspring',[23] he was speaking a mere two years after the publication of a proposal – widely credited to Lord Brougham or to the central Poor Law Commissioners – for 'Limiting Populousness' by gassing poor children.[24]

Such extreme anxieties gradually subsided, but not the practice of vaccinating pauper neonates. Some indirect evidence exists that, from the 1870s and 1880s at least, Whitehall was encouraging this – even outside epidemic periods – rather than let babies loose with their mothers to become untraceable all to soon.[25] In 1881 the 'medical officer at the [Lambeth] infirmary' allegedly told his Guardians that, so far as he was able, he ensured 'that all children born [there] ... were vaccinated within 24 hours'. When in the same year the Holborn Guardians tried stipulating that pauper mothers' consent be sought before their children were vaccinated, their Medical Officer objected that this would in effect mean an end to vaccination, since 'arguing' with paupers was 'useless'.[26]

Enforced vaccination of pauper infants in the workhouse, as one Liberal MP protested during 1881, 'involv[ed]...treatment of the children of the poor...entirely different from that...with respect to...[those] of the rich'.[27] But this was just an extreme example of the discriminations that pervaded public vaccination. The one-clause Act of 1841 declaring that Poor Law vaccination did not pauperize was inadequate to redress the situation. How could potential paupers have confidence that an apparatus they often associated with the 1832 Anatomy Act and the 1834 Poor Law would make an exception for one brief operation? As late as 1878, a 'monstre meeting' of Leeds anti-vaccinationists heard that a male householder whose children had been moved to a smallpox hospital might be struck off the voters' list 'on the ground that he had received "parochial relief"' – a fact denounced in the meeting as 'medical despotism'.[28] But it was not just the threat of disenfranchisement – which anyway remained more or less routine for about a third of adult males until 1918 – that aroused concern. Other stigmas associated with the Poor Law were, in most working-class streets and families, a livelier fear.

The central authorities were not blind here. True, their own vaccination lawyer, D.P. Fry, explained to the 1871 Committee that 'all the way through...[their] great object [had been] to dissociate [vaccination] in the minds of the poor from poor relief'. But he admitted that any such differentiation had become 'a little fanciful', particularly since the Poor Law Board had become responsible for vaccination enforcers – so-called 'vaccination officers'.[29] Meanwhile, many local Boards of Guardians continued to designate Poor Law buildings as stations, while some of their officials doubled as such officers.[30] Other Guardians yearned to divest themselves of the burden of vaccination.[31] Little was done to act on such suggestions, however, and pauper 'taint' continued to haunt public vaccination into at least the 1890s.

Parents' resentment here was exacerbated from the 1860s by the increased insistence on stations. If parents saw vaccination as potentially harmful to their children, they felt even more threatened by the demand to bring them not once but twice, often in weather and along roads or streets not too friendly to the survival of a baby under the legal maximum age of three months. Once at the station they would have to sit for an indeterminate time with other, perhaps infectious, parents and babies, exposed alike to these parents' gaze and to the attentions of a vaccinator who might be both a Poor Law employee and a stranger to them. On returning for inspection, moreover, a 'successfully' vaccinated child might be picked out by the vaccinator, by his (often semi-qualified) deputy, or possibly by some local lymph-monger (many a public vaccinator's unofficial friend or rival), as a source of lymph for further operations. Stational vaccination was thus not only seen to increase the risk for the babies; it also exposed the vaccinator to the risk of being blamed, fairly or not, for childhood morbidity and mortality.[32]

Some medical men, at least, agreed that these risks were real. Stations, argued Finsbury Medical Officer Septimus Gibbon, soon after the 1867 Act, were

> sure to be the means of spreading and keeping alive the very contagious diseases of infancy and childhood, just in the same manner as fairs and markets did the cattle plague....If domiciliary vaccination is good enough for the nobility, gentry and middle classes...[it ought] to be...for the labouring classes.

Accordingly, in an open letter to the Poor Law Board, he denounced stations as intended to 'deter any except the neediest...from seeking vaccination at the public expense'.[33] Gibbon's choice of the word 'deter' was significant. Though public vaccination was not officially supposed to pauperize, he was implying that it nevertheless conformed to the 'deterrent' principles of 1834, according to which all forms of poor relief should be made so unattractive that only the truly desperate would be driven to use them.

At the very least, the fact that the poor had to attend stations widened distinctions between those with incomes sufficient for choice and those without. True, by no means all private vaccination involved persons in any sense well-off. Equally, the well-to-do sometimes chose to make use of stations. While chairing the 1871 Committee, W.E. Forster could boast that his sons and he himself had been vaccinated stationally. He favoured this over the private operation because he could see the source of the lymph.[34] But the point here is surely that Forster had made a free choice that was more or less denied to the mass of people publicly vaccinated. Thus as early as 1854 the *Lancet* argued that the practice of compulsion under the Act of the previous year tended to discriminate between rich and poor: 'to respect the prejudices of the rich, and disregard those of the poor', who were 'compelled' to submit their children to a public vaccinator 'whom they may never have seen before, in whom it is impossible they can feel...confidence and whose selection of lymph they may not question or control'.[35] By 1863 one practitioner was warning that intensified stational operations would 'fan what is now only carelessness respecting vaccination into a bitter hatred against the law and vaccination itself'.[36]

Public and private in the doctor–patient relationship

It was certainly the case that, by the early 1860s, many parents were resisting the demands of the 1853 Act. In 1871, our unlucky Mr Jones was hardly the first to be punished for non-inspection. However, it is remarkable how few such cases seem actually to have been prosecuted at this time. A few had reached the national medical press from the City and from parts of Wales as early as 1854 and 1855,[37] and local magistrates occasionally made defendants into examples. But it is surprising how long the news took to reach some brother justices. Fining a cabman, James Maunders, as late as 1865, one member of the Marylebone bench thought this was 'the first' case of the kind.[38]

The rareness of magisterial attention given to non-attendance for inspections was probably due to vaccinators' reluctance to notify the authorities. While private vaccinators were thought to have a public duty to police parents' observance of the Act, this duty conflicted with a more pressing concern to make a living. Any practitioner informing the authorities that babies had not been vaccinated was risking rejection if not worse from his patients.[39] Thus the fact that, say, the Maunders case came to court at all had perhaps as much to do with the needs of the vaccinator as with the demands of the law. The practitioner, one J.G. Gerrans, complained that the Maunders child had been 'the only' possible vaccinifer he had 'had for a week...and on the day that the mother ought to have brought it I had at least a dozen children waiting in my surgery to be vaccinated'.[40] In this instance, the law actually served the vaccinator's interest. But, more generally, compulsion simply complicated the doctor–patient relationship.

The medical profession reacted to these complications with a profound ambivalence. The most lurid tales of medical officiousness came from doctors themselves – chiefly from private practitioners outraged by this public interference in their relations with patients. Thus one doctor alleged that a Poor Law medical officer had, at Christmas 1853,

> entered the house of a female patient of mine, who was just recovering from...peritonitis....He demanded (in language too unfeeling to be described) whose sick child the woman was nursing. On her telling him that it was her own...he told her he had come to...[vaccinate] it. She remonstrated...telling him she had arranged for her medical adviser to vaccinate it. He threatened to take the child...and, *mirabile dictu*, chased this feeble creature round the room...until she became faint from fear and exertion!!! Such is one among the many scenes that have to be enacted under this legal abortion [i.e. the then new 1853 Act].[41]

State-enforced compulsion thus boosted the anyway enormous Victorian appetite for melodrama, not least where – as allegedly in Stalybridge during the same year – public vaccinators were going 'from house to house...with as much authority as sheriff-bailiffs, representing themselves as the only legally authorized vaccinators'.[42] Not surprisingly, such reports were particularly common while the 1853 Act was fresh,[43] but were not exclusive to that juncture: at any time, professional jealousy could mix unstably with indignation at official officiousness.

On the other hand, where private doctor–patient relationships were not directly threatened – where vaccinators were not dealing with patients from whom they might expect payment – medical spokesmen could look far more favourably on 'compulsion'. Writing from Spitalfields during the 1866 smallpox epidemic, one *Lancet* editorialist argued that 'the poor' were 'more subject to the disease in its worst forms', but were simultaneously 'more indifferent...and more ignorant than the rich. Accordingly they...need to have protection...as it were thrust upon them.'[44] Ten years earlier, Marson had been even more Rousseauan:

> What the educated classes have adopted by choice, after mature deliberation, can hardly, by the most perverted reasoning, be considered improper for the lowest and uneducated class to conform to; it is, in fact, what the latter would most likely adopt, by choice, if they were educated, and a little higher in the scale of society.

Marson had virtually become Jean Jacques with a vaccinal lancet, goading the bovine masses towards health.[45] But other practitioners warned that treating the poor as ill-domesticated herds inevitably led to dangerous abruptness. 'The public vaccinator,' one lecturer reminded the British Medical Association's South London district during 1882,

> attended...for a limited time to possibly a hundred children...he had no acquaintance with their constitution or with that of their parents.... The majority [of the children brought] were more or less diseased....The most favourable pock was selected [for extraction] often without inquiry into the child's family history. If any questions were asked of the mother, they were invariably of the same vague...character: 'Are you healthy? Is your husband a healthy man? Has your child ever had a rash?' Either from ignorance, or from a desire to save time and trouble, or from other equally obvious motives...[she] always [gives] favourable replies –

omitting, for example, symptoms in child or father that might, the speaker suggested, be syphilitic.[46] Such criticisms were sometimes substantiated by vaccinators' own testimony. 'You cannot stop every child that is brought to the station,' A.W. Emms (a public vaccinator near Leicester) reasoned during 1891 to the Royal Commission on Vaccination. True, 'if I had any doubt I should have the child's clothes off'. But, seconds later, came deflation:

> Do you frequently make an examination of that kind? – No.
>
> Do you disturb the clothing at all? – No.[47]

Emms might have been expected to trumpet how careful he was: at that time, he was coming under a cloud over a case of vaccinal contamination. But even he plainly felt little need to disguise how cursory was his treatment of his charges. Most unusually for public vaccinators, he was also a magistrate: conceivably he had grown too used to sitting above criticism.

Even if other vaccinators did not necessarily endorse this cavalier attitude towards vaccinees, some certainly felt that the terms of their employment made it difficult to treat the poor with the same respect as they would extend to private patients. Thus one London surgeon assumed that what he regarded as the peculiarly mean fee of 1s 6d or even 1s per successful vaccination granted by many or most Guardians was 'in great measure' based on the fees 'paid...for examination...of factory children and recruits'. The only way such fees could yield a reasonable recompense, he argued, was by making 'provision for parading all the children of the poor before the vaccinators, as is done in the army' or with 'the factory children'.[48] The point here is not the sheer numbers of vaccinations, running into the hundreds of thousands, that were annually carried out under the Poor Law from the 1840s. Rather, it is that the way in which it was often done had undertones of 'parading'; these echoed military and workhouse discipline. However variable the relationship between doctors and poor patients, its normal co-ordinates were often rudely suspended within public vaccination.

Medicators – often themselves feeling under pressure, exploited or humiliated – could end up reinforcing the discrimination that poor parents felt: via their babies, shoved around as objects of public authority.

Conclusion: the hollowing of stational vaccination

As a result of the tensions inherent in the workings of the public vaccination system, there was by the mid-1890s a massive groundswell of non-compliance by parents. By 1898, relatedly, as many as one-third of all England's Boards of Guardians had ceased even attempting to enforce compulsion (doubtless thanks also to a decade of considerable democratization of local government and to the seven-year deliberations of the Royal Commission on Vaccination). But dissatisfaction with the workings of the vaccination machinery was not confined to the public. Even among leading vaccinators, there was growing recognition that the system of policing the practice of vaccination was not working. The machinery was failing even on its own terms.[49]

The possibilities of mischief within the pre-1898 system had been strikingly formulated in 1882, this time from within Whitehall itself. George Buchanan (Seaton's successor as Chief Medical Officer to the Local Government Board) was eager to overturn his own inspectors' embarrassingly equivocal verdict on an outbreak of post-vaccinal erysipelas (virulent blood-poisoning) in Norwich. Buchanan duly 'solved' the mystery of the outbreak's origins by blaming the vaccinator, Dr William Guy. His penultimate paragraph swatted Guy with a Whitehall file. It detailed why the inspector had seriously faulted Guy in 1876 and 1878, how the inquiry (whose verdict he was now second-guessing) had proved how occasional Guy's grant-winning conformity at the 1880 inspection had been, and how the National Vaccine Establishment had reported him confidentially to the same inspector in readiness for next time: 'a great majority' of Guy's lymph-tubes 'contain[ed] blood, and were not sealed'.[50]

Was the hapless Guy being singled out? The erysipelas had perhaps done that – though not *every* apparent outbreak of erysipelas attracted Whitehall interest publicly. Perhaps this one had become too visible. Certainly, Buchanan was vindicating vaccination at the expense of one vaccinator. Yet, thereby, his account of Guy's misdemeanours (exceptional or not) also revealed a bureaucratic system that could collect, file – but then sit on – information about dangerous practices *for at least six years* before a number of deaths finally prompted a (very rare) official inquiry.

Such revelations thus implicated the system itself. After all, if the National Vaccination Establishment had stopped taking Guy's lymph, why should an indefinite number of unsuspecting Norwich babies still be forced to accept it? And how many other vaccinators had a Whitehall file accumulating merely bureaucratic dirt about physical disasters waiting to overwhelm their vaccinees? True, Buchanan was targeting an individual. But we can perhaps also hear his salvo as symbolizing a growing willingness on the part of officialdom to acknowledge to itself (and, under pressure, to imply publicly) that the system as a whole was failing. Apparently, the honour of some almost abstract 'vaccination' was even more important than that of the (for England) unprecedentedly large apparatus that Buchanan headed. The rite was becoming holier than its hierarchy – evidence of medical certainties under tectonic stress?

The Act of 1898 went far beyond the passage of a 'conscience clause' allowing exemption from vaccination of children whose parents managed to register an objection. It also doubled the maximum age to six months. In general it avowedly sought to alleviate those discriminatory aspects of the system that had rendered so objectionable this intrusion of public authority into the lives of the poor. Workhouse children, for instance, were explicitly protected by Clause 5, which over-rode the rules 'of any lying-in hospital or infirmary' in order to forbid any vaccination before six months without parental consent.[51]

Additionally and crucially, official policy now came to favour the use of glycerinated calf lymph – 'glymph' – over arm-to-arm vaccination. This meant that stational vaccination could now give way to domiciliary, thus doing away with what was seen to be one of the gravest sources of discontent with the old system, namely the discriminatory requirement that the poor attend stations. The poor could now be treated in their homes, just as the rich could. In effect, it meant that universal compulsion applied for the first time to a universally applicable form of the operation, obviating at least some of the discriminatory tensions that had hitherto hindered the workings of this sphere of public authority.

Unfortunately for compulsion, the situation had long been too polarized for concessions from one side to bring calm. Worse, the conscience clause and the switch from stational arm-to-arm operations to home vaccination with glycerinated calf lymph were anyway not necessarily a retreat. Rather, they were embedded within a Bill that displayed some characteristics of a shoddily unilateral truce. The latter word came from the prime-ministerial lips of Lord Salisbury, telling the Upper House that 'a truce and an armistice' would win local authorities back to enforcing vaccination.[52] Worse, there was, first, talk on government benches in both Houses of making adult revaccination compulsory. Second, the whole Act was supposed to lose effect from 1 January 1904: from then, the *status quo ante* would return. True, when the time approached, a still Tory government shrank from chucking this provocative boomerang, just as it (unlike some of its backbenchers) had shrunk from reimposing compulsion against one-third of the Boards of Guardians in England during the summer of 1898. But 'antis' were not necessarily paranoid when warning that those who called attention to their own conscience were fingering themselves for the authorities of 1904. The stalemate persisted until 1907 when the ensuing Liberal government, during its second year, narrowed magistrates' room for manœuvre: where since 1898 objectors had had to convince two amateur magistrates or one stipendiary that they *had* a conscience, from now on they had merely to *declare* a conscience before them.

Third, the response of the magistracy to the Act of 1898 displayed the nonsenses it could spawn. Some magistrates flatly ignored the letter of the law and refused exemption outright; others respected it formally but imposed charges, citing various excuses that they more or less made up on the hoof. Many also harangued applicants or sought to humiliate them in some way. At the other extreme, their colleagues in many boroughs such as Oldham or Northampton made announcements in the local press, triggering multitudinous queuing over several evenings, during which they signed certificates mechanically – virtually till their wrists collapsed. At few times were the tensions inherent within England's centuries of pragmatic centralization-with-delegation-to-amateurs so widely or clearly on display as during November and December 1898.

Fourth, the sudden official love affair with 'glymph' bore many hallmarks of a panicky technical fix – 'much more…a speculative experiment of doubtful efficacy,' the Jenner Society warned, 'than…grappl[ing] comprehensively…with a highly complex problem'.[53] Hectically, the government's Medical Officer, Sir Richard Thorne Thorne, was sent ricocheting back and forth to various continental countries to confirm what more and more medics during the 1880s and 1890s had been telling Whitehall: continental lymph-production was now a veritable laboratory science and no longer some art or lore of squeezing.[54] Thorne's only travelling companion, Dr Sidney Monckton Copeman, had himself been furthering this science since earlier in the decade, and possessed the added propaganda advantage of Britishness. A year later, though, some prominent people were apparently still unaware that 'glymph' was not the only weapon in Continental armouries. Whitehall, in other words, was lurching between crude extremes: from anti-glymph to over-dependence.[55] Rightly, Joseph Lister (the recently baronialized antiseptist) admitted to his fellow Lords that the whole change – not least to glymph – was nothing less than 'a tremendous experiment'[56] ('upon the children of the working classes of England', one East-End trade unionist MP had earlier retorted to similar language from the relevant minister).[57] Not least, laboratory standardization of a pharmaceutical product replaced Whitehall's doomed crusade to standardize local practice.

The new legislation of 1898 thus resolved some of the tensions and contradictions that had been hollowing the vaccination system since 1853: the problems of a system of universal compulsion that made discriminatory provision for the poor; and especially the problem that the poor, as objects of public funding, were required to attend public spaces that they often perceived as dangerous to their children and demeaning to themselves. The Act of 1898 tried to obviate all this by providing a form of vaccination that was universally applicable. Most important, it allowed the publicly funded operation to be conducted in private. Arguably, one lesson here was that public authority could not simply be imposed without making strategic concessions to the demand that all individuals be afforded at least some of the trappings of medical equality with each other.

There is, in sum, no wonder that stational vaccination lay down so late in its dying. It could not be allowed to lie down until 'glymph' could hurriedly be installed in its stead. The tardiness of this was mainly a matter of power-politics between centre and locality: between medical Whitehall (itself a tiny group of experts, often cramped between politician-amateurs and generalist-mandarins), local amateurs (Guardians plus others), local experts (public vaccinators and others) and, not least, parents.

Acknowledgements

Many thanks to Steve Sturdy as Editor, and to Eva Brandt and Thomas Nolte for holding my computer-hand: all exceptionally understanding.

Notes

1 *Lancet*, 1871, vol. 1, p. 833.
2 See for example A. Beck, 'Issues in the anti-vaccination movement in England', *Medical History*, 1960, vol. 4, pp. 310–21; R.S. Lambert, 'A Victorian N.H.S.: state vaccination in 1855–71', *Historical Journal*, 1962, vol. 5, pp. 1–18; the main pioneer, R.M. Macleod, 'The frustration of state medicine 1880–99', *Medical History*, 1967, vol. 11, pp. 15–40; *idem*, 'Law, medicine and public opinion: the resistance to compulsory health legislation, 1870–1907', *Public Law*, 1967, vol. 1, pp. 107–28, 189–211; D. Porter and R. Porter, 'The politics of prevention: anti-vaccinationism and public health in 19th-century England', *Medical History*, 1988, vol. 32, pp. 231–52; E.P. Hennock, 'Vaccination policy against smallpox, 1835–1914: a comparison of England with Prussia and Imperial Germany', *Social History of Medicine*, 1998, vol. 11, pp. 49–71; N. Durbach, '"They might as well brand us": working-class resistance to compulsory vaccination in Victorian England', *Social History of Medicine*, 2000, vol. 13, pp. 45–62; P. Baldwin, *Contagion and the State in Europe, 1830–1930*, Cambridge: Cambridge University Press, 1999, chapter 4. Baldwin's achievement is monumental; I will not hack away at it here. For the non-/queuings, I am currently combing local newspapers in many localities.
3 True, there were also longer-term worries that lymph might 'degenerate' during near-endless series of arm-to-arm operations. Criteria for what constituted either degeneration or contamination remained primitive through much of the century.
4 *British Medical Journal*, 1863, vol. 2, p. 349, summarizing a report by the now late Snow.
5 *Lancet*, 1893, vol. 1, p. 1400, commenting on the Eastbourne Guardians' decision to do just that.
6 As reported via Graily Hewitt, *Lancet*, 1863, vol. 1, pp. 711–12.
7 Epidemiological Society, *Report on Vaccination*, London, 1852, p. 18.
8 'Our Liverpool correspondent, an eminent authority on…vaccination' (surely – from content and style – Steele), *British Medical Journal*, 1871, vol. 1, p. 152.
9 *Lancet*, 1853, vol. 2. pp. 251, 449, 531, emphasis in original.
10 *Lancet*, 1867, vol. 1, p. 721.
11 *Medical Times and Gazette*, 1853, vol. 1, p. 567.
12 Ibid.
13 Epidemiological Society, *Report*, p. 12, paraphrased less sweepingly in *Lancet*, 1853, vol. 1, p. 11.
14 *Association Medical Journal*, 1853, vol. 264, pp. 313–14.
15 For example the anonymous protest in *Lancet*, 1840–1, vol. 1, p. 565.
16 *Lancet*, 1852, vol. 1, p. 416.
17 For example 'in the Midland Counties it [was] the custom' for 'the operative' to resort to such – though our source is merely a London surgeon, William Slyman MRCS of Kentish Town: *Lancet*, 1862, vol. 1, p. 421.
18 Select Committee on the Vaccination Act (1867), *Minutes of Evidence*, PP 1871, vol. 13, q. 5422.
19 *British Medical Journal*, 1863, vol. 2, p. 348. Admittedly, the writer judged 'this feeling' to be 'on the decline'.
20 Dr John Webster, the original physician of the National Vaccine Board (or Establishment), *Report from the Select Committee on the Vaccination Board with the Minutes of Evidence and an Appendix*, PP 1833, vol. 16, q. 1562.

21 Poem in *Boston Guardian and Lincolnshire Independent*, 20 November 1875, n.p.

22 As noted by Richard Griffin (leading activist of the Poor Law Medical Reform Association), *The Grievances of the Poor Law Medical Officers, Elucidated in a Letter to the Members of the Legislature, and a Commentary, on the Proposed Act of Parliament for Redress, &c.*, London: Simpkin, Marshall & Co., 1858, pp. 53–4.

23 *Hansard*, Commons, 17 June 1840, vol. 54, col. 1244–5.

24 R. Richardson, *Death, Dissection and the Destitute*, London: Routledge & Kegan Paul, 1987, pp. 268, 373.

25 Local Government Board, Subject Indexes of Correspondence (giving serial numbers of letters since destroyed, unpaginated and tantalizingly cryptic), Public Record Office (PRO), Kew, MH 15/28 (1872) and MH 15/59 (1882).

26 Dr G.E. Yarrow, *Lancet*, 1881, vol. 1, p. 536.

27 Letter from Mr Blennerhassett, *Times* (London), 24 February 1881, p. 10.

28 *Yorkshire Independent*, 8 November 1878, n.p.

29 Select Committee on the Vaccination Act, 1871, qq. 3973–7.

30 PRO MH15, vol. 46, 1881–2 (premises), 1877 and 1879 (officers).

31 *British Medical Journal*, 1884, vol. 2, p. 128; *Lancet*, 1884, vol. 2, pp. 23, 85.

32 For which see for example *British Medical Journal*, 1883, vol. 1, pp. 438, 538; *Hansard*, Commons, 17 June 1898, vol. 59, col. 570–1.

33 Septimus Gibbon's almost (but not quite) identical letters as reported in *Medical Times and Gazette*, 1868, vol. 1, p. 138, and *British Medical Journal*, 1868, vol. 1, p. 185.

34 Select Committee on the Vaccination Act, 1871, q. 5425.

35 *Lancet*, 1854, vol. 2, p. 404.

36 T.S. Fletcher MRCS of Bromsgrove, *British Medical Journal*, 1863, vol. 2, pp. 684–5.

37 *Lancet*, 1854, vol. 1, p. 408; ibid., 1855, vol. 1, pp. 200, 476.

38 *Medical Times and Gazette*, 1865, vol. 1, pp. 270–1. Not untypically for recalcitrant parents, Mrs and Mr Maunders claimed to have 'already lost three children through vaccination', and James objected further that 'the scabs' on his current vaccinee had anyway 'dried up'.

39 For example 'A Public Vaccinator with his hands tied', *British Medical Journal*, 1859, p. 513.

40 *Medical Times and Gazette*, 1865, vol. 1, pp. 270–1.

41 Anonymous article in *Association Medical Journal*, 1853, p. 1092, emphasis and punctuation as original.

42 M.D.Thompson MRCS, *Lancet*, 1853, vol. 1, p. 236.

43 For example *Lancet*, 1853, vol. 2, pp. 308, 577.

44 *Lancet*, 1856, vol. 2, pp. 263–4.

45 Ibid.

46 Mr J. Brindley James, *British Medical Journal*, 1882, vol. 2, p. 893.

47 Royal Commission appointed to inquire into the subject of Vaccination, *Fourth Report*, C. 6527, PP 1890–91, vol. 44, pp. 14, 615–7.

48 Joseph Curtis of Camden, *Lancet*, 1839–40, vol. 2, p. 910.

49 F.T. Bond, 'Discussion on vaccination with special reference to prospective legislation', *Lancet*, 1898, vol. 2, p. 417.

50 Memorandum by the Medical Officer of the Local Government Board, PP 1882, vol. 57, at p. 653.

51 Ironically, after the 1898 Act passed, Whitehall snarled at Norwich Guardians for proposing to 'apply for exemption certificates for children in the workhouse'. Here, Guardians had surely been intending to consult workhouse mothers in some way: *Daylight*, 10 December 1898, p. 2.

52 *Hansard*, Lords, 8 August 1898, vol. 64, col. 458. The following paragraphs are largely condensed from L. Barrow: 'English vaccination: the 1898 conjuncture' (unpublished paper).

53 Jenner Society, printed 'Memorandum on the Bill...', opening-page '4', in PRO MH 80, vol. 2. That this was the situation was also surmised by the Radical and anti-vaccinationist Norwich weekly, *Daylight*, 10 December 1898, p. 9.

54 *Times* (London), 24 December 1896, p. 5; *British Medical Journal*, 1897, vol. 2, p. 36; 'Glycerinated calf lymph...Report to the Local Government Board', July 1897, PP 1897, vol. 23, p. iii.

55 See, for instance, the editorial in *British Medical Journal*, 1898, vol. 2, pp. 415–16.

56 *Hansard*, Lords, 4 August 1898, vol. 64, col. 37.

57 Ibid., 19 July 1898, vol. 62, col. 381.

11 The shaping of a public environmental sphere in late nineteenth-century London

Bill Luckin

In *The Structural Transformation of the Public Sphere* Jürgen Habermas argues that in the late nineteenth century the most economically advanced European nations underwent a period of radical political and social change. 'Over and above its normal administrative concerns,' he writes, '[the state now] also took over the provision of services that hitherto had been left to private hands, whether it entrusted private persons with public tasks, coordinated private economic activity...or became active itself as a producer and distributor.'[1] From this epoch on, Habermas continues, the classic bourgeois public sphere – which hitherto he supposes to have exercised a restraining surveillance over the activities of the state – was rendered impotent by the emergence of 'administrative', 'social welfare' bureaucracies. As a consequence party political pressure, 'wheeling and dealing' and corporate intrigue replaced open and responsible criticism of public policy.

Habermas's commitment to the idea of a structural transformation of the late nineteenth-century public sphere convinced him that he must take on the task of theorizing the concept of authentic communication in twentieth-century capitalist societies. The resultant and massive body of work, produced between the late 1960s and the present – 'mature' and 'late' Habermas – has been characterized by a retreat from history and a growing preoccupation with the immanent qualities of language and the individual speech act. In this respect, this most prolific of social theorists has suggested that his quest for non-systematically distorted communication constitutes an attempt to reconstruct a late twentieth-century analogue for the classic bourgeois public sphere.[2] Here Horkheimer's formulation is pertinent. 'To speak to someone,' he wrote to Adorno in 1940, 'basically means recognizing him as a possible member of the future association of free human beings. Speech establishes a shared relation towards all forms of existence, according to their capacities. When speech denies any possibilities, it necessarily contradicts itself.'[3]

Habermas's account of the marginalization and decline of an idealized eighteenth-century bourgeois public sphere is superficially convincing. It is noticeably short on detailed empirical substantiation, however. *The Structural Transformation of the Public Sphere* under-specifies differences in rates of structural change within and between individual late nineteenth-century European polities. It communicates little about the specifics of late nineteenth-century government and, in the paradigm case of Britain, fails to demonstrate how, in no more than a genera-tion, largely autonomous sets of governing structures coalesced into a single, semi-modern bureaucratized state apparatus. The Habermasian case is further vitiated by the fact that relationships between centre and periphery are ignored during a period in which local responsibility for community affairs continued to command large-scale elite and popular support.[4] On the related issue of how European capitals – including London, the subject of the present chapter – protected themselves against the chill wind of administrative reform, there is near-silence.[5]

Above all, *The Structural Transformation of the Public Sphere* provides no more than an outline sketch of the day-to-day workings of key institutions of state. Within this context, Habermas's study exaggerates the extent to which, by the later nineteenth century, European legislative bodies had come unequivocally to represent and ratify the interests of distinctive national bourgeois classes. Thus in Britain the profoundly anti-democratic House of Lords repeatedly repudiated 'middle-class' constitutional reform and remained unencumbered by the neces-sity of mollifying increasingly powerful popular electorates. Peers therefore found it possible to adopt surprisingly progressive attitudes towards social issues perceived to be politically over-inflammatory by ministers, backbenchers and party managers. The same was frequently the case in relation to an ever-wider range of scientific and technological concerns.[6]

In the present chapter, an emergent metropolitan – and national – public sphere of environmental debate is examined within the context of the severe air pollution problem that afflicted the capital between the 1870s and the outbreak of the First World War. The chapter begins with a brief overview of these mete-orological episodes themselves. This outline is complemented by an account of the ways in which the problem was perceived and framed by medical men, urban reformers and cultural critics, the great majority of whom were heavily influenced by social-Darwinistic theories of degeneration and 'racial' decline. Here an interpretation is given of ideas contained in the writings of F.A.R. (Rollo) Russell, an influential chronicler of the metropolitan smoke fog phenomenon during the late nineteenth and early twentieth centuries. In a second section, attention shifts to the manner in which reformist solutions were formulated but then failed to be converted into the hard currency of preventive legislation or improved administrative control. These proposals owed much to aristocratic, scientific and middle-class interest groups and to the initiatives of a lone peer – Lord Stratheden and Campbell – within a political context in which the national executive deliberately distanced itself from an increasingly threat-ening pollution crisis. In the final part of the chapter, we re-engage with broadly Habermasian concerns and suggest that the smoke fog problem was partially constituted and fully contested by identifiable interest groups, performing discur-sive roles that, judged according to the normative prescriptions enunciated in *The Structural Transformation of the Public Sphere*, ought to have been undertaken within a generalized political rather than specifically environmental public sphere.[7] In conclusion, comparisons are made between past and present. Does the environmental public sphere of the late nineteenth century resemble that of the present day, and can we learn anything from the past about the terms of modern environmental conflict?

Interpreting the great London fogs

In the late eighteenth and early nineteenth centuries atmospheric pollution in London began to establish itself as a major social and environmental problem. Scientists, medical men and urban reformers such as Thomas Bateman, Robert Willan, William Bent and Luke Howard documented unusual meteorological events and investigated the relationship between bad air and bad health.[8] Nevertheless, they made little headway against a long-established orthodoxy which asserted that, although an insalubrious atmosphere might be capable of further weakening the health of those already suffering from respiratory disease, it could not in itself trigger asthma, whooping-cough or consumption. Adverse social and economic repercussions were thought to be altogether more threatening.

At a social and cultural level, early nineteenth-century newspapers lingered on the details of fatal or crippling fog-induced calamities, street and river accidents, and crime rates that were alleged to soar upwards as noon-time darkness descended on the city. At the same time, smoke fog was theatrically depicted as a unique, and uniquely metropolitan, phenomenon. A 'particular' or 'peasouper' stilled the rush of traffic and commerce, immobilized steamers on the Thames and transformed familiar parks and squares into a ghostly counter-world. When the bad weather lifted, it was as if thousands of tableaux of urban commerce – streets, markets, shops – had been magically reanimated. Little wonder that contemporaries believed that, without an annual fog season, London would have quite simply ceased to be London.[9] During the 1840s and 1850s meteorologists, medical men and urban reformers became more consistently concerned about the severity of the capital's intractable atmospheric problem. 'Rural' white had now been replaced by dirty yellow and, during particularly bad weather, this already unpleasant patina gave way to stifling black. Quantitative techniques that had been used by sanitarians to calculate the 'preventable' costs of fever were now applied to the metropolitan atmospheric problem. Blanketing and increasingly gritty fog over-stretched hospital outpatient provision and medical charities, and traumatically disrupted patterns of working-class casual and street employment. Some commentators claimed that the annual cost might be as high as £5m.[10]

Between the early 1870s and the mid-1890s the capital was repeatedly shrouded in dense smoke fog. There were no fewer than fifty-five serious episodes a year between 1871 and 1891, and sixty-nine between 1882 and 1892, with peaks of eighty-six and eighty-three in 1886 and 1887. The worst of the so-called 'great fogs' in December 1873, January 1882, winter and spring 1886–7, December 1891, December 1892 and November 1901 lasted for between three to four days and a week.[11] Following an as yet unexplained improvement during the Edwardian period, inter-war London was once again intermittently paralysed by fog.[12] There was then an exceptionally severe episode in 1948, and between 5 and 8 December 1952 the capital was enveloped in a smog that may have accounted for what now appears to have been a minimum of around 6,000 excess deaths from respiratory disease.[13]

During the final twenty-five years of the nineteenth century these much feared London fogs gave rise to an intense, anxiety-laden debate about incipient metropolitan – and indeed global – decline. By this juncture a majority of medical men, epidemiologists, sanitarians, meteorologists and social statisticians were convinced that exceptionally black and stifling smoke fog was capable of triggering epidemic-like mortality, with a disproportionate number of deaths occurring among the very oldest and youngest age groups.[14] Expressed in anti-urban and entropic terms, deeply pessimistic environmentalist strands of thought depicted metropolitan atmospheric pollution as both cause and threatening symbol of biological regression in the rapidly depopulating and poverty-stricken inner districts of the capital. During the 1840s sanitarians had pointed to reduced levels of sunlight as a determinant of an inadequate supply of red corpuscles, lankness and a tendency to regress to a phase of development associated with criminality, 'savagery' and mental debility.[15] Thirty years later commitment to social Darwinism generated even grimmer scenarios. Organically and hereditarily damaged by inadequate domestic ventilation and lack of exposure to the vital rays of the sun, working-class cohorts of the 1840s were widely believed to have produced a stock that might be doomed to physiological extinction.[16]

Such morbid visions of degeneration and decline were reinforced by popularized accounts of entropic collapse in the aftermath of the publication of W.S. Jevons's highly influential *The Coal Question* in 1865. This controversial study asserted that acute shortages of energy – and particularly of coal – might condemn metropolitan and indeed all 'advanced' urban civilizations to an arctic future.[17] Twenty years earlier Chadwick's *Sanitary Report* had berated local authorities for failing to introduce by-laws to reduce levels of atmospheric pollution. Not only had such bodies tacitly collaborated with manufacturers who had revealed themselves to be wasteful managers of factories and workshops; they had also set an unacceptable example to the urban working class that should have been taught to appreciate the relationship between thrift and self-improvement.[18] Now, during the final thirty years of the century, the metropolitan elite castigated itself for having failed to disseminate a sense of responsibility in relation to the consumption of domestic fuel. Had more positive attitudes been adopted throughout the social hierarchy, traditional charitable bonds would have been strengthened at precisely the moment when a potentially degenerate 'outcast London' threatened to sever ties with the respectable classes.[19] The final link in the ideological and discursive chain was to suggest that, if the metropolitan working classes were indeed meteorologically and atmospherically doomed, then the environment in which this terrible tragedy would be played out – a spatially over-blown and over-populated capital – must itself be disowned. Hence the powerful strand of anti-metropolitanism and anti-urbanism – accompanied by rural revivalism – which permeated debate of the smoke fog problem in the capital between the 1870s and 1914.[20]

Full crisis struck in December 1873 when, according to the meteorologist James Glaisher, the capital experienced a 'remarkably dense fog, darker in colour, and more dense than I had ever known a fog or cloud to be'.[21] However, it was only following the publication in 1880 of Rollo Russell's *London Fogs* that the metropolitan air pollution problem finally established itself in a manner that would give rise to belated proposals for legislative and administrative control of explicitly domestic consumption of coal in the capital. Rollo Russell was the son of the great Lord John. At an early age he had been appointed guardian to the young and tragically orphaned Bertrand Russell and his older brother Frank. He was educated at Christ Church, Oxford, and, on graduating, entered the Foreign Office. A painfully shy and diffident individual, who was plagued by poor eyesight, Russell was soon compelled to withdraw from public life. He retired to Pembroke Lodge, Richmond, and undertook research into the relationships between atmosphere and disease. During the next twenty-five years, Russell published numerous books, pamphlets and articles on the climatic determinants of infection, the meteorology of cities and rural regeneration. But he also repeatedly revisited the social, economic, environmental and ethical problems associated with metropolitan smoke fog.[22]

Russell was blessed with a simple and vivid prose style that appealed both to the general public and to metropolitan aristocratic, scientific and professional groups who played a crucial role in the establishment of the reformist – and elitist – National Coal Abatement Institution. He succinctly conveyed Londoners' perceptions of and reactions to the increasingly debilitating atmospheric environment in which they were forced to live out their daily lives. *London Fogs* began with a plea for a radical reconceptualization of the environmental and cultural meanings traditionally ascribed to air pollution. In his classic accounts of the events of 1873 and 1880, Russell gave equal weight to meteorological and social and economic concerns. During February of the latter year he noted that 'the ground had been cooled by intense frost, lasting for some days, to a very low temperature, and thereupon a moist southerly current supervened', so that by early morning 'a lamp-post four and a half yards distant was invisible'.[23] There had been no improvement since 1873 when 'it had at times been impossible to see across a street', and in 'perfectly calm conditions, characterized by "great cold" and a "conflict of currents", mortality had exceeded the weekly average by seven hundred'.[24]

Developing social cost-accounting techniques pioneered by Chadwickian sanitarians during the 1840s, Russell identified no fewer than twenty-five interacting variables. In addition to predictable items such as 'extra, year-round gas' and 'additional chimney sweeping', places were now also found for 'loss of time by artists of all kinds, including photographers', 'loss to drapers, dyers and milliners…where delicate colours are used' and 'window cleaning of public and private buildings'.[25] Equally insidious were the moral repercussions of an endemically polluted atmosphere. 'The winter gloom', Russell warned, 'is very unfavourable to sobriety'. Surveying the condition of the inhabitants of the eastern and inner-city districts, he pessimistically concluded that 'owing to the prevalence of westerly winds the eastern portion of the town suffers more from smoke and fog than the western and…its inhabitants present an unhealthy appearance altogether unlike that of the country population'.[26] Potentially irreversible 'moral evils' were bound to flourish in smoke-shrouded and poverty-stricken areas of the city, which deprived the working classes of all contact with 'clear azure' and the 'crisp brilliancy of a [country] winter morning'. These, according to Russell, were the climatic conditions that represented nothing less than a symbolic 'sermon…from nature which humanity has need of'.[27] Emphasizing the inevitable moral fall from grace associated with moving from the countryside to an irretrievably polluted city, Russell insisted that:

> we have the strongest testimony that many who have been good housewives in the country, after an abode of some time in London give up the attempt to keep their houses clean and become quite disheartened in their efforts to make the surroundings of their families bright and pleasant.[28]

More than any other writer of his generation, Rollo Russell conveyed the anxiety experienced by elite metropolitan reformers confronted by the economically depressed and potentially politically unstable eastern and inner-city districts of the capital. Concerned both with meteorological detail and the social and moral implications of London's atmospheric crisis, he nevertheless believed it might be possible to look forward to a half-real, half-imagined future in which the sun would reinvigorate human existence and then itself come to symbolize universal healthfulness and the immanence of godhead within revived rural communities.[29] But how were such objectives to be achieved? How could the 'clear azure' be restored?

The problem of control

The weakness of the central state bureaucracy and continuing commitment to the doctrine of local self-government militated against the implementation of effective national legislation to reduce the severity of atmospheric pollution in mid-nineteenth-century Britain. Only in the case of the alkali industry, the producer of massive quantities of a 'clear, colourless, fuming, poisonous, highly acidic, aqueous solution of hydrogen chloride', did it prove possible to introduce even minimally effective legislation. Following Lord Derby's 'packing' of a House of Lords select committee, the first of a series of Alkali Acts passed on to the statute book in 1863. However, it was the extreme damage experienced by estates, farms and orchards in the vicinity of St Helens rather than preoccupation with working-class health or urban amenity that proved decisive.[30] In this respect, it is worth noting that Derby's report had been signed by a landed elite within an elite – in addition to the chairman, the committee comprised Lord Stanley, the Duke of Richmond, the Early of Shaftesbury and Lords Graham and Grey.

In major cities like Birmingham, Sheffield, Liverpool and Manchester local acts and by-laws, designed to reduce outpourings of soot from factories and workshops, came into operation between the mid-1840s and the 1860s.[31] But few of these measures proved effective. Employers and employees remained convinced that high levels of pollution indicated booming manufacturing conditions, while blue and unsullied skies signalled economic recession. The suggestion that more stringent controls should be introduced to protect health and the quality of the environment provoked even non-dogmatic supporters of mid-Victorian *laissez-faire* to respond that municipal – or even worse, central government – intervention might 'close a town down'. Magistrates who were responsible for the implementation of anti-pollution measures tended to be factory owners or close associates of local manufacturing elites. Punishments were derisory and many successfully prosecuted offenders paid a fine but then failed to adopt the 'best practicable means' for a more effective 'consumption' of smoke. 'Parliament,' one survey has concluded,

> passed laws giving local authorities the power to act; the local authorities, forced to confront the polluters at close quarters in the councils and courts, wavered and passed the responsibility back to central government. In the end, little abatement was achieved.[32]

In the capital in the early 1850s the Home Secretary, Lord Palmerston, had carried the fight to manufacturers who refused to take action to reduce levels of atmospheric pollution. Precisely because they were unconcerned with domestic emissions, Palmerston's Smoke Nuisance Abatement (Metropolis) Acts of 1853 and 1856 uncontroversially passed on to the statute book. Administered by the Home Office in collaboration with the Metropolitan Police, the measures outlawed excessive production of smoke by 'every furnace employed or to be employed in any mill, factory, printing-house, dye-house, iron foundry, glasshouse, distillery, brew-house, sugar refinery, bakehouse, gas works, waterworks, or other buildings used for the purpose of trade or manufacture within the metropolis'.[33] Within less than a decade, however, *The Builder* had become convinced that 'what has been actually achieved [under the Palmerston acts] amounts to very little'.[34] Now, as atmospheric conditions deteriorated, public attention focused ever more intensively on the uncontrolled outpourings of multitudes of residential chimneys. But on this issue the national executive, the Metropolitan Board of Works, and the local vestries and sanitary authorities responsible for the day-to-day administration of individual districts of the capital proved reluctant to intervene. Practical and scientifically authenticated solutions appeared to be unavailable and MPs were unwilling to risk backing a measure that might alienate the great majority of householders. The nettle was finally grasped by Lord Stratheden and Campbell, a maverick peer who introduced no fewer than ten radical but unsuccessful anti-smoke bills into the Lords between the early 1880s and his death in 1893. Before his elevation to the peerage in 1861, William Frederick Campbell had been a member of Parliament for Cambridge between 1847 and 1852, and for Harwich between 1859 and 1860. Campbell possessed no outstanding intellectual or political skills. However, in addition to becoming well versed in the intricacies of the unfathomably complex Eastern Question, he was a vigilant constitutionalist and author of a collection of essays on the 'ministerial position and its dangers'.[35] By the early 1880s Stratheden and Campbell – as he had now become – was convinced that, in the absence of a measure of environmental reform, the increasing frequency and severity of smoke fog would irreparably damage the health and welfare of the entire metropolitan population. In July 1887, Stratheden and Campbell was appointed chairman of a House of Lords select committee to scrutinize one of his own many anti-smoke bills. The measure was probably drawn up in collaboration with the Abatement Institution, whose exceptionally able chairman, Ernest Hart, also appeared as a major witness. Influential editor of the *British Medical Journal* between 1866 and 1898, Hart was a prominent member of the metropolitan reforming elite and had laboured long and hard on issues as diverse as the medical treatment of the sick poor, the abolition of baby farming and improved educational opportunities for apprentice plumbers.[36] In terms of the relationship between high levels of atmospheric pollution and the health and morale of London's working class, Hart was a convinced degenerationist.

When questioned by his predictably sympathetic chairman, Hart suggested that London's local authorities, operating at the level of the vestry rather than the Metropolitan Police, should be made responsible for monitoring and controlling unacceptably smoky emissions from residential dwellings. The underlying principle of the measure, he continued, would be 'educative'.[37] Hart cited numerous examples of aristocratic and upper middle-class households in which a successful shift had been made from reliance on 'soft', smoky fuel from the midland and northern coalfields to Welsh anthracite or a mixture of coke, coal and gas. Sanitary authorities would encourage the adoption of similar strategies in affluent households that had not yet taken preventive action. Thereafter, inspectorial attention would be directed at the respectable poor, with those who could only afford a single, all-purpose grate or fire being made eligible for selective exemption.[38] Hart insisted that individual Londoners must not expect to make major savings on their fuel bills as a result of the changes to be encouraged by the proposed anti-smoke measure. Nevertheless, if grates were modified so as to ensure a more economical burning of each unit of smokeless coal or coke, at an initial outlay of approximately 10s per grate, long-term financial benefits would be achieved. Hart emphasized collective, indirect savings rather than benefits to individual households, and drew on the now standard argument that the energy-conscious resident would be rewarded 'in not having to paint his rooms so often: in not having to wash his linen so often: in not having his books destroyed: and in not having the front of his house destroyed'.[39]

It was Hart's – and Stratheden and Campbell's – misfortune that their proposals should be subjected to rigorous scrutiny by Lord Balfour of Burley. An obituarist recorded that 'without brilliance…[Balfour] represented the best type of public servant – conscientious, purposeful, and with a gift for mastering complicated details and mastering them lucidly and cogently'. Between 1882 and 1917 he chaired inquiries into educational endowments in Scotland, rating and local taxation, national food resources during war and the Royal Commission on Metropolitan Water Supply of 1868–9.[40] Sceptical of the logical underpinning to the Abatement Institution's commitment to 'educative' legislation, Balfour was convinced that the reformist body over-represented the interests of the affluent and the 'scientifically progressive'. Applying the iron laws of the market to choice of domestic fuel, he demanded to know why the alleged attractiveness of modified grates, smokeless fuel and gas had thus far failed to tempt a larger proportion of the middle classes away from traditional methods of heating and cooking.[41] Suggesting that medium- and long-term fuel savings were largely illusory, he claimed that significant sections of London's population were in any case unlikely to be persuaded by arguments that were so heavily dependent on long-term, social rather than immediate, individual financial gain. 'You know what human nature is', he told Hart; '…it will feel the immediate outgoing, and will not so much realize the problematical saving.'[42] Balfour volunteered that his own approach to the problem would have been to acknowledge that 'in gross [the reformist case] is a theory: in the unit it might be reduced to practice: but if you could prove it to be a fact instead of a theory you could further your case'.[43] Ordinary Londoners were disinclined to take action to hasten a 'clearing of the atmosphere'. But they would be ready enough to take steps to reduce their fuel bills and thereby – at some point in the future – play a role in cutting back on the frequency and severity of the capital's perennial pall of winter and spring-time smoke.

Balfour also played a decisive constitutionalist card. He challenged Hart to name any other act of Parliament that 'laid down, as a principle, that a man who lives in a cheap house may commit a nuisance, and that a man who lives in an expensive one must not'.[44] Flustered, Hart fell back on yet another of his favourite sanitary analogies and asserted that 'the bye-laws provide for the thickness of walls, the height of walls – everything is on a more costly scale in the case of the large houses than in the case of the small ones'.[45] Balfour retorted that this was an unsatisfactory example, since it depended on an administrative rather than legislative distinction. Hart had failed to provide a precedent for a measure that would allow a local authority inspectorate to intrude into the houses of the wealthy but ignore potentially illegal behaviour in the dwellings of the poor. Balfour was equally unconvinced by Hart's assurance that the act could be effectively implemented through a mere 'rearrangement' of existing responsibilities within sanitary departments rather than by recruiting and training additional personnel.[46] However admirable its intentions, the elitist Abatement Institution's 'educative' and socially selective solution to the metropolitan smoke fog problem was flawed both in principle and detail. Even had sufficient parliamentary time been made available during the next session, the bill would almost certainly have been subjected to even more scathing criticism in the Commons. Yet another of Stratheden and Campbell's numerous anti-fog initiatives had been stopped in its tracks.

Conservative governments during the 1880s and early 1890s were happy enough to see the controversial issue of domestic smoke control left in the hands of elitist pressure groups and progressive peers. In 1892 the Prime Minister, Lord Salisbury, insisted that any plan to require greater city-wide reliance on larger volumes of anthracite would

> enormously increase the price of that coal, and, consequently the price of living in the whole population: and thus likewise condemn the population to go on for ever, so far as they remained in London, without ever seeing a fire with a flue in it.[47]

The President of the Board of Trade, Sir Michael Hicks-Beach, was dismissively 'thankful to say that [the responsibilities of his department] did not extend to the prevention of fogs in London'.[48] As late as 1920 the anonymous author of a volume celebrating the achievements of the London County Council narrated a continuingly doleful chronology of legislative inaction in relation to the metropolitan fog problem. Emission of black smoke from the chimney of a private dwelling house had not yet been made an offence and 'amelioration in this direction [was to be looked for] in the growing use of gas and electricity for heating and cooking, and in the use of smokeless fuel and grates of the improved kind'.[49] The consolidated Public Health Act (London) of 1891 had made it an offence for trade premises to fail to consume their own smoke, but the relevant clauses were hedged round by qualification, and the maximum fine was a paltry £10. Action had been taken against railway companies under legislation passed as early as 1845 and 1868 but in a single sample year – 1906 – 132 prosecutions had yielded the grand total of £325, or less than £3 per offence.[50] Nevertheless, smoke fog in the capital was significantly less frequent and debilitating between 1900 and 1920 than it had been over the preceding twenty years. In 1905 Rollo Russell concluded that 'forty years ago the kitchen and other chimneys certainly emitted much larger volumes of black smoke than they generally do today and the improvement is chiefly owing to kitcheners [kitchen ranges] and better grates'. Furthermore, 'more general cooking by gas [was] already beginning to purify the London air from…domestic smoke'.[51] In the district served by the Gas Light, South Metropolitan and Commercial companies 58 per cent of 'ordinary' consumers and 79 per cent of those relying on slot meters had shifted away from coal for cooking purposes. But there had been a much slower rate of conversion to gas fires, not least since 'we have been too long used to the cheerful open fire'.[52] Nevertheless, from the 1890s onwards, the capital experienced a working-class gas – and slot-meter – revolution. The chairman of the South Metropolitan Gas Company, Sir George Livesey, estimated that in 1892 fewer than 500 weekly tenants had access to the newer form of fuel via payments of this kind; by 1898 the figure was just over 80,000.[53] Domestic electricity, long idealized as a quasi-magical 'energy of the future', remained something of a luxury in the capital until the 1930s. As early as 1845 a contributor to the *Mining Journal* had 'predicted that the time is not far distant when the globe will be circumnavigated by the agency of electricity'.[54] In 1881 a correspondent in *Nature* asserted that 'in a few years we shall be indebted to the electric light for our source of nightly illumination'.[55] But the early period of mass supply in London was hamstrung by administrative problems, and electric fires in particular were said to make for stuffiness and unhealthiness. In terms of cost, a government inquiry in 1920 concluded that 'we hesitate to advise the adoption [of electricity] on the evidence before us, in view of the high price at present charged for electricity in many localities'.[56] Just as over-expensive gas had inhibited working-class tenants from forsaking the traditional smoky grate, so now in the immediate aftermath of the First World War price considerations continued to militate against mass transition to the 'energy of the future'.

The meteorological record in inter-war London suggests that the pioneering and socially elitist anti-smoke reformers of the 1880s got some things right. Thus, with the exception of two unusually lengthy episodes in February 1927 and November 1936, the great majority of smoke fogs during this period lasted for no more than twenty-four to thirty-six hours.[57] Underlying climatic conditions had remained stable but the slow, cumulative shift from coal to gas ensured that there had been a progressive decline in black, polluting emissions associated with the consumption of 'soft' domestic fuel. 'Education' had been selectively beneficial. But it was pre-eminently a narrowing of price differentials between rival forms of energy that brought novel methods of heating, lighting and cooking unproblematically within the realm of working- as well as middle-class households. As for outpourings from the 15,000 factories and workshops located in the greater London region in the early twentieth century, Rollo Russell was convinced that there had been significant improvement.[58] This may have been the result of more rigorous local authority surveillance and better advice on the 'best practicable means' for the efficient consumption of smoke. But the law still lacked teeth and was very nearly wholly ineffective in cases in which a miscreant paid a fine but then repeatedly failed to undertake required technical modifications.

What kind of public environmental sphere?

It has already been suggested that, far from conforming to Habermas's model of an 'administered' 'social welfare' state, Britain between the 1870s and the outbreak of the First World War continued to be characterized by strong attachment to localism and regionalism. In the field of centralized environmental surveillance, the national Alkali Inspectorate, which concerned itself exclusively with noxious vapours produced by the manufacturing sector, had been established in the early 1860s. However, all other inspectorial bodies continued to report either to sanitary or public health committees or, in London, to longer established and structurally distinctive metropolitan agencies. The intrusion of the Alkali Inspectorate into an ever-wider range of manufacturing activities was associated with the development of specialized technical vocabularies that gradually became more intimately linked to emergent laboratory-based knowledge. Representation and diagnosis of the metropolitan coal smoke problem, by contrast, remained very nearly wholly indistinguishable from a cluster of holistic approaches to the nature of the connections between 'over-urbanization' and racial decline. Nearly every influential medical, scientific or meteorological figure involved in the diagnosis of London's late nineteenth-century atmospheric crisis championed the broadly degenerationist view that chronically high levels of smoke fog constituted a potentially irreversible threat to the vitality and, *in extremis*, continued biological existence of life in the central and eastern districts. This eclectic and seemingly indefinitely flexible discourse was significantly shaped by the collective anxiety and guilt experienced by metropolitan aristocratic and middle-class elites who had, in their own estimation, neglected to repair and sustain charitable bonds with 'outcast London'. Systemic rather than exclusively environmental, this was a multiform discourse that resonated insistently in Parliamentary debates, governmental investigations, the daily and periodical press, and elite and popular poetry, fiction and prose. It constituted nothing less than a newly emergent proto-scientific public sphere during precisely the period characterized, in Habermas's view, by the transformation and degradation of rational critical debate.

In terms of pressure group activity, the National Smoke Abatement Institution remained distanced from the very constituency – the metropolitan working class – that it was determined to recruit and convert. Dominated by progressive peers, socially aware scientists and urban reformers, the Abatement Institution lacked a large and cohesive membership and, as a consequence, found itself socially and politically isolated. As Lord Balfour of Burley emphasized, no organization could have been less well qualified to represent the interests of the great majority of smoke-producing Londoners or to offer credible advice on how much should be spent on heating and cooking and how it should be spent. The views canvassed by so exclusive and elitist a pressure group ensured that it would be marginalized by a national executive intent on ignoring the seemingly insoluble smoke fog problem. The Abatement Institution was therefore forced to make its case at under-attended public meetings and in the poorly reported committee rooms of the House of Lords. Unworldly, underpoliticized and insulated from the highly charged party political atmosphere of the Commons, it possessed few of the characteristics associated with a Habermasian manipulator of inauthentic public opinion. That so socially unrepresentative and politically naïve a body should have successfully predicted aspects of the social ecology of energy use in Edwardian Britain cannot in any way invalidate this judgement.

Finally, there are the issues of disciplinary development, and the accessibility and dissemination of technical information. In terms of meteorological speculation, the later nineteenth century was dominated by research into relationships between climatology, hydrology and physics; the nature of the cyclonic storm; and the potential and limits of forecasting.[59] In applied areas having a bearing on the specifically urban atmosphere, John Herschel and W.J. Russell demonstrated how soot became attracted to and then infiltrated individual droplets of fog vapour.[60] These insights would in due course be integrated into an embryonic science of the man-made climate. Nevertheless, throughout the period considered in this chapter, accounts of the 'naturalness' of rural mist as compared with the 'deviance' of black and yellow urban smoke fog proliferated in the pages of the *Quarterly Journal of the Royal Meteorological Society*, the intellectual reviews and large numbers of popular publications. Framed in the style perfected by Rollo Russell, writings of this kind belonged to a venerable natural historical tradition preoccupied with the detailed characteristics and visual patina of individual weather phenomena.[61]

In general, participants in the great debate about the late nineteenth-century smoke fog crisis eschewed theory. Environmental progressives relied on a *mélange* of long-established empirical knowledge: ventilation studies reaching back to the mid-eighteenth century; comparisons of the merits and demerits of a bewildering array of smokeless stoves and grates that had come on to the market since the 1830s; and evaluations of diverse approaches to the heating of individual aristocratic and upper middle-class residences that made use of 'clean' anthracite, coke and gas. On these and other issues, advocates of anti-smoke legislation were invariably better informed than their opponents. Nevertheless, as Balfour of Burley demonstrated during his questioning of Ernest Hart, a full understanding of proposed anti-air-pollution programmes was less relevant to an effective critique of the reformist stance than an ability to pose basic questions about inter-class differentials in *per capita* income and expenditure, the social determinants of energy use and rival perceptions of what it was that constituted an 'ideal' metropolitan environment.

How does all this compare with the conditions under which environmental politics are conducted in the present day? At the beginning of the twenty-first century, ministries and bureaucracies possess the power and ideological authority to designate which from among a range of publicly contentious issues should be openly discussed and the contexts in which such interchanges are to be constitutionally and administratively located. Juridical and administrative control over the form and duration of public hearings, together with a state-legitimated right to refuse to release crucial technical data into the public domain, frequently enables bureaucracies to neutralize the arguments of those campaigning against government-backed plans to construct nuclear power stations, highway systems and airport runways.[62] Such was emphatically not the case in the late nineteenth-century fog debates. Confrontational interchange was not controlled by representatives of the state holding a gate-keeping monopoly either over scientific and technical data, or over the contexts in which such material might or might not be debated.

In the case considered here, in other words, discursive conditions were quite different from those identified by Habermas in the intimidatingly voluminous body of work that he produced between the late 1960s and the near-present on the theory and possibility of authentic communication under advanced capitalism – conditions that include the role of the state as a deceptively even-handed protector of 'sensitive' material, the removal of an ever-increasing number of topics from the 'non-technical' domain, and legitimation processes that imply a progressive narrowing of informed critical debate.[63] At the same time – and as the opening section of this chapter has sought to demonstrate – the empirical findings of the earlier *Structural Transformation of the Public Sphere* fail to comprehend the astonishing diversity of both differentiated and inter-penetrating political, social, cultural and scientific discourse in late Victorian Britain.

This case study thus calls into question the adequacy of Habermas's attempt to describe and explain the historical background to the current predicament of public debate. It also leads us to doubt whether insight into the conduct of past environmental debates can offer any simple lessons for the pursuit of environmental politics at the present time: discursive conditions in the past were both too dissimilar from and insufficiently deterministic of those that obtain today. It is thus easy to understand Habermas's reasons for abandoning history for the project of formulating a communicative ethics that have occupied the greater part of his career. Nevertheless, despite this and other weaknesses that have been noted in this chapter, Habermas's study of *The Structural Transformation of the Public Sphere* has had the beneficial effect of encouraging historians to redefine the exceptionally important cluster of concepts with which it is concerned. Historical contributions to this project of conceptual clarification may yet prove valuable in rethinking the conditions under which public politics can be reconstituted and revitalised.

Notes

1 J. Habermas, *The Structural Transformation of the Public Sphere: An Inquiry into a Category of Bourgeois Society*, trans. T. Burger, Cambridge, MA: MIT Press, 1989, p. 159.

2 The key works are J. Habermas, *Legitimation Crisis*, trans. T. McCarthy, London: Heinemann, 1975; *The Theory of Communicative Action*, vol. 1: *Reason and the Rationalization of Society*, trans. T. McCarthy, Boston: Beacon Press, 1984; *Moral Consciousness and Communicative Action*, trans. C. Lenhardt and S.W. Nicholsen, Cambridge, MA: MIT Press, 1990; and *Between Facts and Norms: Contributions to a Discourse Theory of Law and Democracy*, trans. W. Rehg, Cambridge, MA: MIT Press, 1995.

3 Quoted by C. Calhoun in 'Social theory and the public sphere', in B.S. Turner (ed.), *The Blackwell Companion to Social Theory*, Oxford: Blackwell, 1996, p. 455.

4 See in particular B. Keith-Lucas, *The Unreformed Local Government System*, London: Croom Helm, 1980; and G. Best, *Mid-Victorian Britain 1851–75*, London: Fontana, 1971, pp. 53–72.

5 See J. Davis, *Reforming London: The London Government System*, London: Oxford University Press, 1998; and D. Owen, *The Government of Victorian London 1855–1889: The Metropolitan Board of Works, the Vestries and the City Corporation*, ed. R. MacLeod, Cambridge, MA: Harvard University Press, 1982.

6 But see D. Zaret, 'Religion, science and printing in the public sphere in seventeenth century England', in C. Calhoun (ed.), *Habermas and the Public Sphere*, Cambridge, MA: MIT Press, 1992, pp. 212–35; Y. Ezrahi, *The Descent of Icarus: Science and the*

Transformation of Contemporary Democracy, Cambridge, MA: Harvard University Press, 1990; and Christopher Hamlin's contribution to the present volume.

7 Calhoun, 'Social theory', p. 457.

8 T. Bateman, *Reports on the Diseases of London and the State of the Weather from 1804 to 1816*, London: Longman, 1819; R. Willan, *Reports on the Diseases of London, Particularly during the Years 1796, 97, 98, 1800 and 1801*, London: R. Phillips, 1801; W. Bent, *A Meteorological Journal: Observations on the Diseases in January 1794*, London: W. Bent, 1794; and L. Howard, *The Climate of London*, second edition, London: Harvey and Darton, J. and A. Arch, Longman, Hatchford, S. Highley (and R. Hunter) 1833.

9 See, on these issues of health and representation, B. Luckin, 'Town, country and metropolis: the formation of an air pollution problem in London, 1800–1870', in D. Schott (ed.), *Energy and the City in Europe from Preindustrial Wood Shortage to the Oil Crisis in the 1970s*, Stuttgart: Franz Steiner, 1997, pp. 77–92.

10 For a classic example of the 'cost accounting' of fever see M.W. Flinn (ed.), *Report on the Sanitary Condition of the Labouring Population of Great Britain by Edwin Chadwick 1842*, Edinburgh: Edinburgh University Press, 1965, pp. 254–76. Neil Arnott, Chadwick's early investigative collaborator and personal physician, was convinced that smoke increased Londoners' washing bills alone by approximately £2.5m a year. For the full argument see Arnott, 'On a new smoke-consuming and fuel-saving fire-place', *Journal of the Society of Arts*, 1852–4, vol. 1–2, pp. 428–35. Chadwick's own approach is summarized in the same article at p. 435.

11 F.S. Brodie, 'On the prevalence of fog during the 20 years from 1871 to 1890', *Quarterly Journal of the Royal Meteorological Society*, 1892, vol. 18, pp. 40–3; R.H. Scott, 'Fifteen years' fogs in the British islands', *Quarterly Journal of the Royal Meteorological Society*, 1893, vol. 19, p. 232; and E. Ashby and M. Anderson, *The Politics of Clean Air*, Oxford: Oxford University Press, 1981, ch. 5.

12 H.T. Bernstein, 'The mysterious disappearance of Edwardian London fog', *London Journal*, 1975, vol. 1, pp. 189–206.

13 Ministry of Health, *Mortality and Morbidity during the London Fog of December 1952*, London: HMSO, 1954; C.K.M. Douglas and K.M. Stewart, 'London fog, December 5–8, 1952', *Meteorological Magazine*, 1953, vol. 82, pp. 67–71; and E.T. Wilkins, 'Air pollution aspects of the London fog of December, 1952', *Quarterly Journal of the Royal Meteorological Society*, 1954, vol. 80, pp. 267–71.

14 *Medical Times and Gazette*, 1873, vol. 2, p. 696; *British Medical Journal*, 1880, vol. 2, p. 254; and A. Carpenter, 'Town smoke and town fog', *Westminster Review*, 1882, vol. 61, pp. 136–7.

15 This remains an underdeveloped theme but see J.W. Burrow, *Evolution and Society: A Study in Victorian Social Theory*, Cambridge: Cambridge University Press, 1966; G. Weber, 'Science and society in nineteenth century anthropology', *History of Science*, 1974, vol. 12, pp. 260–83; and A.S. Wohl, *The Eternal Slum: Housing and Social Policy in Victorian London*, London: Edward Arnold, 1977, pp. 45–73.

16 See for instance J. Cantlie, *Degeneration amongst Londoners: The Parkes Museum of Hygiene Lecture for 1885*, London: Field and Tuer, 1885.

17 W.S. Jevons, *The Coal Question: An Inquiry Concerning the Progress of the Nation*, 3rd rev. edn, London: Macmillan, 1965. The quality of the ensuing national controversy may be adduced from the comments of Sir Robert Peel, *Hansard Parliamentary Debates* (HC 3rd series), 9 March 1866, cols 1811–12. See also P. Brantlinger (ed.), *Energy and Entropy: Science and Culture in Victorian Britain*, Bloomington: Indiana University Press, 1989; and A. Briggs, *Victorian Things*, London: Batsford, 1988, pp. 298–308.

18 Flinn, *Report on the Sanitary Condition*, pp. 355–8.

19 Crucial contextual orientation on late nineteenth-century degenerationism is provided in G. Stedman Jones, *Outcast London: A Study in the Relationship between the Classes in Victorian Society*, Oxford: Oxford University Press, 1971. See also G.E. Searle, *Eugenics and Politics in Britain 1900–1914*, Leyden: Noordhoff, 1976; D. Pick, *Faces of*

Degeneration: A European Disorder c. 1848–1918, Cambridge: Cambridge University Press, 1989; and J. Harris, *Private Lives, Public Spirit: A Social History of Britain 1870–1914*, Oxford: Oxford University Press, 1993, pp. 241–5.

20 See on this under-developed theme, J. Marsh, *Back to the Land: The Pastoral Impulse in England from 1880 to 1914*, London: Longman, 1979; and D. Hardy, *Agricultural Communities in Nineteenth Century England*, London: Longman, 1979. The long-term continuities of the tradition are admirably covered in D. Matless, *Landscape and Englishness*, London: Reaktion Books, 1998.

21 J. Glaisher, *Thirty Sixth Annual Report of the Registrar-General*, London: HMSO, 1873, p. liv.

22 There is little reliable biographical information on Russell but something of his character and religious and ethical preoccupations may be derived from R. Monk, *Bertrand Russell*, vol. 1: *The Spirit of Solitude*, London: Vintage, 1996, pp. 15–19. Russell's anti-fog activities are briefly mentioned in Ashby and Anderson, *Politics of Clean Air*, pp. 55–6. In addition to *London Fogs*, London: E. Stanford, 1880, and numerous periodical articles, Russell wrote *Smoke in Relation to Fogs*, London: National Smoke Abatement Offices, 1889; *Break of Day and Other Poems*, London: T. Fisher Unwin, 1893; *Epidemics and Fever: Causes and Prevention*, London: E. Stanford, 1892; *The Atmosphere in Relation to Human Life and Health*, Washington: Smithsonian Miscellaneous Collections, 1896, vol. 39; 'The artificial production of fog', a paper delivered to the Conference on Smoke Abatement, 1896; and *The Distribution of Land*, London: P.S. King, 1907.

23 Russell, *Smoke*, p. 9.

24 Russell, *London Fogs*, pp. 22–4.

25 Russell, *Smoke*, pp. 24–6.

26 Russell, *London Fogs*, p. 30

27 Ibid., p. 31.

28 Russell, *Smoke*, pp. 21–2.

29 Russell, *Break of Day*, pp. 24–5.

30 A.S. Wohl, *Endangered Lives: Public Health in Victorian Britain*, London: Dent, 1983, pp. 225–32. See also R.M. MacLeod, 'The Alkali Acts administration, 1863–84: the emergence of the civil scientist', *Victorian Studies*, 1965, vol. 9, pp. 85–112.

31 A more detailed account of local environmental legislation is provided by B. Luckin, 'Pollution in the city', in M. Daunton (ed.), *Cambridge Urban History of Britain*, vol. 3: *1840–1950*, Cambridge: Cambridge University Press, 2000, pp. 208–13.

32 C. Flick, 'The movement for smoke abatement in nineteenth century Britain', *Technology and Culture*, 1980, vol. 21, p. 50.

33 Wohl, *Endangered Lives*, p. 220.

34 'Legislative measures for the prevention of smoke nuisance', *The Builder*, 1863, vol. 21, p. 613.

35 *The Times* (London), 24 January 1893.

36 Succinct biographical material is contained in P.W.J. Bartrip, *Mirror of Medicine: A History of The British Medical Journal*, Oxford: Clarendon Press, 1990, pp. 63–8, and Bartrip, 'The British Medical Journal: a retrospect', in W.F. Bynum, S. Lock and R. Porter (eds), *Medical Journals and Medical Knowledge: Historical Essays*, London: Routledge, 1992, pp. 134–40.

37 Select Committee of the House of Lords on the Smoke Nuisance Abatement (Metropolis) Bill, *Report*, Cmd. 321, PP 1887, vol. 12, QQ. 260 and 322, evidence of E. Hart.

38 Ibid., Q. 327, evidence of E. Hart.

39 Ibid., Q. 303, evidence of E. Hart.

40 D. Cannadine, *The Decline and Fall of the British Aristocracy*, New Haven: Yale University Press, 1990, pp. 581–2.

41 Select Committee on the Smoke Nuisance Abatement Bill, Q. 300, evidence of Lord Balfour of Burley.

42 Ibid., Q. 304, evidence of Lord Balfour of Burley.

43 Ibid., Q. 398, evidence of Lord Balfour of Burley.

44 Ibid., Q. 403, evidence of Lord Balfour of Burley.

45 Ibid., Q. 411, evidence of E. Hart.

46 Ibid., Q. 287, evidence of Lord Balfour of Burley and E. Hart.

47 *Hansard Parliamentary Debates* (HL 4th series), 12 February 1892, col. 310.

48 Ibid., 11 February 1892, col. 194.

49 *Report of the London County Council to 31st March 1919*, London: Odhams, 1920, pp. 92–3.

50 Ibid.

51 Russell, 'Artificial production'.

52 Sir G. Livesey, 'Domestic smoke abatement', *Transactions of the Royal Sanitary Institute*, vol. 27, 1906, pp. 58–60.

53 Report of the Select Committee into Metropolitan Gas Companies, Appendix 2, Cmd. 294, PP 1899, vol. 10, p. 359.

54 Cited in *The Builder*, 1845, vol. 3, p. 455.

55 *Nature*, 1881, vol. 25, p. 173.

56 Ministry of Health, *Committee on Smoke and Noxious Vapour Abatement: Final Report*, London: HMSO, 1921, p. 260. The inflexibility of delivery and relative costliness of energy has been fully documented by T.P. Hughes, *Networks of Power: Electrification in Western Society 1880–1939*, Baltimore: Johns Hopkins University Press, 1983, ch. 9. See also J.A. Fleming, 'Official obstruction of electrical progress', *Nineteenth Century and After*, 1900, vol. 49, pp. 348–63.

57 W.A.L. Marshall, *A Century of London Weather*, London: HMSO, 1952, pp. 42–53; J.A. Brazell, *London Weather*, London: Meteorological Office, 1968, pp. 111–114; and T.J. Chandler, *The Climate of London*, London: Hutchinson, 1965, chs 4, 8 and 12.

58 Russell, 'Artificial production'. The estimate of the number of factories and work-shops was made by W.N. Shaw in 'The treatment of smoke: a sanitary parallel', *Transactions of the Sanitary Institute of Great Britain*, 1902, vol. 23, p. 328.

59 Sir W.N. Shaw with the assistance of E. Austin, *Manual of Meteorology*, vol. 1: *Meteorology in History*, Cambridge: Cambridge University Press, 1932, ch. 8.

60 These and related developments are summarized in 'Fogs', *Nature*, 1879–80, vol. 21, p. 356.

61 The early modern origins of this tradition have now been meticulously reconstructed by V. Jankovic, *Reading the Skies: A Cultural History of English Weather, 1650–1820*, Manchester: Manchester University Press, 2000.

62 The larger ideological parameters have been established in Habermas, *Legitimation Crisis*. See also B. Wynne, *Rationality and Ritual: The Windscale Inquiry and Nuclear Decisions in Britain*, Chalfont St Giles: British Society for the History of Science Monographs, 3, 1982; J. Forester, *Planning in the Face of Power*, Berkeley: University of California Press, 1989; S. Chambers, 'Discourse and democratic practices', in S.K. White (ed.), *The Cambridge Companion to Habermas*, Cambridge: Cambridge University Press, 1995, pp. 233–62; and J. Rodger, 'Inauthentic politics and the public inquiry system', *Scottish Journal of Sociology*, 1978, vol. 3, pp. 103–27.

63 Central to an evaluation of this later body of work would be a consideration of Habermas's position in relation to new social movements. For summary accounts see Habermas, 'New social movements', *Telos*, vol. 49, pp. 33–7, and *The Theory of Communicative Action*, vol. 2: *Life World and System: A Critique of Functionalist Reason*, trans. T. McCarthy, Boston: Beacon Press, 1987, pp. 393–6. The Habermasian approach to contemporary environmental activism is cogently assessed in D. Goldblatt, *Social Theory and the Environment*, Oxford: Polity Press, 1992, pp. 112–53. The larger theoretical issue of the potentials of 'discursive democracy' are authoritatively addressed by the contributors to White (ed.), *Cambridge Companion*, part iv.

12 Alternative publics

The development of government policy on personal health care, 1905–11

Steve Sturdy

The years between 1905 and the First World War saw a major expansion of state welfare provision in Britain, including the passage of the National Insurance Act in 1911 and the inception of the National Health Insurance (NHI) scheme two years later.[1] These developments took place against a backdrop of intense debate over the role and responsibilities of the state, prompted by growing concern at the problems of poverty and destitution, and by a widespread perception that nineteenth-century forms of state welfare based in the Poor Law were failing to meet the needs of a modern industrial society. Medical issues loomed large in these debates. Politicians and social reformers expressed concern that high levels of ill health among the working-class population were undermining industrial and military fitness and efficiency, and were thus inimical to the national interest. Most agreed that the poor quality of medical care available to large sections of the working class – be it privately purchased or provided under the Poor Law – was at least partly to blame for such problems. Consequently, a variety of views were formulated on what action the state should take to ensure that the poor were given access to an adequate standard of health care.

This chapter explores three quite distinct sets of proposals for government action on health care put forward at that time – two of which were set out in the Majority and Minority Reports of the Royal Commission on the Poor Laws, which sat from 1905 to 1909,[2] while the third was adopted by the architects of the NHI scheme. These divergent views on the role of government in the provision of medical care are of particular interest in the light of Jürgen Habermas's diagnosis of the growth of state welfare in *The Structural Transformation of the Public Sphere*. Habermas argues that the effect of the intrusion of public authority into private lives through the growth of the welfare services was to erode individual autonomy, turning once-active citizens into passive consumers of corporately produced material and cultural goods. As a result, genuinely independent and critical forms of public action and opinion, pursued by private individuals voluntarily associating as a public, were compromised, while the power of both private and statutory corporations was enhanced.[3] With this diagnosis in mind, what stands out from a re-reading of the medical recommendations put forward by the Majority and Minority Reports of the Royal Commission and by the advocates of

NHI is that each was justified at least in part by an explicit expectation that, contrary to Habermas, it would lead to wider and more active public involvement in self-governing institutions of one kind or another. Government-led developments in health care, in other words, were seen as a way to revive rather than undermine the public sphere.

In what follows I will explore each of these sets of recommendations in turn, to illuminate the different understandings of public life that they embodied, and to show how they supposed that government medical policy might encourage participation in the public sphere. I will also examine how and why the actual implementation of NHI departed from these expectations, and will conclude with a brief discussion of what this enables us to say about Habermas's account of the decline of the structural transformation of the public sphere.

The Charity Organisation Society and organized self-help

One of the most prominent of the organizations involved in Edwardian debates over health policy was the Charity Organisation Society (COS), which was established in 1869 to advance a particularly doctrinaire version of prevailing Victorian views on the ends and means of social welfare.[4] Central to COS policy was the assumption that competent members of society should take responsibility for providing themselves and their families with the necessities of life. This had implications for what sort of support should be available for those who found it difficult to achieve self-sufficiency. The COS were concerned that aid should not encourage dependency and lead to malingering. Properly applied charitable assistance provided a way of confronting that danger head-on. Since charitable aid was given voluntarily, it could be made conditional on the recipient adopting appropriate forms of behaviour. Charity could thus be made into a powerful instrument of moral coercion, aimed at reinforcing rather than undermining the independence and self-sufficiency of its recipients.[5] Indeed, in their more rhapsodic moments, COS philosophers spoke of organized philanthropy as a moral nexus spanning the whole of society, within which the reciprocal responsibilities of the well-to-do and the poor might be realized for the good of society as a whole.[6] They envisaged, in effect, a public sphere of private individuals voluntarily supporting and assisting one another in such a way as to promote both individual self-sufficiency and mutual obligation. The COS accordingly set themselves the task of ensuring that charitable assistance was systematically organized along such lines.[7]

By contrast, the COS saw no such virtue in statutory poor relief as provided under the Poor Law. Since statutory relief was available as a matter of right or entitlement to all who needed it, and lacked the element of personal obligation associated with charitable giving, it embodied no intrinsic influence against the temptations of dependency. Consequently, the COS were strongly inclined to endorse what they called 'the principles of 1834'[8] – that is, the recommendation, written into the 1834 Poor Law Report and embodied in the Poor Law

Amendment Act of the same year, that statutory poor relief be made as unattractive as possible, so that it would only be sought by those who genuinely had no other option. Historians have tended to dwell on the physical and psychological deterrents faced by recipients of poor relief – notably subjection to the harshness of life in the workhouse and the social stigma that went with it.[9] But for the purposes of the present chapter it is important to note also the civil penalties they incurred. Through incarceration in the workhouse and disenfranchisement, recipients of statutory poor relief under the Act of 1834 effectively forfeited their normal rights as citizens. State assistance was thus reserved for, and simultaneously served to identify, a quite distinct category of beings – paupers, or the destitute – whose failure to fend for themselves disqualified them from participating in public life.

Whether or not the practice of deterrence was ever pursued with the rigour that the architects of the Act of 1834 envisaged remains a matter of debate.[10] But whatever the practice, COS activists strongly endorsed the principle of reserving statutory poor relief specifically for those who had shown themselves to be incapable of benefiting from the moral influence of charitable assistance.[11] They carried this view forward into their recommendations to the Royal Commission of the Poor Laws, on which they were strongly represented. The Commission's Majority Report, published in 1909, effectively embodied the COS line on welfare reform.[12] The Report recommended that public assistance should be provided as far as possible through charitable giving. To this end, voluntary aid committees should be established, on a statutory basis but with few statutory restrictions on their actions, to co-ordinate the work of the many different charitable agencies and to oversee applications to them.[13] These would be the bodies to which those in need of assistance applied in the first instance. But the voluntary aid committees would also be able to refer what they regarded as hopeless cases to a separate destitution authority, the public assistance committee, which would dispense statutory poor relief.[14] The principle of reserving such relief for a separate class – the destitute – thus remained intact.[15] Meanwhile, though the deterrent penalties and disqualifications imposed on the recipients of statutory relief need not perhaps be as punitive as those favoured by the architects of the Act of 1834, the Majority Report nonetheless maintained that such assistance should continue to be 'in some way less agreeable than assistance given by the Voluntary Aid Committee'.[16]

The COS's insistence on reserving statutory poor relief for a distinct class of paupers encountered its greatest challenge with the case of medical relief. Under the New Poor Law of 1834, access to statutory medical assistance had been made subject to the same forms of deterrence, including disenfranchisement and a deliberately poor standard of provision, as were applied to other forms of poor relief.[17] Subsequently, however, this tended to be tempered by suggestions that the provision of a better standard of medical care would actually help to reduce Poor Law expenditure. Ill health and infirmity were commonly regarded as contributory causes of destitution, preventing many who otherwise were willing to support themselves by their own labour from doing so. In many such cases, prompt and effective medical treatment would hasten their return to fitness and self-sufficiency. These arguments were taken up and amplified by Poor Law reformers, including many medical officers. As a result, from the mid-nineteenth century onwards, many districts began to provide improved facilities for the treatment of sick paupers.[18] Reformers also argued that, since early intervention was vital if illness was to be arrested before it did permanent harm and caused chronic disability, other forms of deterrence should also be alleviated. Consequently, in 1885 the recipients of medical relief were exempted from the penalty of disenfranchisement.[19] As a result, by the end of the nineteenth century, statutory medical assistance had improved both in quality and in ease of access, to the extent that a witness could tell the Royal Commission on the Poor Laws that the Poor Law infirmaries were 'fast becoming rate-aided hospitals' for the entire working class.[20]

This posed a dilemma for the COS activists who penned the Commission's Majority Report. On the one hand, they were anxious to ensure that provision of medical assistance under the Poor Law should not undermine the incentive to self-help: 'We are not inclined...to make medical assistance so attractive that it may become a species of honourable and gratuitous self-indulgence instead of a somewhat unpleasant necessity resorted to because restoration to health is otherwise impossible', declared the Report.[21] But they also acknowledged that access to good-quality medical care would do much to reduce the incidence of destitution and the burden it imposed on the national economy. The difficulty lay in deciding what balance to strike between deterrence and ease of access – in finding 'the right degree of attractiveness and deterrence for the right class of people'.[22] In the end, the Majority Report abandoned the principle of deterrence altogether, and considered instead whether, in the case of medical care, statutory assistance might not be made into a positive and beneficial moral force. What was needed was some way of rendering medical relief 'attractive to the needy sick, while at the same time stimulating and educating those who, though sick, ought to have themselves made provision against sickness'.[23] '[M]edical assistance, while not being deterrent, should at the same time be such as will encourage rather than discourage independent provision against sickness by every class that is able to afford it', declared the Report.[24]

Following the predilections of the COS, the Majority Report argued that these ends could best be met by interposing voluntary organizations between the needy and the state – though in this instance collective self-help rather than organized philanthropy was cited as the most appropriate form of voluntary activity. The Report recommended that steps should be taken to encourage the formation and co-ordination of a network of provident dispensaries throughout the country.[25] As their name suggests, such dispensaries operated on provident principles. Members paid regular subscriptions into dispensary funds, in return for which they were entitled to receive medical attendance and medication at the dispensary whenever they needed it. In effect, provident dispensaries were a form of non-profit medical insurance, closely akin to the better-known friendly societies.[26] Like the friendly societies, moreover, they were self-governing bodies run by the subscribers themselves. It was this, in particular, that commended provident dispensaries and other provident organizations to the authors of the Majority Report. Not only did such bodies provide an opportunity to save against hard times, but also by involving subscribers in the management of the fund and the distribution of benefits they fostered a sense of mutual responsibility and the need for collective self-discipline among the poor. As the Report put it, provident organizations were 'of great value to the nation, because not only do they aid the growth of thrifty and provident habits but they give an opportunity for the exercise of self-government'.[27]

These moral virtues inspired the authors of the Majority Report to recommend that provident dispensaries should also be made the site for the disbursement of statutory medical assistance for those who could not afford to contribute to the provident schemes. Non-contributors, like contributors, should be allowed to present themselves to the dispensaries for medical treatment. In such cases, however, the destitution authority should follow up with an investigation of the patient's financial affairs. If they were found to be genuinely needy, the authority would then bear the costs of treatment; if not, they would be required to bear the costs themselves.[28] By such means, the Majority Report advised, the deterrent penalties surrounding statutory medical assistance would be removed: the destitute would receive the same standard of medical care and attendance as independent contributors to the dispensaries, and would be spared the social stigma of having to apply in the first instance to the destitution authorities.[29] But at the same time, the recipients of statutory medical relief would be exposed to the beneficial moral atmosphere of collective self-help and self-governance that pervaded the provident dispensaries, and would thereby be encouraged to pursue the same virtues on their own behalf. As a result, concluded the Majority Report, 'The need for deterrence disappears, if the application for medical assistance can be made the introduction, not to pauperism, but to a provident dispensary.'[30]

The Majority Report thus held to a vision of a public sphere of medical welfare organized primarily around voluntary forms of collective self-help and run by financially and morally independent individuals. Statutory agencies were to have only minimal involvement in this voluntary public sphere. Local government would have a duty to encourage the formation of provident dispensaries, but would not determine the terms or conditions on which they provided medical care to their subscribers. Meanwhile, statutory assistance would be restricted to a clearly delimited minority of those attending the dispensaries, who were judged to be genuinely incapable of providing their own medical care. The recipients of statutory medical assistance would not be subjected to disenfranchisement or otherwise deprived of the rights and status of private citizenship (though they might find themselves subject to such penalties if they failed to provide for themselves more generally). But as non-contributors they would occupy a subordinate position within the public sphere of the provident dispensaries, without any say in the management of the medical services or the dispensary funds. The Majority Report anticipated that this would provide the necessary stimulus for the destitute to join the ranks of contributors in their own right, thereby eventually making statutory provision unnecessary. 'We hope that, ultimately, it may be possible to dispense altogether with the service of the district [Poor Law] medical officer,' declared the Report, 'and that his duties will be shared among medical men practising in the district. Meanwhile, arrangements might be made to retain the district medical officer on the staff of the provident dispensary.'[31] For the time being, however, this was merely a hope. Meanwhile, so long as statutory assistance remained a necessity, it would continue to demarcate a specific sub-class of individuals who, as a result of their failure to fend for themselves, were not admitted to full membership of the public sphere of the dispensaries.

Beatrice Webb and state medical services

A very different view of the role of the state in the provision of medical care was presented in the Minority Report of the Royal Commission, whose main author was the Fabian propagandist Beatrice Webb. Webb looked not to the medical services of the Poor Law, as the COS members of the Commission had done, for her model of statutory medical provision, but rather to the public health medical services. In so doing, she drew on a rather different set of assumptions about the purpose of state provision from those adopted by the COS. The public health medical services had expanded dramatically during the last quarter of the nineteenth century, particularly with the establishment of special hospitals to isolate and treat individuals suffering from infectious diseases.[32] Importantly, the provision of such treatment was not understood as a form of statutory assistance for individual patients, but as a way of protecting the health of the community from the spread of disease. Consequently, unlike the Poor Law medical services, public health medical treatment was not restricted to a specific class of paupers, but was available to the entire population – often, indeed, with the force of compulsion.[33] Whereas the Poor Law medical services provided treatment for all forms of illness, however, the public health services dealt only with the relatively small number of scheduled diseases that were seen to threaten the community as a whole. Nonetheless, over the final years of the nineteenth century the facilities of the public health medical services expanded rapidly. By the time the Royal Commission on the Poor Laws reported in 1909, Webb was able to claim that these services provided 'medical advice, attendance or medicine, one way or another, for possibly nearly as many patients – certainly as many acutely sick patients – as are under the care of the Poor Law Medical Service'.[34]

With the support and advice of a number of public health doctors, Webb drew up proposals for a radical reorganization of the state medical services. The facilities of the Poor Law medical services, including both the medical officers who provided domiciliary care and the infirmaries, should be handed over to the public health authorities to create a single medical service that would treat all forms of illness and that would be available to the entire population on a non-deterrent basis. Treatment would be provided free and without penalty to those who could not afford to pay for it, while means-tested fees would be charged to those who could. By proposing to establish a universally accessible state service of this kind, Webb broke decisively with the view that individuals had a moral responsibility to obtain medical care by their own private means, and that state services should therefore be restricted to a specific class of paupers. Indeed, she made it quite clear that she intended the state medical service to replace large sections of the existing market in private medicine. '[T]he very principle of the Poor Law Medical Service…involves…actual refusal of all treatment to persons who are in need of it, but who can manage to pay for some cheap substitute,' Webb wrote in the Minority Report.[35] Universal statutory provision of medical care would ultimately render such 'cheap substitutes' unnecessary. 'In the long run (but this only gradually),' she declared in a memorandum that she submitted to the Royal Commission in 1907, the state medical service 'would substitute for the "sixpenny doctor" and the "club practice" a salaried service of young "dispensary doctors", gaining general experience whilst qualifying for specialism or superior salaried appointments.'[36] By such means, the state would become the main provider of medical care for the working class, including not just the very poor but also a large proportion of those who currently paid for their own private medical attendance.

In Webb's view, a state medical service of this kind would serve the public good far more effectively than the existing market in private medicine. The forms of private medical care affordable by large sections of the working class were generally of poor quality, and often ineffectual in combating illness. As a result, many more cases of disease progressed into chronic debility – and ultimately into destitution – than would have been the case had better treatment been available. The provision of a better quality of care by the state would thus help to reduce the financial and social cost of destitution by ensuring that illness was treated promptly and efficiently, and preventable disability averted.[37] Webb was not just concerned with the quality of treatment, however. The terms on which such treatment was provided were also an issue. As public employees, doctors within a state medical service would be aware of the need to serve the long-term interests of the public as much as the short-term interests of individual patients. Webb saw this orientation exemplified in much of the treatment already available under the public health medical services, which was concerned not just with effecting an immediate cure, but with 'education of the patient in a method of living calculated to minimize the recurrence or spread of the disease'.[38] Indeed, a state medical service was far better suited to providing this kind of treatment than was private medicine. The adoption of an appropriate 'method of living' often involved a measure of self-discipline or self-denial. But private practitioners who insisted too forcefully on such measures risked losing their patients – and hence their livelihood – to more indulgent competitors. Any doctor,

> dependent for a livelihood on a wide popularity among his ignorant patients, cannot be expected to run counter to their prejudices and to offer

them, instead of the 'bottle of physic', stern advice as to the need for physical control, and as to the fatal effects of not altering their careless or
intemperate habits of life. Where the patient chooses the doctor, he chooses
the doctor whose methods and manners he likes best, not the one most likely
to prevent the recurrence of the disease.[39]

By contrast, doctors in salaried state employment would be under no such pressure to pander to their patients' wishes. Their income would be secure, however
much their patients might resent their advice. Even so, there remained a risk that
the strictest practitioners would end up with the fewest patients, and that their
reputations, if not their emoluments, would suffer as a result. To prevent this,
Webb argued that patients under the new state medical service should not be
allowed to choose their doctors. Rather, they would be allocated to a particular
practitioner, and would have no choice but to accept or ignore that doctor's
advice. The result, argued Webb, would be a great improvement in the health of
the population.

The benefits of the state medical service would not end with an improvement
in physical health, however. Arthur Newsholme, one of the public health doctors
who helped Webb to draw up her proposals, made this clear in his evidence to
the Royal Commission:

> The form in which medical aid would be given would be such as constantly
> to enforce on the minds of the patients their duty to the community and to
> themselves in matters of health….They would not be merely passive recipi-
> ents of advice and attention. The influence of the doctor would demand
> from them habits of life and even sacrifices of personal taste in the interest
> of the health of the community, their families and themselves, which would
> leave them conscious of a sensible discharge of duty in return for the atten-
> tion which they receive.[40]

According to Newsholme, the new state medical service would thus have a beneficial effect on more than just the physical health of the population: it would also
inculcate what he called a 'discipline of responsibility', which 'would introduce
into the national life an attitude towards matters of personal health that would
have an indirect effect upon conduct, while directly restricting disease'.[41] Webb
echoed this view in her Minority Report, declaring:

> the essential characteristic of the Public Health Medical Service – that it is
> rendered in the interest of the community and not in order merely to relieve
> the suffering of the individual – actually creates in the recipient an increased
> feeling of personal obligation, and even a new sense of social responsi-
> bility.[42]

Webb and her allies thus claimed for the proposed state medical service much
the same virtues as the COS attributed to voluntary philanthropy. Indeed, the

Minority Report explicitly recommended that various forms of voluntary work and charitable provision should be brought under the direct control of statutory agencies, where they might assist in the public work of surveillance, supervision and treatment of the poor.[43]

In effect, Webb inverted the moral presuppositions that informed the policies put forward by the COS. Where the COS saw statutory provision of medical and other services as a temptation to self-indulgence and malingering, Webb attributed the same weakness to private medicine. Where the COS regarded voluntary forms of philanthropy or collective self-help as the best means of encouraging moral self-discipline among the poor, Webb saw statutory provision as better suited to that aim. These conflicting moral perspectives were also apparent in the different ways that Webb and the COS thought the public sphere should be constituted. The COS envisaged a public sphere made up of private individuals defined by their financial independence, who came together voluntarily to manage their own collective affairs and to exert a salutary discipline over those less independent than themselves. The state, meanwhile, was restricted to providing for that residuum whose persistent failure to achieve independence debarred them from full membership of the public sphere. Webb, in contrast, favoured a sphere of universal public authority and entitlement, mediated by expert state employees, but in turn accountable to an enfranchised public from which no one was to be excluded by dint of destitution. Indeed, she envisaged that the sense of public ownership of the state medical services would actively encourage popular participation in local political life. For Webb, then, the state medical services were to provide a nexus of engagement with a wider public sphere that brought together all sections of society for the purposes of self-governance.

National Health Insurance

In the event, neither the Fabian proposals for a state medical service nor the COS plan for boosting voluntary self-help through the promotion of provident dispensaries became government policy. By 1909, when the Royal Commission on the Poor Laws reported, opinion on the government front bench was already moving in a quite different direction. In particular, Lloyd George and Winston Churchill were unwilling to challenge the powerful vested interests of the Poor Law administration. Instead, they had come to favour a scheme of national insurance as the most expedient way of combating destitution. This scheme, which passed into legislation in 1911 and began operating in 1913, was initially conceived simply as a way of providing against loss of earnings, whether due to unemployment or sickness. To this end, workers who came under the scheme were required to pay regular mandatory contributions into an approved insurance fund, which were then topped up with a combination of compulsory employers' contributions and additional state subsidies. Only belatedly did Lloyd George realize that the insurance fund might also pay for medical treatment – so-called medical benefit – with a view to returning sick workers to gainful employment as quickly as possible.[44]

The national insurance system, and within it the scheme of NHI, satisfied neither the COS nor the Fabians. In certain respects it was much closer to the COS vision of welfare reform than to Beatrice Webb's plans for a state medical service. It was far from universal in its coverage. On the contrary, it was expressly restricted to workers in secure employment. Thus, if anything, it presupposed a moral distinction between the more respectable sections of the working class, who were seen to be worthy of a measure of state assistance, and those in irregular or otherwise marginal jobs – precisely the groups most vulnerable to destitution as a result of sickness or unemployment – for whom self-help or the deterrent mercies of an unreformed Poor Law remained the only options.[45] Nonetheless, the COS maintained their opposition to state subsidies, even when targeted at the respectable working class, for fear that they would undermine the incentive for individuals to fend for themselves. 'The fear of moral injury which state dependence may cause is decreasing,' lamented one COS hardliner in the wake of Parliament's decision to endorse the insurance scheme.[46]

Beatrice Webb and her supporters saw similar dangers in national insurance, and warned that the scheme 'may quite probably (unless very carefully safeguarded) actually increase the evil for which it purports to provide [i.e. destitution]'.[47] They objected on rather different grounds from the COS, however. Their concern was not primarily with the moral consequences of state assistance as such; after all, they had themselves recommended a vast expansion of statutory provision of medical care and other services. Rather, they were worried about the conditions under which medical benefit was provided. Under NHI, patients were at liberty to choose from among all the doctors working the scheme in a particular area. In consequence, the disciplinary dimension that Webb saw as crucial to the operation of their proposed state medical service would be entirely lacking. '[T]he sick man having a "Free Choice of Doctors" is seldom well-informed enough to select the doctor or adopt the treatment – still less lead the life – that will promote his quickest and most effectual recovery,' she warned.[48] Rather, patients would tend to choose those doctors who proved most obliging when it came to granting sick notes or otherwise indulging their patients' wishes.[49] Thus, far from providing a way of promoting healthy living and policing malingerers, Lloyd George's scheme of medical benefit would simply encourage laziness and malingering by postponing the need to return to work.[50]

We should not allow such criticisms to persuade us that the champions of NHI had no interest in matters of morality and public responsibility, however.[51] On the contrary, in its original form at least, the NHI scheme – like the alternative proposals that it supplanted – was justified partly in terms of the expectation that it would foster socially responsible forms of public activity among the working class. Central to the moral justification of NHI was the fact that the scheme was to be administered through the provident friendly societies, and so would bring with it many of the same moral benefits as were associated with voluntary forms of organized self-help. This was the view adopted by W.J. Braithwaite, the civil servant to whom Lloyd George gave much of the responsibility for drafting the National Insurance Bill. As one colleague recalled, Braithwaite's work on NHI was inspired by 'an idealist's belief that the keenness and zeal in the cause of self-government found in the small country Friendly Society...could be developed in the whole working-class population'.[52] Similar views had earlier been expressed by William Beveridge, who looked to the German health insurance system to demonstrate the merits of such a scheme:

> The German system of industrial insurance does not simply dispense benefits. Its elaborate machinery brings men of all sorts into co-operation with one another, in accident insurance associations, in the arbitration tribunals, in the management of sick funds, and in countless other ways. It increases the opportunities of public service. It impresses upon all the sense of the reality of the State and of the claims of the community upon each man's time and thought.[53]

Like Braithwaite, Beveridge attributed these merits to the fact that much of the work of administering the German insurance scheme was undertaken by voluntary organizations. So too did Lloyd George, when he recommended his own National Insurance scheme to Parliament and to the public. Like Beveridge, he pointed to the example of Germany, where 'Insurance has done more to teach the working classes the value of organization than any single thing', and where even the trade unions were forced to acknowledge the popularity of this essentially capitalist institution.[54] NHI would have a similarly beneficial effect on the 'poorer classes' of Britain, he argued:

> It will remove anxiety as to distress, it will heal, it will lift them up, and it will give them a new hope. It will do more than that, because it will give them a new weapon which will enable them to organize, and the most valuable and vital thing is that the working classes will be organized – 15,000,000 of them – for the first time for their own purposes.[55]

Lloyd George's decision to operate the National Insurance scheme through the friendly societies struck an expedient compromise between compulsion and self-governance, and between state support and organized self-help, which did much to help overcome the deep-seated Liberal resistance to statutory assistance, and even won him the support of large sections of the Tory opposition.[56]

For all that he was prepared to repeat his advisers' ideas about the moral and public value of friendly society organization, however, Lloyd George himself inclined towards a more reductively financial view of the scheme. He shared with Churchill a fascination with the actuarial laws on which National Insurance was to be based. Such laws, declared Churchill, would 'bring in the magic of averages to the aid of the million' by providing a means of distributing financial assistance to those who most needed it at any particular time.[57] But that was not all that he believed 'the magic of averages' would achieve. It would also ensure that individual claimants would not abuse the scheme by drawing benefits when they were in fact fit for work – by malingering, in other words. Both Lloyd George and Churchill supposed that the temptation to malinger would be averted once the participants realized that individual abuse would tend to reduce the benefits available to all. As Lloyd George put it:

> The only really effective check [on malingering]…is to be found in engaging the self-interest of the workmen themselves in opposition to it….This Scheme is so worked that the burden of mismanagement and maladminis-tration would fall on the workmen themselves….Once they realise that, then malingering will become an unpopular vice amongst them, and they will take the surest and shortest way to discourage it.[58]

In effect, the 'magic of averages' would bring moral as much as economic bene-fits, by making clear to participants the extent to which their individual welfare depended upon the responsible conduct of all. It would even contribute to the revitalization of civil society more generally. As Churchill put it, National Insurance would help to reinforce 'the stability of our institutions by giving the mass of industrial workers a direct interest in maintaining them…"a stake in the country" in the form of insurance against evil days'.[59]

Indeed, so far as Lloyd George and Churchill were concerned, the moral benefits that would derive from the actuarial logic of the National Insurance scheme would outweigh any beneficial effects that resulted from the involvement of the friendly societies. This became clear when commercial insurance compa-nies began lobbying to be included in the administration of health insurance. The friendly societies objected on the grounds that they would be unable to compete with the aggressive marketing methods employed by the commercial companies. Braithwaite took the side of the friendly societies, reminding Lloyd George that the commercial companies were not self-governing organizations, so would not exert the same moral influence on those they insured. His arguments went unheeded, however. The commercial companies were a powerful force in the business world, and had strong support in Parliament. Moreover, so far as Lloyd George was concerned, there was little reason to exclude them. After all, if morality was primarily a matter of actuarial logic, the commercial insurance companies could administer NHI with as much moral advantage as the self-governing friendly societies.[60]

Besides, Lloyd George had a high regard for the organizational abilities of private businessmen. 'Even before the War,' recalled Braithwaite, 'he was fond of the idea of "business" men running things (as compared with Civil Servants).'[61] Consequently, Lloyd George welcomed the interest that the commercial insur-ance companies were now taking in health insurance, and insisted that they be written into the National Insurance Bill. The result was a disaster for the princi-ples of mutual aid and self-governance represented by the friendly societies, and a triumph for commercial insurance. Looking back from the vantage of the late 1940s, Beveridge acknowledged that the inclusion of the commercial insurance companies in NHI had led to gains in administrative capacity and efficiency, but deplored the fact that 'it was a service bought at the cost of strengthening a form of gain-seeking business'.[62]

As a result, though the inception and growth of NHI undoubtedly led to significant improvements in public welfare, it did so at the expense of efforts to encourage more active participation in public institutions of one sort or another. Patients were given no formal means of exerting collective control over insurance practice, either through the democratic agencies of local government as Webb had hoped, or through self-governing provident organizations as the COS and the early advocates of NHI had envisaged. Their only means of determining the kind of care they received was by exercising their individual right to choose their doctor. In effect, the patient's role under NHI was simply as a consumer of a state-subsidized but still largely private system of commercial medicine.

Conclusion

By compelling large sections of the population to pay regular insurance contributions, the implementation of NHI in 1913 effected a major extension of state authority into private life. And by making private insurance companies responsible for the collection of contributions and the delivery of medical benefits, it militated against direct public involvement in the provision of popular health care. At first glance, these developments appear to confirm Habermas's diagnosis of the decline of the bourgeois public sphere. On closer analysis, however, it becomes less clear that this is the case. Habermas's analysis rests on the assumption that state interference in private affairs tends inevitably to weaken participation in public debate and opinion formation. But political commentators of the early twentieth century would have disputed this assumption. Indeed, many supposed that appropriate forms of state intervention in the organization of health care might do much to encourage rather than undermine active public engagement with various kinds of medical institutions. Since the measures that these commentators advocated were not in the end put into practice, it is impossible to tell whether or not they would have been proved right. But in the absence of empirical evidence one way or the other, it seems unreasonable to dismiss their claims a priori, particularly in view of the demonstration by other contributors to the present volume that in certain instances state institutions had provided an effective locus for the mobilization of public opinion and action.[63]

In Habermas's defence, it might be argued that, whatever alternatives were proposed, the government nonetheless adopted a form of medical welfare that denied the public any active role in the organization or management of their own health care. But it would seem that this too was far from inevitable. The specific form of medical provision enacted in 1911 was a consequence of particular historical contingencies, including the influence that the commercial insurance companies enjoyed in Parliament, Lloyd George's peculiar regard for businessmen and the inability of philanthropic voluntarists and Fabian propagandists to agree on the fundamental principles of state action. Moreover, it is doubtful whether these contingencies can be assimilated to Habermas's broader structural-functional understanding of the alignment of social forces in late nineteenth and early twentieth-century society. Habermas supposes that state intervention in hitherto private matters such as personal health care was primarily a response to the fragmentation of a once homogeneous and consensual bourgeois public sphere into conflicting interest groups defined by wealth and class, and was intended to moderate such conflict, chiefly by countering the worst excesses of industrial exploitation of the working class. In support of this view, it is certainly the case that Edwardian welfare initiatives were prompted at least in part by the expansion of the franchise and the need to accommodate the new-found electoral power of the working class.[64] But in the case of the specifically medical policy developments discussed in this chapter, it would appear that working-class demands were of far less concern than employers' and politicians' anxiety over the impact of poor public health on industrial and military efficiency.[65] Again, overarching structural-functional explanations seem to take second place to more local and contingent accounts of the policy process in this instance.

Consequently, if we are to understand just how and why public life has declined since the high point of the early nineteenth century, we cannot rest content with the broad generalities that Habermas offers. His overview of the transformation of the bourgeois public sphere is an insightful and suggestive one, which raises many questions for more detailed historical investigation. But his explanatory framework is overly deterministic and pays insufficient attention to the contingencies of political negotiation and the possibility of alternative lines of historical development. In particular, his view of the state is reductionist and monolithic, and fails to recognize both the variety of institutional forms that state intervention might take, and the opportunities that such institutions might have provided for the regeneration of public life. Thus, while we might share Habermas's disappointment in the fate of the bourgeois public sphere, we need not follow him in assuming that this was the only route that history could have taken.

Acknowledgements

The research on which this chapter is based was conducted during my tenure of a Wellcome Trust University Award in the History of Medicine. I gratefully acknowledge the Trust's generous support of my work. I am grateful also to Bernard Harris for insightful comments on earlier drafts of this chapter.

Notes

1   B.B. Gilbert, *The Evolution of National Insurance in Great Britain: The Origins of the Welfare State*, London: Michael Joseph, 1966; E.P. Hennock, *British Social Reform and German Precedents: The Case of Social Insurance 1880–1914*, Oxford: Clarendon Press, 1987. On the wider context of social welfare reforms at this time, see D. Fraser, *The Evolution of the British Welfare State*, 2nd edn, Basingstoke: Macmillan, 1984, ch. 7: 'Liberal social

policy, 1905–14'; M. Freeden, *The New Liberalism: An Ideology of Social Reform*, Oxford: Clarendon Press, 1978; and J. Harris, *Private Lives, Public Spirit: Britain, 1870–1914*, Harmondsworth: Penguin, 1994, ch. 7: 'Society and the state'.

2 The politics and personalities of the Royal Commission are examined at length in A.M. McBriar, *An Edwardian Mixed Doubles: The Bosanquets versus the Webbs: A Study in British Social Policy 1890–1929*, Oxford: Clarendon Press, 1987.

3 J. Habermas, *The Structural Transformation of the Public Sphere: An Inquiry into a Category of Bourgeois Society*, trans. T. Burger with the assistance of F. Lawrence, Cambridge: Polity Press, 1989, section V: 'The social-structural transformation of the public sphere'.

4 J. Lewis, *The Voluntary Sector, the State and Social Work in Britain: The Charity Organisation Society/Family Welfare Association since 1869*, Aldershot: Elgar, 1995.

5 R.J. Morris identifies this as a common aspiration behind the formation of many philanthropic bodies from the late eighteenth century onwards: 'Voluntary societies and British urban elites, 1780–1850: an analysis', *Historical Journal*, 1983, vol. 26, pp. 95–118. See also P.K. Gilbert, 'Producing the public: public medicine in private spaces', this volume.

6 The most refined expressions of this view are to be found in the writings of the COS philosopher, Bernard Bosanquet; see, for instance, his discussion of 'The meaning of social work', *International Journal of Ethics*, 1900–1, vol. 11, pp. 291–306. See also G. Stedman Jones, *Outcast London: A Study in the Relationship between Classes in Victorian Society*, Harmondsworth: Penguin, 1976, pp. 256–61.

7 This was particularly evident in the system of 'casework' that is often seen as the COS's most lasting legacy: K. Woodroofe, *From Charity to Social Work in England and the United States*, London: Routledge & Kegan Paul, 1968, ch. 2: 'The C.O.S. and social casework'.

8 On COS activists' adoption of this phrase in the context of the debates that followed on the publication of the reports of the Royal Commission on the Poor Laws, see below, n. 16.

9 F.M.L. Thompson cites 'The drab workhouse clothing, deliberately intended to destroy individuality, and the standard workhouse haircut, which made paupers instantly recognizable if they went out in public', as serving to publicize their membership of the general class of paupers: *The Rise of Respectable Society: A Social History of Victorian Britain, 1830–1900*, London: Fontana, 1988, p. 350. Anne Digby enlarges on this aspect of deterrence when she argues that the threat of the workhouse 'did not reside in its material deprivation but in its psychological harshness', which had the effect of 'depersonalising the individual' especially through the practice of 'classifying inmates' into specific categories of pauperism: *The Poor Law in Nineteenth-century England and Wales*, London: The Historical Association, 1982, p. 17.

10 See for example K. Williams, *From Pauperism to Poverty*, London: Routledge & Kegan Paul, 1981; L.H. Lees, *Solidarities of Strangers: The English Poor Laws and the People, 1700–1948*, Cambridge: Cambridge University Press, 1998.

11 H. Bosanquet, *Social Work in London, 1869–1912: A History of the Charity Organisation Society*, Brighton: Harvester Press, 1973, orig. pub. 1914, pp. 266–71. This functional division of labour remained implicit through several shifts in the terms that the COS used to designate, respectively, the proper recipients of charity and of statutory poor relief – first the 'deserving' and 'undeserving' poor, then 'likely' and 'unlikely to benefit', and later 'helpable' and 'unhelpable': G. Himmelfarb, *Poverty and Compassion: The Moral Imagination of the Late Victorians*, New York: Alfred A. Knopf, 1991, pp. 188–94; G. Finlayson, *Citizen, State, and Social Welfare in Britain 1830–1990*, Oxford: Clarendon Press, 1994, pp. 142–3; McBriar, *An Edwardian Mixed Doubles*, pp. 57–8. Also R. Humphreys, *Sin, Organized Charity and the Poor Law in Victorian England*, London: Macmillan, 1995.

12 The strong COS presence on the Commission is profiled in McBriar, *An Edwardian Mixed Doubles*, pp. 179, 181–7.

13 The officers of each County and County Borough Council would be responsible for ensuring that a Voluntary Aid Council was established, which would then appoint and supervise the work of the Voluntary Aid Committees. All registered voluntary societies with offices in a particular county or county borough would retain the right to nominate members to the Voluntary Aid Councils and Committees. The Voluntary Aid Councils would be responsible chiefly to the Charities Commission, rather than to local government. Royal Commission on the Poor Laws, *Majority Report*, Cd. 4499, London: HMSO, 1909, vol. 2, pp. 103–5.

14 Royal Commission on the Poor Laws, *Majority Report*, vol. 1, pp. 539–40; vol. 2, pp. 98–100, 104.

15 Beatrice and Sidney Webb sought to portray the Majority Report's proposals to alleviate certain deterrent penalties as marking a decisive break with earlier Poor Law philosophy. But as Karel Williams points out, this was as much a rhetorical attempt to undermine the Majority Report's claim to historical precedent as a reflection of the principles behind the report: *From Pauperism to Poverty*, pp. 92–3. Meanwhile the COS insisted that, while they were prepared to shift their ground on precisely what forms deterrence and less eligibility might take in practice, the 'principles of 1834' themselves had not been and should not be abandoned. B. Bosanquet, 'Charity organisation and the Majority Report', *International Journal of Ethics*, 1909–10, vol. 20, pp. 395–408, at p. 403; H. Bosanquet, 'The historical basis of English Poor Law policy', *Economic Journal*, 1910, vol. 20, pp. 182–94, at pp. 187–9.

16 Royal Commission on the Poor Laws, *Majority Report*, vol. 1, p. 542. The Majority Report accepted that some of the deterrent penalties currently imposed on the recipients of poor relief should be relaxed, most notably the franchise disqualification, which should be lifted for paupers of less than three months standing: ibid., p. 552. It also suggested that the conditions under which public assistance was provided might even be modified so as to exert a restorative effect 'even when applied to the relief of the able-bodied': ibid., p. 54. But while these conditions might not be particularly punitive in the first instance, the Report also recommended that the government should set up a series of increasingly strict disciplinary procedures and institutions for dealing with the longer-term destitute: ibid., pp. 542–4, 548–9.

17 M.W. Flinn, 'Medical services under the New Poor Law', in D. Fraser (ed.), *The New Poor Law in the Nineteenth Century*, London: Macmillan, 1976, pp. 45–66; R.G. Hodgkinson, *The Origins of the National Health Service: The Medical Services of the New Poor Law, 1834–1871*, London: Wellcome Historical Medical Library, 1967; *idem*, 'Poor Law Medical Officers of England 1834–1871', *Journal of the History of Medicine*, 1956, vol. 11, pp. 299–338.

18 By the late 1850s a handful of provincial Boards of Guardians had begun to construct infirmaries that met the highest current standards of hospital design, and even to employ trained nurses to care for the inmates. Meanwhile, campaigners brought pressure to bear on central government for such improvements in medical provision to be made an article of official Poor Law policy. This resulted in the passage of the Metropolitan Poor Law Amendment Act of 1867 and the Poor Law Amendment Act of 1868, both of which officially encouraged local unions to provide improved infirmary accommodation. See J.E. O'Neill, 'Finding a policy for the sick poor', *Victorian Studies*, 1963–4, vol. 7, pp. 265–84; B. Abel-Smith, *The Hospitals 1800–1948*, London: Heinemann, 1964, ch. 4: 'Sick paupers', and ch. 6: 'The creation of pauper hospitals'; M.A. Crowther, *The Workhouse System 1834–1929: The History of an English Social Institution*, London, Methuen, 1983, pp. 156–81; J.V. Pickstone, *Medicine and Industrial Society: A History of Hospital Development in Manchester and its Region, 1752–1946*, Manchester: Manchester University Press, 1985, pp. 122–7.

19 B. Rodgers, 'The Medical Relief (Disqualification Removal) Act 1885: a storm in a political teacup', *Parliamentary Affairs*, 1955–6, vol. 9, pp. 188–94.

20 Royal Commission on the Poor Laws, *Minority Report*, London: HMSO, 1909, pp. 197–8.
21 Royal Commission on the Poor Laws, *Majority Report*, vol. 1, p. 379.
22 Ibid., p. 379.
23 Ibid.
24 Ibid., p. 384.
25 Ibid., pp. 387–8. The public assistance authority in each county or county borough council would be required to appoint a medical assistance committee, which would include members of the local authority public health committee and of the local branches of the British Medical Association, to co-ordinate any existing provident dispensaries or establish new ones within the relevant administrative areas.
26 Provident dispensaries are discussed in Hodgkinson, *Origins of the National Health Service*, pp. 610–19. For more general discussion of the friendly societies and other forms of provident and mutual aid schemes in the early to mid-nineteenth century, see: P.H.J.H. Gosden, *The Friendly Societies in England, 1815–1875*, Manchester: Manchester University Press, 1961; Finlayson, *Citizen, State, and Social Welfare*, pp. 24–45; J.C. Riley, *Sick, not Dead: The Health of British Workingmen during the Mortality Decline*, Baltimore: Johns Hopkins University Press, 1997.
27 Royal Commission on the Poor Laws, *Majority Report*, vol. 1, pp. 370–1.
28 Ibid., pp. 384–8. The proposal was not entirely novel; from as early as the 1840s some Boards of Guardians had chosen to subscribe to local provident dispensaries instead of appointing their own medical officers, though the practice was not widespread: Flinn, 'Medical services under the New Poor Law', pp. 50–1. The Majority Report also argued that the quality of institutional care in the Poor Law infirmaries might in many cases be improved, chiefly by expanding the medical and nursing staffs: *Majority Report*, vol. 1, pp. 351–2.
29 Ibid., pp. 383–4.
30 Ibid., p. 384.
31 Ibid., pp. 358–9.
32 W.M. Frazer, *A History of English Public Health, 1834–1939*, London: Baillière, Tindall & Cox, 1950, pp. 153, 288, 318; Abel-Smith, *The Hospitals*, pp. 127–9; Pickstone, *Medicine and Industrial Society*, ch. 8: 'Infectious diseases and hospitals, 1860–1910'; J.M. Eyler, 'Scarlet fever and confinement: the Edwardian debate over isolation hospitals', *Bulletin of the History of Medicine*, 1987, vol. 61, pp. 1–24.
33 No deterrent penalties were imposed where treatment was conducted in municipal facilities. A significant amount of sanitary work, including isolation of infectious disease cases, was also initially carried out under the auspices of the local Poor Law authorities, however. Initially such treatment carried the same penalty of disenfranchisement as ordinary medical relief. This was removed with the passage of the Disease Prevention Act of 1882 and Disease Prevention (Metropolis) Act of 1883, thus preceding and paving the way for the same alleviation of deterrence for medical relief in general. Rodgers, 'The Medical Relief (Disqualification Removal) Act', p. 189, n. 1. As a consequence, the number of patients treated in such institutions – for instance the metropolitan isolation hospitals, which officially fell under the Poor Law – grew rapidly during the closing decade of the nineteenth century: A. Hardy, *The Epidemic Streets: Infectious Disease and the Rise of Preventive Medicine, 1856–1900*, Oxford: Clarendon Press, 1993, pp. 277–8.
34 Royal Commission on the Poor Laws, *Minority Report*, p. 212.
35 Ibid., p. 231.
36 B. Webb, 'The medical services of the Poor Law and the public health departments of English local government, in their relation to each other, to the public, and to the prevention and cure of disease', in Royal Commission on the Poor Laws, *Minutes of Evidence*, vol. 12, Cd. 4983, PP 1910, li, pp. 261–311.

37 Ibid. For a succinct statement of this view, see Sidney Webb's address to the 1909 Annual Dinner of the Society of Medical Officers of Health, reported in *Public Health*, 1909–10, vol. 23, pp. 62–71.

38 Webb, 'The Medical Services of the Poor Law', p. 301.

39 Ibid., p. 309.

40 Royal Commission on the Poor Laws, *Minutes of Evidence*, vol. 9, Cd. 5068, PP 1910, xlix, pp. 164–5.

41 Ibid., p. 165.

42 Royal Commission on the Poor Laws, *Minority Report*, pp. 224–5.

43 Ibid., pp. 416–18.

44 Gilbert stresses that Lloyd George's main aim in promoting health insurance was 'to replace lost income, not cure sickness': Gilbert, *Evolution of National Insurance*, pp. 314–16.

45 This has been argued by T. Novak, for instance, in his *Poverty and the State: An Historical Sociology*, Milton Keynes: Open University Press, 1988, pp. 134–8.

46 C.S. Loch, quoted in S. Collini, *Public Moralists: Political Thought and Intellectual Life in Britain 1850–1930*, Oxford: Clarendon Press, 1991, p. 117. Loch stands out as one of a small group of COS activists who persisted in opposing the insurance scheme as Lloyd George succeeded in winning more widespread public support: McBriar, *An Edwardian Mixed Doubles*, pp. 334, 338.

47 S. Webb and B. Webb, *The Prevention of Destitution*, London: Longmans, Green & Co., 1911, p. 162.

48 Ibid., p. 187.

49 Ibid., pp. 187–8.

50 Ibid., pp. 166–7, 174–5.

51 Stefan Collini, for instance, draws on C.S. Loch's comments to conclude that the adoption of NHI as a central plank of government policy was symptomatic of a wider decline in concern with the maintenance of character and moral health among the working-class population. Collini, *Public Moralists*, pp. 117–18.

52 H.N. Bunbury, 'Biographical note', in W.J. Braithwaite, *Lloyd George's Ambulance Wagon: Being the Memoirs of William J. Braithwaite 1911–1912*, ed. Bunbury, London: Methuen, 1957, at p. 14.

53 William Beveridge, 'Social reform: how Germany deals with it', *Morning Post*, October 1907, quoted in Hennock, *German Precedents*, p. 137. See also Jose Harris, *William Beveridge: A Biography*, Oxford: Clarendon Press, 1977, pp. 97–103.

54 Lloyd George speaking to the Commons, 19 July 1911, quoted in J. Grigg, *Lloyd George: The People's Champion 1902–1911*, London: Eyre Methuen, 1978, p. 337. Like Beveridge, both Lloyd George and Churchill were also careful to point out that the German health insurance scheme was in large part run by voluntary organizations: Hennock, *German Precedents*, pp. 136, 144.

55 Lloyd George speaking to the Commons, 19 July 1911, quoted in Grigg, *The People's Champion*, p. 338.

56 Hennock, *German Precedents*, pp. 130–1, 171–2, 187–91, 206–11; Finlayson, *Citizen, State, and Social Welfare*, pp. 185–6.

57 Winston Churchill, speech in support of Part II of the Insurance Bill, 25 May 1911, quoted in P. Addison, *Churchill on the Home Front, 1900–1955*, London: Cape, 1992, p. 147.

58 Lloyd George, National Insurance Bill, Memorandum Explanatory of the Bill, quoted in Hennock, *German Precedents*, p. 191.

59 Churchill, quoted in J. Harris, *Unemployment and Politics: A Study in English Social Policy, 1886–1914*, Oxford: Clarendon Press, 1972, p. 365.

60 The commercial companies had not hitherto taken an interest in the relatively unremunerative field of health insurance, which they were content to leave to the non-profit friendly societies. Their demands for a part in NHI were prompted by

fears that the friendly societies' involvement would give them an edge in competing for more profitable forms of insurance, chiefly widows' pensions and death benefits. Lloyd George had initially excluded the commercial companies from NHI because of the high administration costs involved in employing large numbers of salesmen and collectors, but he now accepted that the scheme would be able to bear such costs. Gilbert, *Evolution of National Insurance*, pp. 318–43.

61 Braithwaite, *Lloyd George's Ambulance Wagon*, p. 260. He added: 'I did not know what this [i.e. the idea of "business" men running things] meant (nor did he!)....He never discussed it with me, and I don't know with whom he did in fact discuss it.' On Lloyd George's later drafting of businessmen into government administration, see P.K. Cline, 'Eric Geddes and the "experiment" with businessmen in government', in K.D. Brown (ed.), *Essays in Anti-Labour History*, London: Macmillan, 1974, pp. 74–104. On the influence of organized business in Liberal politics, see G.R. Searle, 'The Edwardian Liberal Party and business', *English Historical Review*, 1983, vol. 98, pp. 28–60.

62 W. Beveridge, *Voluntary Action: A Report on Methods of Social Advance*, London: G. Allen & Unwin, 1948, pp. 79–83, quoting p. 82. Friendly society membership actually rose as a result of NHI, and remained high through the inter-war years: as late as 1938 almost as many workers were insured through the societies as through the commercial insurance companies. But the nature of the friendly societies changed markedly during this period. In competition with the commercial companies, economies of scale and competitiveness become crucial to survival. As a result, smaller societies failed while larger ones grew bigger still. Opportunities for contributors to participate in the management of the societies declined accordingly, to be replaced by more business-oriented forms of management preoccupied with staying afloat in a competitive market. See P. Johnson, *Saving and Spending: The Working-Class Economy in Britain 1870–1939*, Oxford: Clarendon, 1985, pp. 67–8. Thanks to Bernard Harris for bringing these references to my attention. In deference to Braithwaite's and others' advocacy of the friendly societies, Lloyd George had initially agreed that the commercial companies should be required to establish some form of democratic and representative local organization along the lines of the friendly societies. Little of this remained when the Bill finally passed into legislation, however. Gilbert, *Evolution of National Insurance*, pp. 341–2, 378–83; Grigg, *Lloyd George: The People's Champion*, pp. 344–5.

63 Particularly D. Brunton, 'Policy, powers and practice: the public response to public health in the Scottish city', and N. Pfeffer, 'Fertility counts: from equity to outcome'.

64 See the extensive literature on the so-called New Liberalism of this period, e.g. H.V. Emy, *Liberals, Radicals and Social Politics, 1892–1914*, Cambridge: Cambridge University Press, 1973, and Freeden, *The New Liberalism*.

65 Searle, 'The Edwardian Liberal Party and business', expressly challenges what he sees as historians' excessive emphasis on the direct or indirect impact of organized labour on Liberal policy formation at this time.

13 Fertility counts

From equity to outcome

Naomi Pfeffer

The Structural Transformation of the Public Sphere was published in Germany in 1962 when the command and control model of the social-welfare state was enjoying a heyday. In the late 1970s, this model of social-welfare state began to be undermined and replaced by what is called a regulatory state.[1] While Habermas might claim the regulatory state as a further development of the social-welfare state, nonetheless the landscape of the political public sphere has undoubtedly been transformed by its establishment.

Some crucial differences between the two models of social-welfare state are captured by the words 'government' and 'governance'. The former is associated with the command and control model, and the latter with the regulatory model of social-welfare state. 'Government' speaks of an administrative ideology and practice conducted at a functional centre by a hierarchical, classic bureaucracy whose task is to allocate to citizens their entitlement of welfare benefits meted out according to principles of equity and redistribution. Government is paternalistic; politicians, civil servants and professionals hand down benefits to deferential and grateful citizens. Because regulatory states are associated with developments such as post-colonialism, globalization and identity politics, they require 'governance', a system of negotiation between decentralized, self-steering organizations bent on satisfying the demands of individual consumers. Although governance is associated with privatization and deregulation, surveillance and regulation of reconfigured providers of benefits have increased through audit and the measurement of outcomes such as performance indicators. The reasons for this paradox are complex and include a succession of scandals and the management of heightened perceptions of risk.[2]

This chapter contrasts the kinds of engagements and debates in the public sphere provoked and permitted by the two models of social-welfare state. It does so by comparing the history of data monitoring in the implementation of the Abortion Act 1967 and the Human Fertilisation and Embryology Act 1990, both of which were introduced to contain and survey the rate of destruction on medical grounds of human foetuses and embryos. Both Acts are controversial. The material culture of debates preceding and following their passage has included many things, among them the testimony of police, medical professionals, coroners and women, and photographs of a solitary human foetus conveying the misleading impression that a foetus is capable of existing independently of its mother's body. This chapter focuses on statistics because increasingly numbers have formed the working materials of opinion-forming associations – groups which, according to Habermas, operate within the public sphere, challenging conventional wisdom and proposing alternative policies.[3] Because the collection and analysis of data for the production of statistics is a major undertaking, demanding in the first instance the capacity to command their submission, rational criticism of the state has increasingly come to depend on and has been limited by the data collected and published by the state, or by a body to which the state has delegated its powers. As a result of this dependence on the state for what is considered authentic evidence, the kinds of political public debates which opinion-forming associations can conduct can be facilitated or constrained by it.

Intentional abortion in the inter-war period: guessing numbers

In the inter-war period, the birth rate fell below replacement level. Opinion-forming organizations concerned about the consequences of the apparent diminution in the fertility of the British population were hampered by a lack of statistical data on its causes. No one was certain if the retreat from motherhood had been effected through more conceptions being prevented or the deliberate termination of more pregnancies. Numerical data on both were unavailable.[4] Although contraception was morally frowned upon, the extent of its use had not yet been documented.[5] Because termination of pregnancy was illicit (outwith exceptional circumstances discussed below), it was naturally carried out in secret and came to official notice mostly when a woman died. There were few data on how many women suffered and survived the sequelae of an abortion. Doctors refused to collect them on the grounds that it contravened the duty of confidence owed to patients. They were supported by the British Medical Association (BMA), which claimed disclosure was against the public interest: fear of prosecution would make women needing treatment for a botched abortion reluctant to seek medical help.[6] Because of the legal obligation to notify police of a felony, few hospital management committees allowed patients' notes to distinguish between women admitted to hospital for completion of an intended abortion and women undergoing similar treatment for a miscarriage. Some hospitals simply did not record intentional abortion cases.

Police prosecutions and maternal mortality data, the only officially collected statistics on illicit abortion, were of little help. Each year between 1925 and 1935, a maximum of 116 and a minimum of fifty-five cases came to the attention of the police in England and Wales, and about two out of every three of these cases led to a prosecution.[7] Prosecutions and convictions were relatively rare where a woman survived because life imprisonment, the maximum sentence for procuring an abortion, was considered too severe a penalty. Around 500 women were thought to die each year as a result of an intentional abortion, many more than came to the attention of the police. Ironically, although women who died following an intentional abortion were trying to avoid motherhood, their deaths were categorized by the Registrar General's Office as maternal deaths. Thirteen per cent of all the maternal deaths occurring in 1934 were attributed to intentional abortion, while more than a quarter of total maternal deaths from sepsis, one of the classes under which maternal mortality data were analysed, were attributed to sequelae of abortion. Furthermore, according to confidential enquiries undertaken by the Committee on Maternal Mortality and Morbidity set up by the Ministry of Health in 1928, the proportion of maternal deaths attributable to intentional abortion had risen from 10.5 per cent in 1930 to 18.2 per cent in 1935.[8] Although the data on which these statistics were based were known to be incomplete, they were taken as suggesting that rates of abortion were increasing.

After 1929, an increasing number of pregnancy terminations fell within the law. The Infant Life (Preservation) Act of 1929 provided doctors with a *mens rea* – the intention of saving a woman's life – through which they might escape prosecution under Section 58 of the Offences against the Person Act of 1861. Women who could afford it paid for what became known as a 'therapeutic' abortion, a relatively safe operation carried out under medical supervision. As a safeguard in case of court proceedings, most doctors would insist women obtain a second opinion from another medical man.

Most operations carried out under the 1929 Act were reputed to be carried out in nursing homes. A fictional account of this world is presented in A.J. Cronin's *The Citadel*, in which Ivory, the surgeon, specializes in 'Love's labour lost'. He is described as 'nothing but a damned abortionist....There's a couple of nursing homes...where they do nothing else – all very pretty and above board of course – and Ivory's the head scraper!'[9] Although they provided other kinds of care including maternity care, the reputation of nursing homes was sullied by abortion. The problem was that the significance of abortions in relation to other kinds of procedures carried out in nursing homes was unknown. The 1929 Act did not impose a legal requirement for data on therapeutic abortion to be collected. The Nursing Homes Registration Act of 1927 had made local authorities responsible for their oversight. However, they lacked the authority to inspect records, and hence were unable to ascertain how many and what kinds of patients were being cared for.

The judgement in R. v. Bourne in 1939 widened further the grounds under which a doctor might escape prosecution to include circumstances where she or he believed the woman's mental as well as physical health would suffer if the pregnancy continued to term. Mr Aleck Bourne, a consultant obstetrician-gynaecologist at St Mary's Hospital, London, had performed an abortion on a 14-year-old girl who had been raped by four soldiers. The abortion was carried out not to save the mother from immediate death but because in Bourne's opinion, formed after consultation with colleagues, if the girl had had to continue with the pregnancy it would have severely damaged her mental health. Bourne made no attempt to conceal the operation but rather reported the matter to the police so that it became a test case. From then on, alienists enjoyed a lucrative source of income in providing a second opinion on the effect of a woman's pregnancy on her mental health.

During the 1930s, opinion-forming associations began to complain about the legislation on abortion, albeit for wholly divergent reasons. Their pressure on the government led in 1937 to the establishment of an inter-departmental committee

> to enquire into the prevalence of abortion, and the law relating thereto, and to consider what steps can be taken by more effective enforcement of the law and otherwise to secure the reduction of maternal mortality and morbidity arising from this cause.[10]

Called the Birkett Committee after its chairman, Lord Birkett, the committee's report was published in 1939. The committee provided the various protagonists with ample opportunity to put their case.

Prominent amongst those arguing for decriminalization was the Abortion Law Reform Association (ALRA) established in 1936. Its founders included feminists such as Stella Browne and Dora Russell who believed abortion represents 'the right of every woman...to decide what should happen to her body'.[11] The ALRA sought to redress the social class inequalities in access to safe and legal abortion that had been exacerbated by the 1929 Act. Its propaganda focused on the plight of impoverished women encumbered by drunken husbands, debts and sickly children, women who would not be deterred from seeking an abortion when, in their judgement, a pregnancy was a disaster. ALRA used death-bed confessions and coroners' enquiries to reveal such women's 'desperation'. They make gruesome reading. A list of cases examined by the coroner for the Northern District of the County of London included a 27-year-old milliner married for two years with no children who was found dead in her bathroom with an enema syringe in her vagina; and a 21-year-old chambermaid, unmarried, who died after undergoing a septic instrumental abortion carried out by a Dr A who had already served eighteen months in prison for abortion.[12]

Ironically, in describing women as desperate, ALRA fell into the trap of suggesting that domestic and personal circumstances cloud women's capacity for reason – an argument similar to that put forward by those seeking a tightening of the regulations, who claimed many women were terminating a pregnancy for flippant reasons, for example because pregnancy is inconvenient when on holiday or playing golf. Equally reprehensible were women who had conceived as a result of an adulterous relationship irrespective of whether it was they or the man who was married. Some witnesses appearing before the Birkett Committee condemned intentional abortion as a sin as had been restated in December 1930 by Pope Pius XI in his encyclical *Casti Connubii*.

Statistics were seen as weapons in the struggles around abortion. Some anti-abortionists favoured compulsory registration of therapeutic abortion, on the ground that it would discourage intentional abortion by making unscrupulous doctors afraid of performing the operation. Registration had been introduced for this purpose by the German Reich Medical Services, who claimed it had worked.[13] In compulsory registration, an abortion would be reported to the office of the Registrar General following a procedure similar to that of births and deaths. However, representatives of the Ministry of Health opposed it on the grounds that using compulsory registration as a deterrent was at odds with the values that registration was meant to foster in relation to birth. In initiating the provision of child health services by a local authority, compulsory registration of birth was meant to be beneficial to both women and children whereas compulsory registration of intentional abortion was meant to act as a deterrent and sometimes to initiate a criminal prosecution. Furthermore, it was unlikely that all abortions would be registered. In particular, working-class women would be over-represented in the data; abortions receiving public hospital attention were more likely to find their way on to the register than 'minor surgical procedures' carried out in a private nursing home.

An alternative considered by the Birkett Committee was compulsory notification of abortion to the local public health authority, a procedure similar to that of a notifiable contagious disease. In effect, notification would have construed intentional abortion as a public health problem, reflecting its role as a contributory factor in Britain's scandalously high rates of maternal mortality at that time. Notification was supported by working-class organizations such as trade unions and the Women's Co-operative Guild who sought valid and reliable statistical data to help explain and develop policies that might lower the toll on women's lives exacted by botched illegal abortions.

Public health officials had another reason for supporting notification: it would allow them to distinguish between sepsis following an abortion and puerperal fever.[14] The Midwives Act 1936, which had established a salaried midwifery service, had made midwives responsible for visiting expectant women. Occasionally they found a woman with a fever that looked suspiciously like the result of a botched or successful, illegal abortion. The Act obliged a midwife to notify the local supervising authority (LSA), usually the Medical Officer of Health, who had to pay an attending doctor's fees. If advised by the doctor that the fever was the result of an intentional abortion, the LSA was legally obliged to inform the police. However, Medical Officers of Health increasingly resented the financial cost incurred and the imposition on them of quasi-police and detective functions, and looked to notification as a way of pre-empting at least some such cases.

A contrary view was taken by the Ministry of Health who claimed that both registration and notification would make women less willing to seek treatment for the sequelae of abortion whether self-induced or induced by other people, and that their reluctance would show up in maternal mortality data.[15] Both schemes were also forcefully opposed by the BMA on public interest grounds: if the duty of confidentiality was removed by compulsion, all patients' trust in their doctors would be damaged.

The Birkett Committee recommended placing on the statute book the judgement in the Bourne case and decided in favour of notification and making failure to do so an offence. The data would be treated as confidential, except that police might have access to them in order to investigate an unusually high rate of abortion in their area.[16] However, the Second World War put paid to any official response to the Birkett Committee's report.

Abortion in the 1960s: regulation by premises

The creation of a National Health Service (NHS) in 1948 involved the establishment of the machinery of government associated with the command and control model of the social-welfare state, including the routine collection of data. From one such data-gathering instrument, the hospital inpatient enquiry, a rate of abortion was estimated; for example, in 1959, the number of women discharged from NHS hospitals after a dilation and curettage (D&C) was 56,900, of whom 1,800 had had a therapeutic abortion and 55,100 had the operation for other reasons.[17] What these other reasons might be was unspecified; the data did not separate women undergoing a D&C after suffering a miscarriage from those who needed it to complete an illegal intentional abortion. No data were collected from private nursing homes and hospitals where it was thought most therapeutic abortions were performed.

Shortly after the Second World War ended, the ALRA renewed its campaign for a woman's right to abortion.[18] However, neither the BMA nor the Royal College of Obstetricians and Gynaecologists (RCOG) supported a change in legislation, claiming that the 1929 Act afforded reputable doctors – and hence, the public – sufficient protection. This argument was seen to be justified in 1958 when Dr Louis Newton was convicted for manslaughter of a woman who died from renal failure after he had injected utus paste (a medicated soap, widely used as an abortifacient) into her uterus in his consulting room; Newton was found to have been struck off the medical register for five years in 1942 for issuing certificates of epilepsy to enable men to evade serving in the forces.[19] Six attempts at introducing legislation by private members of Parliament were defeated mostly by the tactics of a group of Roman Catholic MPs. The seventh attempt, David Steel's Medical Termination of Pregnancy Bill, succeeded in 1967, mostly because of public outrage provoked by thalidomide, a drug developed to counter the effects of nausea in early pregnancy, which had led to a number of children being born with serious deformities.[20] Abortion was no longer understood simply as a solution to immorality and flightiness: it began to be acknowledged as a public health measure. Steel's Bill was not intended to legislate for abortion on demand; women were not given the 'right to choose'. The Bill sought to place on the statute book the judgement in Bourne and, in including a new 'social' clause, extend the circumstances under which a doctor might escape prosecution for performing what otherwise remained – and still remains – an illegal operation.

In the committee stage, Steel explained why his Bill included a proposal for compulsory notification. Opponents of the Bill insisted that 'professionals' –

doctors who did little other than perform abortions in private clinics – undergo a process of approval before they could practice. Steel countered that notification would identify any practitioner undertaking more than a reasonable number of abortions, and would provide evidence sufficient for a criminal prosecution where justified. In addition, he advocated approving places, not doctors, which he claimed would prevent racketeering by the private sector.[21]

Steel's proposals passed into legislation. The requirement for notification included the NHS because abortion was understood as a public health measure and data were required for epidemiological and other research purposes. The Registrar General's Office had suggested the following should be ascertained: name of institution; woman's maiden name; date of birth; NHS number; marital status; number of live children; date of any previous abortion; occupation of husband or, if unmarried, her own or the father's occupation.[22] The form prescribed in Schedule 2 of the principal regulations also asks for grounds for termination and the woman's usual address. Statutory Instrument 1968 No. 390 states that notification of any termination under the Act must be made within seven days and the forms sent to the local Medical Officer of Health by the medical practitioner who terminates a pregnancy. The forms are sent on to the Chief Medical Officers of the health departments in England and Wales and in Scotland. Up until 1974, notifications were published in supplements to the Registrar General's Statistical Review. From 1974, data relating to England and Wales were published quarterly by the Office of Population Censuses and Surveys (OPCS), the government statistical service.[23]

According to the terms of the Act, non-NHS abortions could only be carried out in premises that met with ministerial approval. NHS premises did not require prior approval because, as a civil servant from the Department of Health explained:

> the difference between the independent sector and the NHS is that the NHS has a whole series of checks and balances with respect to management and there is the ultimate responsibility to the Secretary of State. That is not shared, except only in part, as far as the independent sector is concerned. It is these checks and balances which make it unnecessary to apply the same sort of structure to the public sector.[24]

Contrary to Steel's assertion, the system of approving premises, not doctors, did allow some 'professionals' to prosper under the Act. As one critic put it, they 'were driven from the back-streets not into obscurity but in a Rolls-Royce to more fashionable accommodation in the High Street or Ascension Square'.[25] However, 'professionals' were not the only doctors performing abortions in nursing homes: a survey carried out in the early 1970s found that consultants who did high numbers of NHS abortions supplemented their income with relatively large numbers at private clinics. For example, those doing over forty in a private nursing home did more than 100 in the NHS. One reason for this was that the private sector filled the gap in services in the

NHS, where demand for abortion had to be met out of existing resources – an impossible requirement as demand outstripped everyone's expectations and because the Act was not backed up by any specific allocation of money or facilities within the NHS.[26]

Drawing up rules and procedures for approval of places was delegated to civil servants in the Department of Health. Initially, these were similar to those used to register nursing homes. However, as evidence of abuse came to light, they were tightened up and more questions were asked about the suitability of premises and facilities. When the application form was revised by civil servants in 1972, it included a question on financial backing of the clinic.[27] If approval was granted, it was for a limited period only. Inspections of approved places were made without notice. In 1971, the Department of Health recruited on secondment two police officers from Scotland Yard. Some nursing homes were closed.[28]

The passage of the Act galvanized into action both anti- and pro-abortion lobbies. The anti-abortion lobby had been poorly organized before the introduction of Steel's Bill. The Society for the Protection of the Unborn Child (SPUC) was launched in January 1967, initially to prevent the Bill's passage. LIFE, the second of the two major anti-abortion interest groups, was founded in 1970. Pro-abortion groups were formed to support the ALRA in its defence of the Act. The biggest of these was the National Abortion Campaign (NAC), formed in 1975 with a strong feminist agenda.[29]

Both SPUC and LIFE are locally based organizations. Some of their strength lies in the capacity of local groups to put pressure on constituency MPs. Almost from the moment the Act was on the statute book, MPs sympathetic to the anti-abortion lobby began asking questions in Parliament. Between 1969 and 1980, nine attempts were made to have the legislation amended.[30] The working of the Act was reviewed by four parliamentary select committees and a committee appointed by Sir Keith Joseph, Secretary of State for Social Services, under the chairmanship of Justice Elizabeth Lane and known as the Lane Committee of Enquiry.[31] Attempts to introduce new legislation and reviews of the Act provided pro- and anti-abortion activists with ample opportunities to voice their opinions about the kinds of social problems caused or remedied by intentional abortion, including relief of the suffering of individual women, mitigating the threat of over-population, undermining the sanctity of foetal life, encouraging promiscuity, spreading venereal diseases, reducing the number of babies available for adoption, degrading the medical specialty of obstetrics and gynaecology, and exacerbating overcrowding of NHS hospitals.[32]

Statistics played a key role in these debates. Because of a lack of data, no one could anticipate the size of the demand for abortion when the Act came into force on 27 April 1968. In the first six years of the Act's implementation, the number of pregnancies terminated on residents of England and Wales rose from 49,800 in the last eight months of 1968 (equivalent to an annual rate of 74,700) to 110,600 in 1973. The data were broken down according to the type of premises – NHS and non-NHS – in which the procedure was carried out. In 1969, the first full year of the Act, two out of every three abortions were performed within the NHS; five years later, the NHS was responsible for just over half. Public awareness of these figures in particular led both pro- and anti-abortion campaigners to concentrate on issues of private as opposed to public provision.

The pro-abortion lobby used the data on premises to highlight inequalities in NHS provision. In some parts of the country, they argued, the NHS was failing in its duty to provide for citizens according to their medical needs and, as a result, women entitled to have an abortion free at the point of delivery were being compelled to pay for it. For example, it was twice as easy to get an abortion on the NHS in Newcastle as in Birmingham. The Lane Committee agreed the NHS has a responsibility to provide abortion on the grounds that it fell within the wording of Section 1(1) of the 1946 Act, which imposed a duty on the Secretary of State to promote the establishment in England and Wales of a comprehensive health service designed to secure improvement in the physical and mental health of people. In effect, Committee members associated citizenship with entitlement to free health care from the NHS and with a right to therapeutic abortion – an association confirmed in 1979 by the Royal Commission on the NHS, which recommended that the health service should aim to provide at least 75 per cent of local abortions within the next few years.[33]

Pro-choice campaigners undertook research to find out why, in some areas, an NHS abortion was difficult to obtain. If it was because of pressure on beds, local groups could demand that more resources be made available, sometimes through the offices of community health councils, set up in 1974 as the 'patient's voice' within the NHS. Little could be done where difficulties arose because of the anti-abortion views held by consultants and other medical practitioners because the 1967 Act had included a 'conscience clause' that acknowledged their right to refuse to carry out abortions. In areas such as the West Midlands, where several Catholic gynaecologists held sway, activists sought ways of helping women obtain an abortion at low cost. Two major charities were set up in 1968 for this purpose: the Birmingham Pregnancy Advisory Service, now called the British Pregnancy Advisory Service (BPAS); and the London Pregnancy Advisory Service, now called the Pregnancy Advisory Service (PAS). In addition to offering women advice on where to obtain an abortion, both charities operated a loans and grants system so that no woman who is legally entitled to an abortion is turned away because of lack of money. Both organizations set up their own private facilities.

The anti-abortion lobby also exploited the belief then widely held that payment for treatment represented a flaw in the pure crystal of the NHS.[34] However, instead of calling for improved public provision, they drew a different moral inference. Women who were ambivalent about whether or not to terminate a pregnancy were, they claimed, being persuaded to do so by doctors operating in the private sector who were eager for the fees. As Bernard Braine, a Conservative MP, put it in the evidence he submitted to the Select Committee on the Abortion (Amendment) Bill in April 1975:

With great respect, it is contrary to common sense to suggest that somebody who is in this business for money is going to forego his fee by suggesting that another course of action is open…in a system where there are fees, and where for example, the more dangerous the condition the higher the fees, there seems to be no guarantee whatsoever that the right kind of advice will be given.[35]

Braine went on to make the following point:

Let me say that in the National Health Service one would normally expect the doctor to give you the right advice to the best of his judgement and ability. What we are concerned with in this Bill is to clear up abuses in the commercial private sector where the whole emphasis is upon giving an abortion in return for a fee.[36]

The anti-abortionists' solution was to insist on 'independent' counselling for women. Taking a leaf out of the pro-abortion lobby's book, in the mid-1970s LIFE began to provide services that, it claimed, would help women avoid abortion. These included offering advice and accommodation before and immediately after the birth of the child.[37]

Anti-abortionists' arguments too struck a chord with the Lane Committee, which agreed that 'activities within the private sector had resulted in scandal and disgrace to the British medical profession'.[38] It expressed concern about the safety of facilities in nursing homes, and singled out for special mention the 'trade' in abortion to foreign women that had been sensationalized in newspaper reports of touts finding 'customers' for clinics amongst young women travellers arriving at railway stations serving ports and of travel agents arranging 'package deals'.[39] The Committee's recommendations were on the whole a disappointment to anti-abortionists however. When some of the worst abuses of the private sector were addressed by changes in the regulations and criminal prosecutions, the anti-abortion lobby began to focus its energies on having the legislation amended to prevent the destruction of foetal life.

'Government', of the kind exercised by social-welfare states, aptly describes the method of implementation of the 1967 Act: civil servants at the centre of government drew up rules and monitored compliance. Professional discretion was unquestioned: doctors approved patients, deciding which women might and which might not undergo a pregnancy termination.[40] Above all, the Act and its implementation embodied a widely shared assumption that public provision of contentious services such as abortion was morally preferable to private provision, and that the latter must be subject to public oversight and regulation if it was to be permitted at all. In disputing the merits and demerits of intentional abortion, both pro- and anti-abortion lobbies projected their fantasies of social evil onto private for-profit health care.[41] However, although their challenges to government policy absorbed a considerable amount of Parliamentary and extra-Parliamentary time and energy during the 1970s, neither side could claim a victory. The overall number of pregnancies terminated under the Act increased every year, and a diminishing proportion of them were carried out in NHS premises. Nonetheless, abortion had become a safe procedure: after the 1967 Act, police prosecutions and convictions for illegal abortions fell to single figures and most young doctors trained in Britain have never seen a woman suffering or dying from the effects of a criminal abortion.[42]

The regulatory state: from premises to practice

Seasoned in campaigns against the 1967 Act, the anti-abortion lobby responded to the news of the birth in July 1978 of Louise Brown, the first baby conceived *in vitro*, by extending its protection of the human foetus within a woman's body to the human embryo on a petri dish. In *in vitro* fertilization (IVF), more embryos are created than are implanted in a woman's uterus. Anti-abortionists objected both to the destruction of 'spare' embryos and to their use as research material. However, although destruction of foetal life outwith the law was a crime, destruction of the human embryo was not. Anti-abortionists suggested filling this legal vacuum by defining an embryo as a potential foetus, which, they claim, is a potential person. According to this logic, destruction of a human embryo is tantamount to murder. Supporters of the new technology countered that fertilization of a human egg by a sperm does not start an individual baby but rather initiates cell-division in the egg, a process which can also be started in unfertilized eggs by a variety of electrical or chemical stimuli. Furthermore, they argued that an embryo is little more than a cluster of cells until it is about fourteen days old; only then can it be considered a 'foetus-in-the-making', and, even then, its development depends largely on its environment, specifically upon conditions in the uterus into which it has arrived.[43]

The argument over the moral and legal status of the human embryo was made more urgent by the competition heating up between investigators and practitioners. Louise Brown's birth was the result of the collaboration of gynaecologist Patrick Steptoe and embryologist Robert Edwards in the development of human IVF and embryo transfer. In the United States, Australia and Britain, the potential of the techniques began to be explored. A crude measure of research interest in human IVF is the number of publications: these rose from a handful in 1966 to over 300 in 1985.[44] In these studies, 'success' rates measured the capacity of a technique to produce a live birth. However, anti-abortionists understood these data in a negative light, as a measure of the rate of attrition or 'waste' of human embryos created *in vitro*.

In exploiting human embryos for research, anti-abortionists claimed, potential persons were being treated like laboratory animals. (Ironically, rules and regulations governing the conduct of medical research afford far more protection to animals than to human subjects.) Investigators defended their use of human embryos: research would lead to more effective and efficient techniques that would reduce 'wastage' and bring happiness to many hitherto 'desperate' women. Desperation, once said to characterize pregnant women seeking an abortion, was now attributed to involuntarily childless women.[45]

IVF revitalized some gynaecologists' interest in the treatment of involuntary childlessness that hitherto had been professionally unrewarding. However, like abortion, treatment available on the NHS fell short of demand in terms of resources and quality of care, forcing people who could afford it to seek treatment in the private medical sector. Medical and patient enthusiasm for IVF coincided with the election in 1979 of a radical Conservative government under the leadership of Margaret Thatcher. Among the first policies it implemented were the removal of impediments to private health care and the encouragement of income-generating schemes within the NHS. While these measures did not signal a renunciation of a commitment to the availability of comprehensive health care free at the point of delivery, they were ideologically driven, designed to challenge British antipathy to the profit motive in medicine and to encourage initiative and effort in supplementing the state's finite resources.[46] Their impact on the diffusion of IVF was considerable in that they allowed quasi-private clinics to be established within the NHS. By 1986, there were twenty-three IVF clinics in the UK, only one of which was supported by the NHS.[47] In effect, most IVF was carried out in the private medical sector.[48]

The BMA, Medical Research Council (MRC) and the RCOG, among others, set up committees of inquiry into the ethics and regulation of such procedures. Recommendations published during 1983 included licensing of practitioners and monitoring of treatment. Moreover, because opponents of the techniques were questioning the moral status of people who countenanced undergoing them, various approaches to the approval of patients were suggested.[49] These and many other recommendations were submitted to the committee of inquiry into human fertilization and embryology set up by the government in 1982 under Mary Warnock, a philosopher. Published in 1984, the committee's report – the Warnock Report as it is now called – rehearses some of the concerns expressed in earlier debates on abortion, notably deficiencies in statistical data on the prevalence and epidemiology of infertility and the inadequacy of NHS provision.[50] In effect, like the Lane Committee on abortion, the Warnock committee assumed involuntarily childless women and men were entitled to NHS treatment. Its recommendations to the government included that funding be made available for the collection of adequate statistics on infertility and infertility services, and that the government include infertility services in its plans for the NHS.

The Warnock Report also recommended the establishment of a statutory licensing authority that would use licensing and inspection to regulate investigators and clinicians creating and working with human embryos. Many leading investigators and clinicians welcomed this recommendation because, if the authority's rules were formulated in their favour, regulation would be permissive while at the same time giving their work a semblance of oversight that would allay public fears about the motives and consequences of work with human reproductive material.[51] To their dismay, the government procrastinated. Consequently, when Enoch Powell introduced his Unborn Children

(Protection) Bill to Parliament on December 1984 in an attempt to prohibit human embryo research, the MRC and RCOG responded by setting up the Voluntary Licensing Authority (VLA), which held its first meeting in March 1985.

Perforce, the licensing system was a voluntary one: the VLA had no authority to impose rules or punish offenders. Significantly, investigators and practitioners in both the NHS and private-sector clinics were included in the licensing arrangements. Structural regulation – that is, the checks and balances of the NHS – was no longer considered a sufficient safeguard against abuse. Furthermore, in the shift from government to governance which had begun in the late 1970s, regulation by premises was being replaced by regulation of practice, irrespective of where it took place. The VLA specified the conditions under which human embryos created *in vitro* might be kept, used as research materials and disposed of. Clinics would be granted a licence on condition that medical, nursing and technical staff were appropriately trained, detailed records were kept, and clinics had access to an ethical committee that would review clinical and research programmes.[52] The VLA was committed to the traditional family structure and demonstrated its intention to safeguard it from the threat of unconventional social relationships, made possible by the technology, by requiring patients to undergo a process of approval by clinicians assisted by counsellors and ethical committee members.[53]

The VLA was effectively an IVF industry body representing the views of investigators and clinicians. In its first years, it devoted considerable time to countering the argument that human life begins at fertilization. It coined the term 'pre-embryo' to describe the cluster of cells that develops following fertilization, on the grounds that it does not always form an embryo and, even when it does so, only a small portion of the total cluster is involved.[54] The VLA permitted research on the pre-embryo, a rule supported by Progress Educational Trust, an alliance of scientists, clinicians, politicians and patient support groups, set up in 1985 to defend in public and Parliament the use of human gametes and embryos in research.

In its second annual report, the VLA began to publish statistics on success/attrition rates achieved for every treatment cycle undertaken at licensed clinics.[55] But although the Authority held success/attrition rates of each individual clinic, these were never released; the data were aggregated because the clinics had agreed to provide data on condition that they remained anonymous. The success/attrition rate had acquired commercial significance. Some clinics had not yet achieved an IVF pregnancy and, it was rumoured, others were inflating their proficiency in promotional material.[56] Competition was at the root of the problem. Almost all the clinics were private and needed customers, volume being crucial to financial viability.[57] In an attempt to bring into line clinics refusing to submit data, the VLA made providing it a condition of a licence. In 1987, the *Independent* newspaper published *Choosing a Test Tube Baby Clinic*, which provided information on clinics licensed by the VLA for would-be customers.[58]

Save for total number, the VLA's statistics reveal nothing about the women who underwent the procedures. Yet other countries, notably Australia, New Zealand and France, were collecting more detailed information including epidemiological data.[59] Because of anxieties about possible deleterious effects of fertilization *in vitro* on resulting children, in 1983 the MRC had agreed to sponsor a register of babies born following IVF.[60] The VLA also published crude statistics on multiple pregnancies, a potentially hazardous outcome of the technology that was provoking increasing concern amongst parents and medical professionals. A more elaborate monitoring exercise was begun in 1989 by the OPCS (now the Office of National Statistics) in collaboration with the VLA. The information collected was a compromise agreed between the Authority, which wanted comprehensive data, and the clinics who were reluctant to provide it.[61] The data were organized according to size of clinic – small, medium or large – and allowed calculation of success/attrition rates by women's age, indications for treatment, number of previous attempts and UK or overseas residency.

Concerned primarily with measuring practice, none of these monitoring exercises included information on who paid for or profited out of treatment. Yet by the mid-1980s, there was growing public concern about the low level of NHS funding of IVF. Stories about the lengths to which some women went to raise money for treatment began to feature regularly in newspapers and the broadcast media. Campaigners began to collect data that might demonstrate inequalities in NHS provision. The first such survey was undertaken in 1986 by Frank Dobson, a Labour Party Member of Parliament and at that time Shadow Health Minister.[62] It was repeated in 1990 by Harriet Harman, his successor.[63] Both found that NHS provision was haphazard and unsatisfactory. Inevitably, the data were incomplete. Both lamented the lack of routine information about the availability of infertility services on the NHS. At the same time, in the light of the poor pregnancy rates then being reported – around one out of every ten treatment cycles led to a live birth – an argument began in medical circles about whether or not the NHS could or should afford IVF. Not only were the medical and social consequences of IVF worrying, but its revenue consequences were considered excessive, indeed more than the NHS could afford.[64] As champions of the market and the regulatory power of consumerism and individual agency even within the state medical service, the Conservative government did not engage in the debate on whether or not the NHS should fund IVF. In effect, the debate represented the final gasps of the command and control way of thinking about health care. In 1990 the Human Fertilisation and Embryology Act was passed, and the Human Fertilisation and Embryology Authority (HFEA) was established to develop and administer its rules. The HFEA was little better than the VLA, the regulatory system it superseded. A quasi-autonomous non-governmental organization (quango), it did little more than put on a statutory and compulsory basis the licensing activities of the VLA.[65]

As a quango, the HFEA is immune to challenge by public opinion. Its rules can only be challenged on a case-by-case basis by individuals pursuing the process of judicial review. In the shift from government to governance, parliament's rule-making capacity is devolved. Politicians who in the previous forty years or so had spent much time and effort adjudicating over the ethics of destroying human gametes, embryos and foetuses are no longer susceptible to public pressure.

The HFEA inherited the VLA's responsibility for data collection.[66] In its first years, it simply used the system developed by the OPCS for IVF.[67] Greater transparency only came about when commercial data became important within the NHS itself. In 1991, in a major restructuring of the NHS, the centralized command and control structure was destroyed and replaced by a quasi-market. As a result of subsequent restructuring, the NHS now consists of a network of different kinds of organizations, some holding purse strings and with the power to determine entitlements to health care according to their own criteria, some providing health care and some doing both.[68] In place of administrative fiat, control is now exercised through contracts drawn up by NHS purchasers for services provided by both public and commercial organizations. Purchasers began to seek information on the success/attrition rates of individual clinics, and in 1995 the HFEA agreed to publish indicators of their performance.

The data are published in the HFEA's *Patients' Guide* to donor insemination and IVF clinics in a format which acknowledges that IVF is a business with customers (the same data are provided for NHS purchasers and private individuals). Some clinics do better than others; poorly performing clinics are unhappy about publication of individual clinic success rates, claiming that disclosure of poor results might lead to a loss of business – a curious argument suggesting that providers but not customers can justly claim protection from the vicissitudes of competition.[69] The data are opaque and extremely difficult to make sense of.[70] Each successive version of the guide contains a more elaborate explanation of how to interpret them. The HFEA also advises individual prospective patients to look beyond the figures:

> Your decision on the best clinic for you should not be based solely on the live birth rate. You should also consider: the treatments offered; how comfortable you feel with the staff and the surroundings; what information and counselling is offered; the cost; and the location of the clinic.[71]

If the data published by the HFEA are unhelpful as a basis for consumer choice, they are even less informative about the extent to which the NHS is meeting the needs of citizens. The 1999 edition of the Patients' Guide includes information on whether or not a clinic would accept what are called 'non-fee paying' patients, presumably a euphemism for patients whose treatment is paid for by an NHS purchaser. Opinion-forming associations concerned with inequalities in access to treatment have begun to collect their own data; in 1993, the first survey of how many women undergoing IVF had their treatment paid for out of taxation was sponsored by ISSUE, the National Fertility Association.[72] However, because voluntary bodies lack the authority to command them, the data are incomplete.

Because of the timing of their emergence, IVF and related techniques have been in the vanguard of a tendency developing under the regulatory state characterized by abandonment of the view that private provision and the pursuit of the profit motive in public services is morally repugnant. Government is increasingly reluctant to interfere with commercial providers in the name of the public interest, promoting instead a system of regulation that pursues public acceptability rather than facilitating public oversight. Paradoxically, despite claims that this system of regulation promotes the interests of consumers, even when it is put on a statutory footing, little useful information is made available to the public, particularly where such information is of a commercial nature.

Conclusion

The transformation of the social-welfare state from the command and control model to a regulatory one has involved abdication on the part of the state of its previously publicly sanctioned role in facilitating and enacting public opinion. Habermas supposes that the growth of the social-welfare state tended inevitably to weaken and marginalize public debate. At least in the case of abortion, however, the growth of state services involved a system of oversight that facilitated debates in the public sphere about what constitutes the public good and the nature of entitlements. By contrast, as the case of IVF shows, the growth of the regulatory as distinct from the social-welfare state has involved the expansion of private provision and the introduction of a system of regulation that recognizes commercial interests and defends them against hostile public opinion. Information is made available to the public in such a way as to minimize opposition to the manipulation and destruction of human embryos; such information is generally unhelpful in facilitating public oversight and opinion formation on entitlements.

This shift has had profoundly conservative and misogynistic consequences. Women who make use of both abortion and IVF tend to be construed as desperate and irrational, and as therefore inclined to act in ways that are damaging to both their own and the public good. However, at least under the command and control model of the social-welfare state, women had the opportunity to contribute to the processes of opinion formation, and thereby circumvent some of the disqualifications that are otherwise imposed on them. Under the regulatory state, such opportunities for public representation are significantly curtailed, and women seeking IVF are largely confined to the role of consumers. In April 1995, the front page of the *Daily Mail* was emblazoned with the headline 'Shame of test tube mother'. Underneath, it told the story of a woman who had stolen £20,000 from her employer for treatment. Inside was a description of how her inability to obtain NHS treatment had driven her to crime. Once again, the theme of desperation was rehearsed. However, whereas in the command and control model of the social-welfare state, women's desperation was a public concern dealt with by public provision, in the regulatory state it is now a private matter, to be resolved only by honest or dishonest consumerism.

Habermas's pessimism about the pernicious consequences of the growth of the social-welfare state has been vindicated – not, however, because of any inherent tendency for public welfare to undermine active citizenship, but because the state has itself withdrawn from its role in facilitating public opinion, and has sided instead with the interests of private business.

Acknowledgements

Thanks to Steve Sturdy and Susan Kerrison for helpful discussion in formulating my analysis.

Notes

1 There is a growing literature on the regulatory state. A useful starting point is G. Majone, 'From the positive to the regulatory state: causes and consequences of changes in the mode of governance', *Journal of Public Policy*, 1997, vol. 17, pp. 139–67.
2 M. Moran, 'From command state to regulatory state', *Public Policy and Administration*, 2000, vol. 15, pp. 1–13.
3 J. Habermas, *The Structural Transformation of the Public Sphere*, trans T. Berger, Cambridge: Polity Press, 1989, p. 241.
4 For a discussion of the surveys carried out into the diminished fertility of the English, see N. Pfeffer, *The Stork and the Syringe: A Political History of Reproductive Medicine*, Cambridge: Polity Press, 1993, pp. 3–29.
5 An attempt by someone other than the pregnant woman to induce an abortion after 'quickening' – the first time a pregnant woman feels the foetus move – had become a felony in 1803 with the passage of Lord Ellenborough's Wounding and Maiming Act. Self-induced abortion became a felony with the passage of the Offences against the Person Act of 1861.
6 See the chapter by Morrice in this volume.
7 Memo by Sir Leonard Dunning, HM Inspector of Constabulary (England and Wales), to the Inter-Departmental Committee on Abortion, Public Record Office (PRO), Kew, HO 326/29.
8 A. Oakley, *The Captured Womb: A History of the Medical Care of Pregnant Women*, Oxford: Blackwell, 1986, p. 91.
9 Barbara Brookes, *Abortion in England 1900–1967*, London: Croom Helm, 1988, p. 65.
10 Quoted in Interdepartmental Committee on Abortion, *Report*, London: HMSO, 1939.
11 Brookes, *Abortion in England*, p. 95.
12 Coroner for Northern District of County of London. Joint Council of Midwifery, Interim Report of the Committee of Enquiry into Non-Therapeutic Abortion, April 1937. Part II: Appendices: Appendix B. PRO HO 326/29.
13 Joint Council of Midwifery, Interim Report.
14 J. Lewis, *The Politics of Motherhood: Child and Maternal Health in England, 1900–1939*, London: Croom Helm, 1980, p. 209.
15 Evidence of the Ministry of Health, 26 May 1938, PRO HO 326/31.
16 Interdepartmental Committee on Abortion, *Report*, p. 123.
17 B. Botting, 'Trends in abortion', *Population Trends*, 1991, vol. 64, pp. 19–29.
18 D. Marsh and J. Chambers, *Abortion Politics*, London: Junction Books, 1981.
19 J.D.J. Havard, 'Therapeutic abortion', *Criminal Law Review*, 1958, pp. 600–13.
20 Marsh and Chambers, *Abortion Politics*.
21 PRO MH 156/142.
22 General Register Office, 10 October 1967. PRO MH 156/143.

23 Office of Population Censuses and Surveys. Abortion statistics: England and Wales, Series AB, OPCS.
24 Department of Health and Social Security witness, 'Witness evidence', in Select Committee on the Abortion (Amendment) Bill, *Special Reports and Minutes of Evidence together with the Proceedings of the Committee, Session 1974–75*, London: HMSO, p. 64.
25 A. Horder, *Legal Abortion: The English Experience*, Oxford: Pergamon Press, 1971, p. 106.
26 Editorial, 'The first year of the Abortion Act', *Lancet*, 26 April 1969, pp. 867–8.
27 Department of Health and Social Security witness, 'Witness evidence', in Select Committee on the Abortion (Amendment) Bill, *Special Reports*, p. 63.
28 Ibid., p. 19.
29 Marsh and Chambers, *Abortion Politics*.
30 Norman St John-Stevas Bill, 1969; Bryant Godman Irvine Bill, 1970; John Hunt Bill, 1971; Michael Gryll Bill, 1974; James White Bill, 1975; William Benyon Bill, 1977; Sir Bernard Braine Bill, 1978; John Corrie Bill, 1979/80; David Alton Bill, 1980.
31 Abortion (Amendment) Bill, *Proceedings of Standing Committee C*, London: HMSO, 1974, 1976–7, 1979–80; Select Committee on the Abortion (Amendment) Bill, *Special Reports*; Abortion (Amendment) Bill: Committee on the Working of the Abortion Act, *Report*, Cmnd 5579, London: HMSO, 1974; Abortion, Select Committee, *Report*, *Evidence* and *Second Report*, London: HMSO, 1975–6.
32 Committee on the Working of the Abortion Act, *Report*, p. 6.
33 Royal Commission on the NHS (Chairman Sir Alec Merrison), *Report*, Cmnd 7615, London: HMSO, 1979.
34 R. Klein, *The Politics of the NHS*, London: Longman, 2nd edn, 1989, p. 118.
35 B. Braine, 'Witness evidence', in Select Committee on the Abortion (Amendment) Bill, *Special Reports*, p. 59.
36 Ibid., p. 52.
37 J. Lovenduski, 'Parliament, pressure groups, networks and the women's movement: the politics of abortion law reform in Britain (1967–83)', in J. Lovenduski and J. Outshoorn (eds), *The New Politics of Abortion*, London: Sage, 1986, pp. 499–66.
38 Abortion, Select Committee, *Report*, p. 8.
39 Ibid., p. 132.
40 S. Macintyre, 'Who wants babies? The social construction of instincts', in D. Leonard Barker and S. Allen (eds), *Sexual Divisions and Society: Process and Change*, London: Tavistock, 1976, pp. 150–73.
41 K. Figlio, 'Unconscious aspects of health and the public sphere', in B. Richards (ed.), *Crises of the Self: Further Essays on Psychoanalysis and Politics*, London: Free Association Books, 1989, pp. 85–100.
42 D. Munday, C. Francome and W. Savage, 'Twenty one years of legal abortion', *British Medical Journal*, 1989, vol. 298, pp. 1231–4.
43 P. Leach, 'Human in vitro fertilisation', in Voluntary Licensing Authority for Human In Vitro Fertilisation and Embryology, *The First Report*, London: Medical Research Council, Royal College of Obstetricians and Gynaecologists, 1986, p. 39.
44 S. Fishel, 'IVF – historical perspective', in S. Fishel and E.M. Symonds (eds), *In Vitro Fertilisation: Past, Present, Future*, Oxford: IRL Press, 1986, pp. 1–16.
45 N. Pfeffer, 'Artificial insemination, in-vitro fertilization and the stigma of infertility', in M. Stanworth (ed.), *Reproductive Technologies: Gender, Motherhood and Medicine*, Cambridge: Polity Press, 1987, pp. 81–97.
46 J. Mohan, 'Privatization in the British health sector: a challenge to the NHS?', in J. Gabe, M. Calnan and M. Bury (eds), *The Sociology of the Health Service*, London: Routledge, 1991, pp. 36–57.
47 Voluntary Licensing Authority, *The First Report*.
48 N. Pfeffer, 'From private patients to privatisation', in M. Stacey (ed.), *Changing Human Reproduction: Social Science Perspectives*, London: Sage Publications, 1992, pp. 48–74.

49 J. Gunning and V. English, *Human In Vitro Fertilisation: A Case Study in the Regulation of Medical Innovation*, Aldershot: Dartmouth, 1993, pp. 30–1.
50 Committee of Inquiry into Human Fertilisation and Embryology, *Report*, Cmnd 9314, London: HMSO, 1984.
51 N. Pfeffer, 'Regulating reproduction', in A.R. Saetnan, N. Oudshoorn and M. Kirejczyk (eds), *Bodies of Technology: Women's Involvement in Reproductive Medicine*, Columbus: Ohio State University Press, 2000, pp. 254–77.
52 Voluntary Licensing Authority, *The First Report*.
53 King's Fund Centre Counselling Committee, *Counselling for Regulated Infertility Treatment*, London: King's Fund Centre, 1991.
54 M. Mulkay, *The Embryo Research Debate: Science and the Politics of Reproduction*, Cambridge: Cambridge University Press, 1997.
55 Voluntary Licensing Authority for Human In Vitro Fertilisation and Embryology, *The Second Report*, London: Medical Research Council, Royal College of Obstetricians and Gynaecologists, 1987.
56 R.J. Lilford and M.E. Dalton, 'Effectiveness of treatment for infertility', *British Medical Journal*, 1987, vol. 295, pp. 155–6.
57 M.R. Soules, 'The in vitro fertilization pregnancy rate: let's be honest with one another', *Fertility and Sterility*, 1985, vol. 43, pp. 511–13.
58 S. Benady, *Choosing a Test Tube Baby Clinic*, London: The Independent, 1987.
59 Gunning and English, *Human In Vitro Fertilisation*, p. 94.
60 V. Beral, P. Doyle, S.L. Tan, B.A. Mason and S. Campbell, 'Outcomes of pregnancies resulting from assisted conception', *British Medical Bulletin*, 1990, vol. 46, pp. 753–68.
61 Gunning and English, *Human In Vitro Fertilisation*, p. 94.
62 F. Dobson, *Infertility Services in the NHS: What's Going On?*, London: House of Commons, 1986.
63 H. Harman, *Trying for a Baby: A Report on the Inadequacy of NHS Infertility Services*, London: House of Commons, 1990.
64 R.M.L. Winston and R.A. Margara, 'Effectiveness of treatment for infertility', *British Medical Journal*, 1987, vol. 295, p. 785; M. Burke, 'Effectiveness of treatment for infertility', *British Medical Journal*, 1987, vol. 295, pp. 784–5.
65 G. Drewry, 'The civil service: from the 1940s to "Next Steps" and beyond', *Parliamentary Affairs*, 1994, vol. 47, pp. 583–95.
66 R.G. Lee and D. Morgan, *Human Fertilisation and Embryology: Regulating the Reproductive Revolution*, London: Blackstone Press, 2001.
67 The HFEA also collects data on donor insemination, a procedure which falls within its purview.
68 C. Webster, *The National Health Service: A Political History*, Oxford: Oxford University Press, 1997, pp. 182–205.
69 Human Fertilisation and Embryology Authority, *The Publication of Centres' Success Rates for In Vitro Fertilisation and Donor Insemination: Consultation Document*, London: HFEA, 1995, p. 2.
70 E.C. Marshall and D.J. Spiegelhalter, 'Reliability of league tables of in vitro fertilisation clinics: retrospective analysis of live births', *British Medical Journal*, 1998, vol. 316, pp. 1701–5.
71 Human Fertilisation and Embryology Authority, *A Patients' Guide to IVF Clinics*, London: HFEA, 1999, p. 2.
72 ISSUE, *Report of the National Survey of the Funding and Provision of Infertility Services*, London: College of Health, 1993.

Index

Note: figures are indicated by italicized page numbers

Milton Keynes UK
Ingram Content Group UK Ltd.
UKHW040448071024
449327UK00020B/1082

9 780415 863049